EXERCISE in Cardiovascular Health and Disease

EDITED BY

EZRA A. AMSTERDAM, MD
JACK H. WILMORE, PhD
ANTHONY N. DeMARIA, MD

EXERCISE IN CARDIOVASCULAR HEALTH AND DISEASE

Printed in the United States of America.

First Edition

Third Printing

Library of Congress Catalog Card Number: 77-82741

International Standard Book Number: 0-914316-11-7

EXERCISE in Cardiovascular Health and Disease

Edited by

Ezra A. Amsterdam, MD
Associate Professor of Medicine
Chief, Coronary Care Unit
Section of Cardiovascular Medicine
University of California
School of Medicine
Davis, California

Jack H. Wilmore, PhD
Professor and Head
Department of Physical Education and Athletics
University of Arizona
Tucson, Arizona

Anthony N. DeMaria, MD
Associate Professor of Medicine
Director, Echocardiography
Section of Cardiovascular Medicine
University of California
School of Medicine
Davis, California

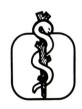

YORKE MEDICAL BOOKS
666 FIFTH AVENUE, NEW YORK, NEW YORK

To our wives and children,
for their love, understanding,
support and forbearance

CONTENTS

PART III

CORONARY HEART DISEASE DIAGNOSIS: METHODOLOGICAL AND INTERPRETIVE ASPECTS

PART IV

PREVENTIVE ASPECTS OF CORONARY HEART DISEASE

Contributors

WILLIAM C. ADAMS, PhD
Associate Professor
Department of Physical Education
Human Performance Laboratory
University of California
Davis, California

EZRA A. AMSTERDAM, MD, FACC
Associate Professor of Medicine
Chief, Coronary Care Unit
Section of Cardiovascular Medicine
University of California
School of Medicine
Davis, California

NAJAM AWAN, MD, FACC
Assistant Professor of Medicine
Section of Cardiovascular Medicine
Department of Medicine
University of California
School of Medicine
Davis, California

DANIEL BERMAN, MD, FACC
Assistant Professor of Medicine
Director, Nuclear Cardiology
Cedars-Sinai Medical Center
Los Angeles, California

EDMUND M. BERNAUER, PhD
Professor and Chairman
Department of Physical Education
Human Performance Laboratory
University of California
Davis, California

ASHOK K. BHAN, PhD
Assistant Professor of Medicine and
  Biochemistry
Division of Cardiology
Montefiore Hospital and Medical Center
  of the Albert Einstein College
  of Medicine
New York, New York

C. GUNNAR BLOMQVIST, MD, FACC
Professor of Medicine and Physiology
Southwestern Medical School
Dallas, Texas

JOSEPH A. BONANNO, MD, FACC
Director, Cardiac Catheterization
  Laboratory
San Dieguito Hospital
Encinitas, California
Assistant Clinical Professor of Medicine
University of California
San Diego, California

NEMAT O. BORHANI, MD, FACC
Professor and Chairman
Department of Community Health
University of California
School of Medicine
Davis, California

JOHN L. BOYER, MD, FACC
Medical Director
Exercise Physiology Laboratory
San Diego State University
San Diego, California

ROBERT A. BRUCE, MD, FACC
Professor of Medicine
Co-Director, Division of Cardiology
University of Washington
School of Medicine
Seattle, Washington

GERALD DAVIS, PhD
Assistant Professor of Health Science
College of Pharmacy and
Allied Health Professions
Northeastern University
Boston, Massachusetts

ANTHONY N. DeMARIA, MD, FACC
Associate Professor of Medicine
Director, Echocardiography
Section of Cardiovascular Medicine
University of California
School of Medicine
Davis, California

CARLYLE H. FOLKINS, PhD
Assistant Professor in Residence
Department of Psychiatry
University of California
School of Medicine
Davis, California

VICTOR F. FROELICHER, JR, MD, FACC
Assistant Professor of Medicine
University of California
School of Medicine
San Diego, California

PHILIP D. GOLLNICK, PhD
Professor
Department of Physical Education
Washington State University
Pullman, Washington

FRED HARRIS, MD
Assistant Professor of Medicine
Section of Cardiovascular Medicine
Department of Medicine
University of California
School of Medicine
Davis, California

WILLIAM L. HASKELL, PhD
Co-Director, Stanford Cardiac
Rehabilitation Program
Stanford University School of Medicine
Palo Alto, California

JAMES L. HUGHES, III, MD
Associate Director
Cardiac Catheterization Laboratory
Cooper Medical Center
Camden, New Jersey
Assistant Clinical Professor
of Medicine
Jefferson Medical College
Philadelphia, Pennsylvania

ALBERT A. KATTUS, MD, FACC
Professor of Medicine
Division of Cardiology
Department of Medicine
University of California
School of Medicine
Los Angeles, California

TERESA LaFAVE
Student Fellow
California Heart Association
Section of Cardiovascular Medicine
University of California
School of Medicine
Davis, California

GARRETT LEE, MD
Assistant Professor of Medicine
Director, Cardiac Catheterization
  Laboratory
Section of Cardiovascular Medicine
University of California
School of Medicine
Davis, California

DEAN T. MASON, MD, FACC
President, American College
  of Cardiology
Professor of Medicine and Physiology
Chief, Cardiovascular Medicine
University of California
School of Medicine
Davis, California

MALCOLM M. McHENRY, MD, FACC
Director, Cardiac Catheterization
  Laboratory and Coronary Care Unit
Cardiopulmonary Laboratory
Sutter Memorial Hospital
Sacramento, California
Assistant Clinical Professor of Medicine
University of California
School of Medicine
Davis, California

RICHARD R. MILLER, MD, FACC
Professor of Medicine
Chief, Section of Cardiology
Baylor College of Medicine
Houston, Texas

JOHN NAUGHTON, MD, FACC
Dean, School of Medicine
Professor of Medicine
State University of New York
Buffalo, New York
Director, National Exercise and Heart
  Disease Project
Rehabilitation Services Administration
National Institutes of Health
Department of Health, Education
  and Welfare
Bethesda, Maryland

WILLIAM A. NEILL, MD
Chief, Cardiology Section
Veterans Administration Hospital
Professor of Medicine
Tufts University School of Medicine
Boston, Massachusetts

RALPH S. PAFFENBARGER, JR, MD
Preventive Medical Health Officer
California State Department of Health
Berkeley, California

SOMSONG PENPARGKUL, MD, PHD
Assistant Professor of Medicine
Division of Cardiology
Montefiore Hospital and Medical Center
  of the Albert Einstein College
  of Medicine
New York, New York

JAMES E. PRICE, MD
Assistant Professor of Medicine
Section of Cardiovascular Medicine
Department of Medicine and Physiology
University of California
School of Medicine
Davis, California

KAY RIGGS, BS
Research Associate
Section of Cardiovascular Medicine
Department of Medicine and Physiology
University of California
School of Medicine
Davis, California

JAMES SCHEUER, MD, FACC
Professor of Medicine
Director, Division of Cardiology
Montefiore Hospital and Medical Center
  of the Albert Einstein College
  of Medicine
New York, New York

LEIGH D. SEGEL, PhD
Research Biochemist
Section of Cardiovascular Medicine
University of California
School of Medicine
Davis, California

WALTER L. SEMBROWICH
Research Associate
Department of Physical Education
  for Men
Washington State University
Pullman, Washington

KARL G. STOEDEFALKE, PhD
Associate Dean for Academic Affairs
College of Health, Physical Education
  and Recreation
The Pennsylvania State University
University Park, Pennsylvania

ZAKAUDDIN VERA, MD
Assistant Professor of Medicine
Director, Clinical Electrophysiology
Section of Cardiovascular Medicine
University of California
School of Medicine
Davis, California

JACK H. WILMORE, PhD
Professor and Head
Department of Physical Education
  and Athletics
University of Arizona
Tucson, Arizona

Preface

Interest in exercise as a means of promoting health dates from antiquity. However, it was not until this century that scientific efforts were devoted to the systematic elucidation of physiological responses and adaptations to the stress of exercise.[1] Since then, greater understanding of exercise physiology has provided a more rational basis for application of habitual aerobic activity in the treatment of cardiac disease. Paralleling the development of this area was the introduction almost 50 years ago of analysis of the circulatory response to exercise as a test of cardiac function,[2] with subsequent extension to the detection of myocardial ischemia.[3]

Exercise is now playing an increasingly important role in the diagnosis and functional evaluation of cardiac disease as well as in its treatment. This book reviews the current status of exercise testing and training in terms of physiological bases and clinical applications. Many of the authors are important contributors to the expanding knowledge in this field. The book is divided into five parts: general concepts of coronary heart disease, physiologic aspects of exercise, application of exercise testing, the potential of exercise training in maintenance of cardiovascular health, and exercise therapy in cardiac rehabilitation.

Part I begins with a review by Borhani of the epidemiology of coronary heart disease (CHD). He notes that CHD is the leading cause of mortality in the technologically developed societies. The basic pathologic process, coronary artery atherosclerosis, is still not well understood but certain metabolic and personal characteristics, known as the coronary risk factors, have been identified which are associated with increased incidence of CHD. Because the relationship between the coronary risk factors and CHD is thus far one of association and not causality, the capacity of risk factor modification to reduce the occurrence of the disease is not known at this time. The clinical features of CHD and their underlying pathophysiology are discussed by Amsterdam and Mason in the second chapter. Obstructive coronary artery disease results in myocardial ischemia, the fundamental physiologic defect which produces the clinical manifestations of CHD. Myocardial ischemia usually indicates coronary luminal narrowing of 70% or more and the vast majority of patients with overt CHD have severe, multivessel coronary involvement. Cardiac pump dysfunction in CHD is typically the result of myocardial damage due to infarction. The important issue of the relation between physical activity and risk of developing CHD is reviewed by Paffenbarger in the closing chapter of the first section. His findings indicate a strong inverse correlation between high occupational energy expenditure and fatal myocardial infarction. He emphasizes that this negative relationship reflects a protective, rather than selective, effect of physical activity. This conclusion is supported by a rigorous analysis of the data in which high energy expenditure emerges as an independent factor associated with reduced risk of death from myocardial infarction.

Part II is introduced by Wilmore's review of the physiology of exercise. Methodologic problems and approaches are described and the cardiocirculatory, respiratory and metabolic alterations associated with acute and chronic exercise are considered, as well as the relation of these changes to augmented oxygen transport. Maximum oxygen consumption ($\dot{V}O_2$ max) is presented as the index of physical working capacity in terms of cardiorespiratory function. Exercise training raises $\dot{V}O_2$ max and results in reduced heart rate and elevated stroke volume during submaximal exertion. The succeeding papers in this section explore the effect of exercise on specific aspects of physiological function. Gollnick and Sembrowich discuss the response of human skeletal muscle to physical conditioning. These investigators indicate the remarkable ability of skeletal muscle to adapt to different patterns of use and to undergo alterations in metabolic character during training, despite lack of demonstrable change in the contractile properties of muscle fibers induced by such exertion. The contribution of enhanced skeletal muscle performance to the overall increase in exertional capacity induced by physical training is emphasized. Segel critically reviews the experimental data on myocardial adaptations to chronic exercise, noting the variations in methodology which may contribute to the often contradictory findings. Important functional and structural alterations include bradycardia and cardiomegaly. There is also evidence, although inconsistent, of augmented coronary vasculature, enhanced mechanical function under stress and increased cardiac myosin ATPase activity.

Scheuer and colleagues synthesize their significant investigations on the cardiac effects of exercise training in which they provide experimental evidence of partial protection of myocardial performance during hypoxic stress. This effect is associated with improved coronary blood flow and oxygen delivery and increased levels of cardiac actomyosin and myosin ATPase. The complex effects of physical activity on hemostatic mechanisms, including blood clotting, fibrinolysis and platelet function, are analyzed by Lee and co-workers. Exercise increases blood coagulability while exercise-associated changes in fibrinolysis vary with age, intensity of effort and time of day; alterations in platelet function related to activity are dependent on intensity of exertion. Exercise conditioning appears to reduce the hypercoagulable state induced by exercise without altering the increase in fibrinolytic activity. In the final chapter in this section, Neill discusses the contributions of alterations in skeletal muscle, myocardial oxygen demand and myocardial oxygen supply to the enhanced exertional capacity and increased anginal threshold following exercise conditioning. Although increased metabolic capacity of trained skeletal muscle and hemodynamic changes consistent with reduced myocardial oxygen demand during submaximal exertion have been associated with exercise training, the effect of the latter on myocardial oxygen delivery remains unresolved.

In the first paper in Part III, Bruce discusses exercise testing in terms of indications, methods and various physiological modalities. He focuses on assessment and clinical implications of functional aerobic impairment as well as upon electrocardiographic evidence of ischemia. Kattus addresses the frequent and important clinical problem posed by interpretation of ST-segment abnormalities in evaluating the presence of myocardial ischemia. Emphasized in this exposition are causes of ST-segment changes other than myocardial ischemia in the exercise electrocardiogram. The role of the computer in exercise stress testing is assessed by Blomqvist. Computer technology may be of value methodologically by reduction of artifact and in interpretation, through alleviation of the problem of inter- and intra-observer variability. Further, computer analysis has been demonstrated by some investigators to enhance the sensitivity and specificity of exercise electrocardiography in the diagnosis of ischemic heart disease. The influence of disease prevalence upon the significance of exercise-induced ST-segment changes is emphasized by Froelicher. He points out that the sensitivity and specificity of the exercise electrocardiogram in the identification of coronary disease is closely related to its prevalence in the population being evaluated. The prevalence of CHD in asymptomatic patients is low. Therefore, the majority of asymptomatic subjects with this electrocardiographic abnormality will have normal coronary arteries despite the identification, by ischemic ST depression, of a group at increased risk for coronary disease.

DeMaria and associates discuss arrhythmias and conduction defects occurring during exercise stress testing and review current knowledge regarding the diagnostic, prognostic and therapeutic implications of these electrophysiologic events. The authors note that exercise may be associated with both provocation and abolition of ventricular arrhythmias and emphasize that the response of ventricular ectopic beats to exertion does not reliably discriminate between normal individuals and patients with cardiac disease. Amsterdam and colleagues analyze the use of exercise testing to determine pathophysiologic severity and therapeutic mechanisms in angina. They stress the distinction between external work, performed by the skeletal muscles, and internal work or cardiac performance. The latter parameter is critical to the assessment of angina and can be conveniently evaluated by the use of indirect hemodynamic indices of myocardial oxygen consumption such as the heart rate–blood pressure product. The authors stress that meaningful evaluation of the mechanisms and therapy of angina can be achieved within the limits of this method.

Harris and co-workers discuss the value and limitations of exercise testing in patients with valvular heart disease. They indicate that exercise may be utilized as a challenge by which to assess the degree of compensation of cardiac function, or may be applied in an attempt to objectively assess functional impairment consequent to valvular heart disease. However, at the present time, the precise value of exercise stress testing in determining the hemodynamic severity of cardiac valvular lesions remains undefined. This section is completed by Berman and associates who assess the rapidly expanding role of nuclear cardiology in the detection of myocardial ischemia. Myocardial stress scintigraphy provides an accurate means of evaluating left ventricular regional perfusion and in early studies has surpassed exercise electrocardiography in accurate identification of ischemia due to coronary disease. The broad application of this technique in the diagnosis and management of syndromes presenting as myocardial ischemia is emphasized.

Part IV deals with the role of exercise training in the prevention of CHD. Wilmore begins with a discussion of the exercise prescription and directs attention to the importance of individualizing the exertional regimen for each subject. He notes that endurance activity for at least 20 to 30 minutes, three times weekly at a target heart rate 75% of that associated with maximal oxygen consumption, renders a significant training effect upon functional cardiovascular parameters. Bonanno discusses the effect of such exercise programs upon coronary risk factors. Beneficial effects have been demonstrated on elevated blood pressure and hypertriglyceridemia, while it appears that exercise does not alter. serum cholesterol. Folkins and Amsterdam explore the potential of habitual physical activity to favorably modify stress and tension. They discuss the role of psychological stress in the genesis of coronary heart disease and review data indicating that physical conditioning is associated with decreased stress emotions and improved psychological state.

Stoedefalke discusses the requisite features of a successful adult fitness program. He emphasizes the importance of an imaginatively designed and individually tailored training regimen in maintaining participant adherence, and underscores the value of having a program which is designed and supervised by an individual who is well versed in the theory and practice of exercise training. Boyer and Wilmore emphasize that exercise programs should be implemented in childhood in order to promote long-term cardiac health. They indicate that an exercise fitness program for children should strive not only to eliminate coronary risk factors, but also to achieve adherence to patterns of endurance activity during the formative years and thereafter.

The final section is opened by McHenry, who indicates that selection of subjects for training programs entails systematic evaluation to eliminate patients at excessive risk, determine the potential for benefit, and assess motivation. Adams and co-workers review the long-term physiologic adaptations of the cardiovascular system to exercise and present their experience with a training program in normal individuals and in those who have had myocardial infarction or aortocoronary bypass surgery. Both exercise training and surgery can improve functional capacity and when applied together, can increase the separate benefits of each. Haskell considers the subject of physical activity after myocardial infarction, particularly in the hospital and during the early post-discharge period. He emphasizes that a training program should begin with early ambulation during the hospital phase of the illness. Gradually progressive activity minimizes the adverse cardiovascular and psychological effects of prolonged bed rest. In the final chapter, Naughton describes the basis, objectives and methods of long-term cardiac rehabilitation. Aimed at restoring the patient with cardiac disease to optimal physical performance, rehabilitation is implemented through a systematic program involving functional evaluation, exercise prescription and graduated, supervised activity. The individual patient's specific problems and needs in a rehabilitation program are stressed.

Acknowledgment—The production of this book was facilitated by a number of people to whom the editors wish to express their appreciation. Particular acknowledgment is made to Kristen Cowan for her tireless and efficient administrative and secretarial assistance and to the publishers, Yorke Medical Books, for their aid and support.

EZRA A. AMSTERDAM, MD
JACK H. WILMORE, PHD
ANTHONY N. DeMARIA, MD

References

1. Amsterdam EA, Wilmore JH, DeMaria AN: Introduction. Symposium on Exercise in Cardiovascular Health and Disease. *Amer J Cardiol* 33:713-714, 1974.
2. Master AM, Oppenheimer ET: A simple exercise test for circulatory efficiency with standard tables for normal individuals. *Amer J Med Sci* 177:223-243, 1929.
3. Master AM, Friedman R, Dack S: Electrocardiogram after standard exercise as a functional test of the heart. *Amer Heart J* 24:777-793, 1942.

PART I

Coronary Heart Disease: An Introduction

Epidemiology of Coronary Heart Disease

Nemat O. Borhani, MD

Cardiovascular diseases have a worldwide distribution. Some disease entities, such as hypertensive heart disease, rheumatic heart disease, vascular lesions affecting the central nervous system (stroke) and certain congenital abnormalities are found in practically every part of the world. Others are distributed predominantly in certain geographic areas. Foremost among the latter group is coronary heart disease, which comprises the major portion of mortality due to cardiovascular diseases in the United States and most Western societies. According to the World Health Organization, analysis of vital statistics data from 29 technologically advanced countries (including the United States) shows that in 1967, 39% of deaths in 25 to 64-year-old men were due to cardiovascular diseases; coronary artery diseases accounted for about 75% of these deaths.[1] In 50 countries that maintain vital statistics, cardiovascular diseases account for about 37% of all deaths each year. In the United States, these diseases account for approximately 54% of all deaths (Figure 1). Despite the fact that there is some indication of a downward trend in mortality from coronary heart disease, at least in the United States since 1968,[2] this disease continues to be the leading cause of death in this country. Further, mortality rate from coronary heart disease recently has been increasing more rapidly among the younger age groups than those in their sixth or seventh decades of life. Between 1951 and 1961, the average coronary heart disease death rate among 35 to 54-year-old men increased by 50%, as compared to a 20 to 25% increase in the older age groups. Every year nearly one million men and women in the United States succumb to either acute fatal and nonfatal myocardial infarction or sudden death. Coronary heart disease kills more Americans each year than any other disease including cancer. Thus, the death toll inflicted by coronary artery disease has become a challenge not only to the medical profession, but to society as a whole. Indeed, this disease has reached an epidemic stage and casts a much larger shadow on our civilization

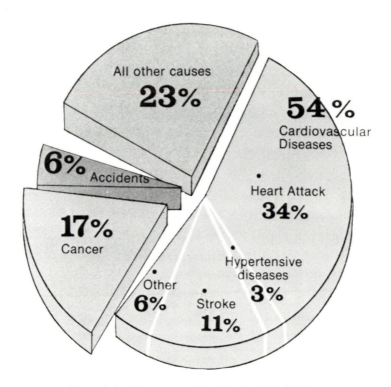

Figure 1. Leading causes of death in the United States.

than its rates of mortality indicate. Fears engendered by its existence reduce the potentials of our society.

Clinical manifestations of coronary heart disease are sudden death (which constitutes about 50 to 60% of all deaths due to coronary artery disease), acute fatal and nonfatal, as well as silent and clinically unrecognized, cases of myocardial infarction and angina pectoris. Although clinical manifestations of coronary heart disease vary among different population subgroups and in different geographic areas, the basic pathophysiologic mechanism remains the same (see Chapter 2). The basic and fundamental pathogenic process of the disease is thought to be atherosclerosis of the coronary arteries, about which we know very little.

Even though during the past 200 years, we have amassed a substantial body of knowledge about the clinical features and natural history of coronary artery disease,[3-7] a great deal remains unknown. At the very least we must learn more than we now know about the biochemistry and physiology of the arterial wall, the mechanism of development of atherosclerosis and the formation of atheroma. Nevertheless, it is important to note that epidemiologic data, accumulated in recent decades, have provided a wealth of knowledge about the natural history and dynamics of this disease and the factors that determine its distribution in different populations.[8-17] The totality of these observations gains greater significance than ordinarily appreciated by many, in that it is so very consistent with the results of the clinicopathologic investigations of Heberden, Jenner and Herrick,[4-7] and the laboratory and experimental investigations of Anitschkow, Rosenthal and others.[18-21] Relating available epidemiologic data not only to each other but to results of other studies in different fields of medical research, has enabled us to establish a theory known as "the multiple risk factor hypothesis"; this theory constitutes a firm scientific basis for our understanding of the dynamics of coronary heart disease. Although the strength of association between the factors implicated in the incidence of coronary heart disease (CHD risk factors) is almost overwhelming, these associations *do not* indicate causality. That is, we know very little about the etiology of atherosclerosis or myocardial infarction. Therefore, it should be emphasized that from the point of view of primary prevention of coronary heart disease, it remains to be seen whether or not risk factor modification will favorably influence the incidence of the disease. Experimental epidemiologic studies (community clinical trials) on the efficacy of risk factor intervention (MRFIT) currently under way in the United States and elsewhere, should provide needed information with regard to the efficacy, feasibility and indeed safety of community primary prevention programs of coronary heart disease, based on risk factor alteration (eg, dietary modification).

Coronary Heart Disease Risk Factors

One of the major contributions of the prospective epidemiologic studies of the past 25 years has been the identification of certain personal characteristics and socioenvironmental factors that are associated with the incidence of coronary heart disease. These factors, commonly known as coronary heart disease risk factors, include such parameters as age, sex, familial history of coronary heart disease, the levels of serum cholesterol and triglyceride, the level of systolic and diastolic blood pressure, cigarette smoking, impaired vital capacity, obesity, abnormal glucose tolerance and diabetes mellitus, hyperuricemia and gout, hypothyroidism, sociopsychological stress, certain personal behavioral patterns, and physical inactivity and sedentary life. Basic information about these factors is reviewed on different occasions. Through the use of refined statistical methods of analysis (ie, multiple logistic function analysis), we are now capable of using the combined information about these factors and can make powerful predictions in terms of probability of the occurrence of coronary heart disease among population subgroups.[22] The available evidence strongly suggests that among all known coronary heart disease risk factors, the most powerful predictors of coronary heart disease are age, sex, level of blood pressure, level of serum cholesterol, cigarette smoking and physical inactivity. Other than age and sex, three of these risk factors (cigarette smoking, serum cholesterol and blood pressure) stand out consistently in their association with the incidence of coronary heart disease in all epidemiologic studies.

Age and Sex

The incidence of coronary heart disease increases with age in both sexes and in all races. Mortality data indicate that coronary heart disease death rate rises rapidly with age, in an exponential manner, in both sexes and among different races (Figure 2). Although in the past the incidence of coronary heart disease deaths under the age of 35 was low, in recent years more and more younger individuals have succumbed to this malady. It should be noted, therefore, that coronary heart disease is no longer a "degenerative" disease of the elderly, as it was once considered.[12, 13]

Men over the age of 45, both whites and nonwhites, have a higher death rate from coronary heart disease than women. The male to female ratio, however, diminishes progressively from a maximum of 6:1 in those under the age of 40, to about unity in the very elderly.[13, 14]

Arterial Blood Pressure

Both mortality and morbidity from coronary heart disease show a positive association with the levels of systolic and diastolic blood pressure. Indeed, the rate of death from all causes (*ie*, total mortality) increases proportionally to an increase in the level of blood pressure. Findings of all prospective epidemiologic studies indicate a regular and continuous positive gradient between the level of blood pressure and the probability of future incidence of clinical manifestations (*ie*, acute myocardial infarction) of coronary heart disease (Figure 3). As can be seen from the data in Figure 3, this relationship is continuous; it exists even in the range not generally considered extreme by clinical criteria. It is important to note that there is no line of demarcation in the distribution of blood pressure (either systolic or diastolic) above which a group of individuals is at high risk of coronary heart disease and below which such a group is immune to it. Arterial blood pressure is a biologic quantity, and its adverse effects are numerically related.[23]

Based on multiple logistics function analysis of data derived from prospective epidemiologic investigations, arterial blood pressure is one of the most powerful predictors of coronary heart disease. In the presence of the other coronary heart disease risk factors (eg, cigarette smoking and overweight), elevated blood pressure assumes a much more dangerous position as a precursor of coronary heart disease. For example, a 35-year-old white man who does not smoke cigarettes has a six-year probability of 0.5 per 100 to develop coronary heart disease when the level of his systolic blood pressure is 135 mm Hg and his serum cholesterol is 185 mg/dl (Figure 3). Yet, the same probability increases to approximately 4.5 when systolic blood pressure is 180 mm Hg and serum cholesterol 310 mg/dl. If, in addition, the individual smokes more than one pack of cigarettes a day, his probability of developing an acute event of coronary heart disease rises to about 6.9 per 100.

Obviously, the contribution of the levels of systolic and diastolic blood pres-

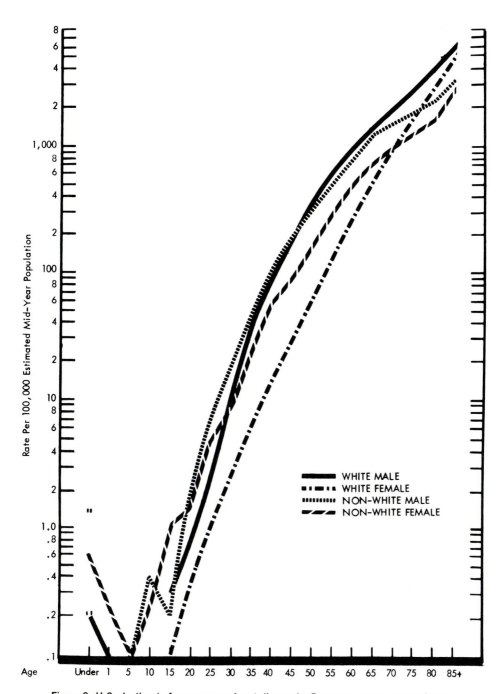

Figure 2. U.S. death rate from coronary heart disease by 5-year age group, sex and race.

6   *Borhani*

35-YEAR-OLD MAN

NON CIGARETTE SMOKER, NO LVH, NO GLUCOSE INTOLERANCE

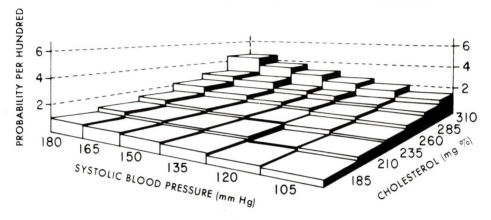

CIGARETTE SMOKER, LVH, GLUCOSE INTOLERANCE PRESENT

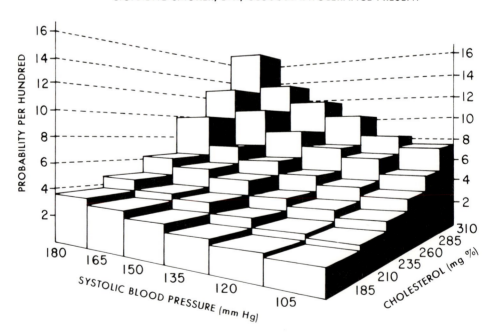

Figure 3. Probability of developing coronary heart disease in 6 years by systolic blood pressure, cholesterol, left ventricular hypertrophy by ECG, cigarette smoking and glucose intolerance (the Framingham study).

sure to the risk of coronary heart disease depends very much on the presence of other risk factors. This particular epidemiologic observation has a tremendous clinical application in the treatment of coronary heart disease complications among susceptible individuals, especially in view of the fact that the findings of clinical trials on hypertension have demonstrated that judicious medical treatment of hypertension reduces not only the level of blood pressure but the mortality and morbidity associated with it.[24, 25] It should be noted, however, that our present knowledge regarding the efficacy of antihypertensive therapy is based only on the results of clinical trials conducted among a selected group of male patients with sustained elevation of blood pressure. There are three certain assumptions inherent in the application of the results of these clinical trials to the control of hypertension in the community: (1) Antihypertensive therapy will be effective in reducing the level of blood pressure among *all* hypertensive patients (men and women), not only those selected men who participated in the clinical trials; (2) Effective antihypertensive therapy will reduce the risk of coronary heart disease to the level of risk naturally occurring among those who never had hypertension; and (3) No mortality or significant morbidity (eg, side effects) will result from large scale administration of antihypertensive agents in the general population to offset the expected benefits of treatment. These assumptions need careful scrutiny, before applying our present knowledge to community programs of prevention.

Serum Lipids

The term hyperlipidemia refers to the elevation of serum cholesterol and triglyceride, both of which have been demonstrated to be associated with an increased risk of coronary heart disease. As in the case with arterial blood pressure, there is no cutoff point in the distribution of serum cholesterol (or triglyceride) above which people are at high risk of coronary heart disease and below which they are free from it. The higher the level of serum cholesterol, the greater is the risk (Figure 3). Numerous laboratory and experimental studies have established the role of cholesterol in atherosclerosis, and have uncovered the nature of lipid metabolism and dietary fats in the pathogenesis of atherosclerosis.[18-21] Recent epidemiologic investigations have confirmed this relationship.[8-17] It is now generally accepted that in atherosclerosis, arterial lesions cannot be produced experimentally in laboratory animals without a modification of the diet, involving high intake of saturated fat, leading to elevation of serum cholesterol. Similarly, international epidemiologic studies have documented the fact that, with a few exceptions, populations consuming diets high in saturated fats and cholesterol have elevated levels of serum cholesterol and high incidence of coronary heart disease, and vice versa. Notwithstanding the persuasive force of these data implicating elevated serum cholesterol in the incidence of coronary heart disease, the nature of the development of atherosclerosis remains unknown and the role of serum cholesterol and different fractions of plasma lipoproteins (*ie*, high and low density lipoproteins) in the incidence of coronary heart disease continues to be controversial. Available epidemiologic data are not by themselves sufficient to warrant mass public health programs for prevention of coronary heart disease by dietary manipulation. These data are consistent, however, in demonstrating the increased level of risk that is associated with the increment in the level of serum cholesterol (and triglyceride). What remains to be done is demonstration that alteration in the level of serum cholesterol will result in a reduction of mortality and morbidity from coronary heart disease.

There is another question that surrounds the cholesterol issue. It has been reported that significantly higher low density lipoprotein (LDL) is present in white men (with high incidence of coronary heart disease) whereas increased high density lipoprotein (HDL) is found among black men (with low incidence of coronary heart disease).[26] Low density lipoprotein (LDL), commonly known as beta lipoprotein, results from the catabolism of very low density lipoprotein (VLDL), and includes over one-half of the total serum cholesterol. The HDL, or alpha lipoprotein, comprises the smallest portion of lipoproteins. It is thought that, perhaps, high density lipoproteins exert an inhibitory (and protective) influence on the development of atherosclerosis, and thus the incidence of coronary heart disease.

Cigarette Smoking

Cigarette smoking is possibly the most significant and important risk factor associated with the incidence of coronary heart disease.[9, 12-14] This is because all the scientific conditions prerequisite to launching effective programs in prevention have been met. It has been demonstrated that cigarette smoking is associated with an increase in the incidence of coronary heart disease and that the habit can be altered; once the smoker stops the habit, after a few years (perhaps as long as ten years) his risk reverts to almost that of a nonsmoker.

Epidemiologic data indicate that total mortality among cigarette smokers is twice as high as in nonsmokers. Although the relationship of cigarette smoking has been emphasized more in its association with lung cancer, it is of interest to note that only 19% of the excess mortality among smokers is due to lung cancer, while 37% of this excess is due to coronary heart disease. Further, cigarette smoking considerably accentuates the influence of other coronary heart disease risk factors (Figure 3). Obviously cigarette smoking is a much more dangerous risk factor if it is associated with other coronary heart disease risk factors (eg, hypertension or obesity). The adverse influence of cigarette smoking on the incidence of coronary heart disease is quite independent of other risk factors. This particular observation, along with the consistency of findings among all epidemiologic studies, makes cigarette smoking a very powerful risk factor indeed. Unfortunately, and perhaps ironically, one of the most important pieces of evidence against cigarette smoking is the fact that the death rate from coronary heart disease among young women is increasing almost parallel to the rate of increase in their average consumption of cigarettes in recent years. Similar data can be obtained from those countries which until recently enjoyed a relatively low incidence of coronary heart disease (eg, Italy), and suddenly began to report a sharp and dramatic rise in the rate of coronary heart disease as the rate of cigarette consumption among their citizens (especially women) increased.[27] It is now universally accepted that cigarette smoking is a very strong additive factor in the mosaic of multiple risk factors implicated in the incidence of coronary heart disease. Cigarette smoking is a factor that lends itself most readily to programs for primary prevention of this dread disease.

Other Risk Factors

The relationship between physical inactivity and the incidence of coronary heart disease is discussed in Chapter 3. Other than physical inactivity and/or sedentary life as a risk of coronary heart disease there are other factors (in addition to sex, age, levels of blood pressure and serum cholesterol and cigarette smoking) associated with the incidence of coronary heart disease, which should be discussed, albeit briefly, in this chapter.

Foremost among these factors are obesity, social and psychological stress, patterns of personal behavior and some metabolic abnormalities such as glucose intolerance, gout and hypothyroidism. Excellent reviews on the role of these factors, and other factors as well, are available [8-17]; only a few selected factors will be reviewed here.

Obesity—Although the gradient between the incidence of coronary heart disease and obesity is a modest one, it is generally accepted that overweight, especially weight gain in middle age, contributes to the risk of coronary heart disease.[28] Perhaps it is the association of obesity with the level of blood pressure (and the level of serum triglyceride) that mediates the effect. In the presence of hypertension or diabetes mellitus, obesity assumes a much stronger position as a risk of coronary heart disease and should not be dismissed lightly. It should be noted, however, that we have at present no evidence that a systematic weight reduction program will reduce the incidence of coronary heart disease. Those who advocate weight reduction, do so purely on an empirical basis and because it favorably influences other coronary heart disease risk factors, as well as enhances a sense of well being.

Family History—It is a well known clinical observation that coronary heart disease exhibits a strong familial aggregation in its clinical manifestation. Those with positive family history are considered at high risk; these individuals are more vulnerable to the ravages of the disease when they possess one or more of the conventional risk factors (eg, cigarette smoking). To the extent that familial tendency of coronary heart disease would be interpreted as hereditary, it should be noted that coronary heart disease is a multifactorial disease entity, and that the genetic factors involved in it are multiple. In other words, coronary heart disease is "a polygenic trait."[29]

Stress and Behavioral Patterns—One of the generally accepted definitions of the word "stress" is an individual's response to occupational and other environmental situations inducing emotions such as frustration, fear, hostility and insecurity. Based on empirical clinical experience, this response varies among individuals and relates, in some instances, to the incidence of coronary heart disease. Foremost among epidemiologic and clinical studies on this subject is the observation that certain patterns of personal behavior are positively associated with the incidence of coronary heart disease. What is commonly known as "Type A Behavior" (characterized by excessive sense of time urgency, preoccupation with deadlines, aggressiveness and competitive drive) is reported to be an independent risk of coronary heart disease that aggravates the influence of other risk factors (eg, hypercholesterolemia and hypertension).[30] The estimated logistics coefficient for behavior pattern (as a coronary heart disease risk factor) is reported around 0.6 and 0.7 respectively for men in the age groups of 30 to 49 and 50 to 59 years.[31] When type A behavior factor is removed from the constellation of risk factors under observation, there remains, however, an additional residue of risk. Therefore, the behavioral pattern is considered, at best, as one of many risk factors found to be associated with the incidence of coronary heart disease.

There are other aspects of social or psychological stress that relate to the incidence of coronary heart disease. Among factors other than personal behavior, the role of social and cultural incongruities has been stressed the most.[32] It has been reported that the incidence of coronary heart disease is high among those who have marked discrepancies between their social background and present status in society, or among those who migrate to an unfamiliar social and cultural milieu, and are forced to adapt quickly to their new environment.

Glucose Intolerance—We have known for years that the main complication of diabetes mellitus is premature atherosclerosis. Recently the role of diabetes mellitus, especially in its early stages, has been emphasized as a strong coronary heart disease risk factor.[33] The prevalence of abnormal response to glucose tolerance test in a community should be expected to be around 2 to 3%, with an additional 10% with "borderline" response. The risk of coronary heart disease increases parallel to this pattern of response to the glucose tolerance test. It should be noted that abnormal glucose tolerance (and clinically manifest diabetes) is associated with other coronary heart disease risk factors, ie, obesity and hyperlipidemia. Thus, glucose intolerance should be considered as one of the significant coronary heart disease risk factors because of its association with other factors.

Summary

Coronary heart disease remains the leading cause of death in the United States and most of the technologically advanced countries in the world, despite indications of a decline in mortality since 1968. Clinical manifestations of coronary heart disease include sudden death (which comprises about 60% of all coronary heart disease deaths), acute fatal and nonfatal infarctions and angina pectoris. The basic pathogenic process of the malady is atherosclerosis, about which we know very little.

Epidemiologic studies in recent years have sharpened our focus on the natural history and dynamics of coronary heart disease. Certain personal characteristics and socioenvironmental factors, collectively called the "coronary heart disease risk factors," are found to be associated with risk of the disease.

Foremost among these factors are age, sex, positive family history, levels of serum cholesterol and blood pressure, cigarette smoking, impaired vital capacity, glucose intolerance, overweight and physical inactivity. Among all known coronary heart disease risk factors, age, sex, levels of serum cholesterol and blood pressure, cigarette smoking and physical inactivity are the most powerful predictors, in terms of a conditional probability, of developing coronary heart disease.

References

1. Myocardial Infarction Community Registers, Public Health in Europe, W.H.O. Report No. 5, 1976.
2. Gordon T, Tom T: The recent decrease in coronary heart disease mortality. *Prev Med* 4:115-125, 1975.
3. Morgan AD: Some forms of undiagnosed coronary disease in nineteenth-century England. Cit. No. 34 73207, *Med Hist* 12:344-358, 1968.
4. Leibowitz JO: *The History of Coronary Heart Disease*, London: Wellcome Institute of History of Medicine, 1970.
5. Fothergill J: A case of angina pectoris with remarks. *Med Obsns Inquir* 5:233-235, 1776.
6. Jenner E: "Letter to W. Heberden," in Jacobs HB: *Edward Jenner—A Student of Medicine, as illustrated in his letters*, New York: Hoeber, 1919.
7. Herrick JB: Clinical features of sudden obstruction of the coronary arteries. *JAMA* 59:2015-2020, 1912.
8. Epstein FH: The epidemiology of coronary heart disease, a review. *J Chronic Dis* 18:735-774, 1965.
9. Borhani NO: "The Magnitude of the Problem of Cardiovascular Diseases," in Lilienfeld A. Gifford AJ (Eds): *Chronic Diseases and Public Health*, Baltimore, Maryland: Johns Hopkins Press, 1966.
10. *Build and Blood Pressure Study*, Vol 1, Chicago: Society of Actuaries, 1959.
11. Dawber TR, Moore FE, Mann GV: Coronary heart disease in the Framingham study. *Amer J Physiol* 47:4-24 1957.
12. Acheson RW: The etiology of coronary disease. A review from the epidemiologic standpoint. *Yale J Biol Med* 35:143-170, 1962.
13. Primary Prevention of Atherosclerotic Diseases. Report of the Intersociety Commission for Heart Disease Resources (abstract). *Circulation* 42:55-95, 1970.
14. Epstein FH: "Coronary Heart Disease Epidemiology," in Stewart GT (Ed): *Trends in Epidemiology*, Springfield, Illinois: Charles C Thomas, 1972.
15. Blackburn H: "Progress in the Epidemiology and Prevention of Coronary Heart Disease," in Yu PN, Goodwin JF (Eds): *Progress in Cardiology*, Philadelphia: Lea and Febiger, 1974.
16. The Framingham Study: An Epidemiological Investigation of Cardiovascular Diseases, Diet and the Regulation of Serum Cholesterol; Section 23, Washington, D.C.: Government Printing Office, 1970.
17. Keys A (Ed): Coronary heart disease in seven countries. *Circulation* 41 (suppl 1): 1-51, 1970.
18. Antischkow NN: "A History of Experimentation on Arterial Atherosclerosis," in Blumenthal HT (Ed): *Cowdry's Arteriosclerosis*, ed 2, pp 21-44, Springfield, Illinois: Charles C Thomas, 1967.

19. Rosenthal SR: Studies in atherosclerosis, chemical experimental and morphological. *Arch Path* 18:473-506, 660-698, 1934.
20. Fredrickson DS, Lees RS: A system for phenotyping hyperlipoproteinemia. *Circulation* 31:321-327, 1965.
21. Fredrickson DS, Levy RI, Lees RS: Fat transport in lipoproteins—an integrated approach to mechanisms and disorders. *New Eng J Med* 276:34-42, 94-103, 148-156, 215-225, 273-281, 1967.
22. Truett J, Cornfield J, Kannel W: A multivariate analysis of the risk of coronary heart disease in Framingham. *J Chronic Dis* 20:511-524, 1967.
23. Borhani NO: "Implementation and Evaluation of Community Hypertension Programs," in Paul O (Ed): *Epidemiology and Control of Hypertension*, Miami, Florida: Symposia Specialists, 1975.
24. Veterans Administration Cooperative Study Group on Antihypertensive Agents. Effects of treatment on morbidity in hypertension, results in patients with diastolic blood pressures averaging 115-129 mm Hg. *JAMA* 202:1028-1034, 1967.
25. Veterans Administration Cooperative Study Group on Antihypertensive Agents. Results in patients with diastolic blood pressures averaging 90-114 mm Hg. *JAMA* 213:1143-1152, 1970.
26. Tyroler HA, Hames CG, Krishan I, et al: Black-white differences in serum lipids and lipoproteins in Evans county. *Prev Med* 4(4):541-549, 1975.
27. Reid DD: "Smoking and Ischemic Heart Disease," in Anguissola AB, Puddu CG (Eds): *Cardiologia d'Oggi*, pp 233-243, Turin: C.A. Edizioni Medico-Scientifiche, 1975.
28. Rabkin SW, Mathewson FAL, Hsu PH: Relation of body weight to development of ischemic heart disease in a cohort of young north American men after a 26-year observation period: the Manitoba study. *Amer J Cardiol* 39:452-458, 1977.
29. McKusick VA: "Genetic Factors in Atherosclerosis With Particular Reference to Atherosclerosis of the Coronary Arteries," in Blumenthal HT (Ed): *Cowdry's Arteriosclerosis*, ed 2, pp 551-575, Springfield, Illinois: Charles C Thomas, 1967.
30. Friedman M, Rosenman RH: Association of specific overt behavior pattern with blood and cardiovascular findings. *JAMA* 169:1286-1296, 1959.
31. Brand RJ, Rosenman RH, Sholtz I, et al: Multivariate prediction of coronary heart disease in the western collaborative group study compared to the findings of the Framingham study. *Circulation* 53:348-355, 1976.
32. Syme SL, Borhani NO, Buechley RW: Cultural mobility and coronary heart disease in an urban area. *Amer J Epidemiol* 82(3):334-346, 1966.
33. Ostrander LD, Lamphiear DE: Coronary risk factors in a community; findings in Tecumseh, Michigan. *Circulation* 53:152-156, 1976.

2

Coronary Artery Disease: Pathophysiology and Clinical Correlations

Ezra A. Amsterdam, MD
Dean T. Mason, MD

Severe coronary artery disease results in impairment of the coronary circulation and thereby deprivation of adequate oxygen supply to the myocardium. This fundamental physiologic deficit is the basis for the spectrum of clinical disorders comprising coronary heart disease, currently the single greatest cause of mortality in the industrialized societies. This chapter will discuss the anatomic and physiologic aspects of the normal coronary circulation, and the functional and clinical consequences of derangements in this system.

Coronary Artery Anatomy

The coronary vessels originate directly from the aorta as two main trunks, the right and left coronary arteries, through which the blood supply to the myocardium is delivered. The anatomy of these vessels in the human heart has been fully described by James.[1] Figure 1 depicts the general anatomic relationships of the coronary arteries and their major branches. The distribution of these vessels and relative mass of myocardium supplied by each are generally consistent within a limited degree of variation. Familiarity with coronary artery anatomy is of clinical relevance, since the site of disease in the coronary circulation is an important determinant of the location, extent and nature of the functional abnormalities and myocardial damage consequent to pathology in these arteries.

The left coronary artery divides into its major divisions, the left anterior descending and left circumflex arteries, within 2 cm of its origin. The left anterior descending artery runs in the anterior interventricular sulcus and through

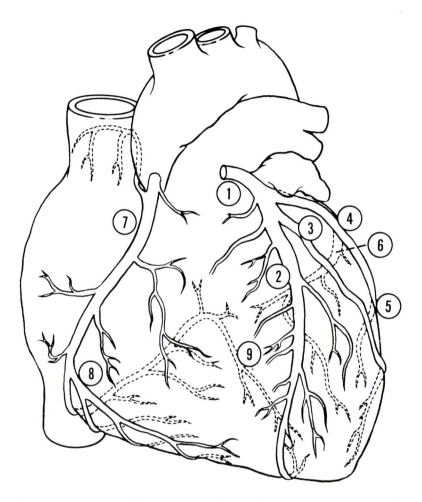

Figure 1. Coronary artery (CA) anatomy. 1-Left main CA; 2-Left anterior descending CA; 3-Diagonal branch of #2; 4-Left circumflex CA; 5-Marginal branch of #4; 6-Posterior circumflex CA; 7-Right CA; 8-Marginal branch of #7; 9-Posterior descending artery.

branches along this course supplies the free wall and apex of the left ventricle and interventricular septum. It also provides some branches to right ventricular myocardium adjacent to the interventricular septum. As a rule, the distal portion of the anterior descending artery continues around the apex, ascending for a short distance in the posterior interventricular sulcus where, before terminating, it issues branches to the proximal inferior areas of both ventricles and the apex. The left circumflex artery circles in the left atrioventricular sulcus to the obtuse margin of the left ventricle and continues beyond toward the posterior interventricular sulcus. Along its course it supplies branches to the lateral and inferior walls of the left ventricle as well as the left atrium. In about 10% of cases the circumflex artery crosses the crux of the heart and is the source of the posterior descending artery, which continues anteriorly in the posterior inter-ventricular sulcus toward the apex to meet the terminal branches of the anterior descending artery.

The right coronary artery descends in the right atrioventricular sulcus toward the acute margin of the right ventricle. In approximately 90% of human hearts it continues beyond this point and crosses the crux to ascend in the left atriovent-ricular sulcus toward the terminal portion of the left circumflex artery. Along its course it provides branches to the right atrium and the right ventricle, and in those hearts in which it crosses the crux it gives off the posterior descending artery and branches to the inferior wall of the left ventricle.

The arterial supply of the inferior wall of the left ventricle and certain of the specialized conducting tissues is variable. In the approximately 90% of in-stances in which the distal right coronary artery extends beyond the right atri-um and ventricle to the left side of the heart, it provides the posterior descend-ing artery and the vascular supply to half or more of the inferior surface of the left ventricle. In these hearts the artery to the atrioventricular node, which also supplies the His bundle and origins of the bundle branches, originates from the distal right coronary artery. In approximately 10% of cases the atrioventricular nodal artery is a branch of the distal left circumflex artery, in which cases the latter provides the major supply to the inferior left ventricle. In a certain pro-portion of cases the blood supply of the inferior left ventricular wall is de-rived in varying or equal degrees from both the right and left circumflex arter-ies. The sinoatrial node receives its blood supply from the right coronary artery in 55 to 60% of human hearts and from the left circumflex artery in 40 to 45%. The bundle branches, to a large extent, receive their blood supply from the same sources as the interventricular septum within which they originate. In this trifascicular conducting system the right bundle branch and the anterior fascicle of the left bundle branch are supplied by septal branches of the anterior descending artery. The posterior fascicle of the left bundle branch possesses a dual blood supply from the anterior and posterior descending coronary arteries.

In the context of coronary artery disease, the blood supply to the left ventricle is most relevant, since significant myocardial injury consequent to coronary disease and productive of functional derangement chiefly involves the left ven-tricle. From the preceding discussion it can be seen that the left coronary sys-tem is predominant in the human heart in terms of total mass of myocardium and of left ventricle supplied. In summary, except for its inferior surface, which is generally supplied by both right and left coronary arteries, the left ventricle receives its blood supply from the left coronary artery.

Physiology of the Coronary Circulation and Myocardial Metabolism

The functional burden of the heart surpasses that of all other organs, and its metabolism is accordingly adapted to support its intense energy requirements.

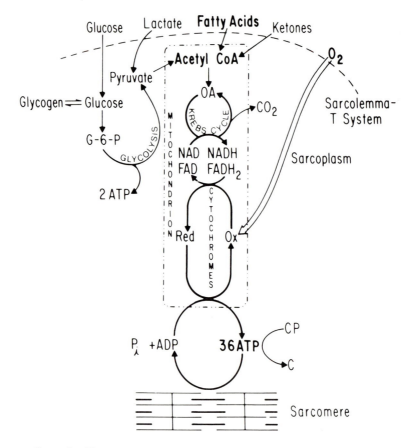

CORONARY CIRCULATION

Figure 2. Diagram of metabolic pathways of energy (adenosine triphosphate) production within the cardiac cell. Complete oxidation of a substrate such as glucose yields a total of 38 moles of adenosine triphosphate per mole of glucose, whereas glycolysis alone provides only 2 moles of adenosine triphosphate. Fatty acids are the preferred substrate. ADP = adenosine diphosphate; ATP = adenosine triphosphate; C = creatine; CP = creatine phosphate; CoA = coenzyme A; FAD and FADH = flavin adenine dinucleotide and its reduced form, respectively; G-6-P = glucose-6-phosphate; NAD and NADH = nicotinamide adenine dinucleotide and its reduced form, respectively; OA = oxaloacetic acid; Ox = oxidation; P_i = inorganic phosphate; Red = reduction.

Myocardial metabolism is essentially exclusively aerobic, thereby providing an efficient means for production of energy in the form of adenosine triphosphate (ATP). Further, this metabolic pattern, which is dependent on continuous delivery of oxygen to the myocardium, is sustained by a high level (near maximal at rest) of oxygen extraction from perfusing blood. Finally, because there is little capacity to augment oxygen extraction, increases in myocardial oxygen requirements are met by elevation of coronary blood flow, with alterations in the latter under the control of exquisitely sensitive autoregulatory mechanisms. In these aspects of function, myocardial muscle differs fundamentally from other organs, as indicated by comparison with skeletal muscle. Thus, oxygen extraction by skeletal muscle is relatively low at rest, increased oxygen demand is met by elevation of oxygen extraction as well as augmentation of blood flow, and anaerobic metabolism occurs when increased energy demand exceeds oxygen availability, a normal accompaniment of vigorous activity.

Cardiac muscle utilizes a number of substrates, principal among which are free fatty acids (Figure 2). The importance of continuous adequate oxygen delivery to the myocardium is indicated by the relative contributions of aerobic and anaerobic pathways to production of ATP, to which myocardial energy metabolism is primarily directed. Complete metabolism of one molecule of glucose, which includes cytoplasmic glycolysis (an anaerobic process) and mitochondrial oxidation, yields a net production of 36 ATP molecules (Figure 2). By contrast, glycolysis alone results in a net synthesis of two ATP molecules from each glucose molecule. Anaerobic metabolism, in itself, is therefore inadequate to sustain cardiac function. However, during severe limitation of myocardial oxygen supply and depression of oxidative processes, the potential is greater for a significant contribution to energy production and maintenance of cell viability through glycolysis.[2]

The energy requirements of the heart are reflected by its oxygen needs, which exceed by threefold or more those of other organs.[3] However, while 10% of total body oxygen consumption is cardiac, the myocardium receives only 4% of total cardiac output.[4] Thus, myocardial oxygen extraction in the basal state is approximately 70%, in contrast to 10 to 20% by other organs.[3] This mechanism, as previously noted, provides little reserve for augmenting oxygen supply and results in a fundamental dependence on alterations in coronary blood flow to meet changes in myocardial oxygen requirements. The function of this system is thus critically related to the structural integrity of the coronary circulation, and in the presence of significant disease of the coronary vasculature, the basic relationships between myocardial energy demand and supply cannot be maintained. Under normal conditions coronary blood flow can increase fivefold.[5] These changes in coronary blood flow are effected by modulation of coronary vascular resistance through autoregulatory mechanisms responsive to variations in the metabolic requirements of the heart as well as neurohumoral and metabolic influences. Predominant among these factors is myocardial oxygen demand which, through its major hemodynamic determinants, significantly influences coronary circulatory dynamics.

Because of the obligatory aerobic nature of cardiac metabolism, myocardial energy utilization correlates closely with the oxygen consumption of the heart $(M\dot{V}O_2)$.[6] The major determinants of $M\dot{V}O_2$ are heart rate, intramyocardial tension (a function of the product of ventricular systolic pressure and volume), and contractility; there are also several minor factors, among them external

TABLE I

Determinants of Myocardial Oxygen Consumption

Major	Minor
Heart rate	External work (load × shortening)
Intramyocardial tension	Activation energy
ventricular systolic pressure	Basal energy
ventricular volume	
Myocardial contractility	

cardiac work (Table I).[6] These hemodynamic variables are altered by mechanical, neural, humoral and metabolic factors regulating cardiac performance in relation to systemic blood flow requirements. The overall oxygen needs of the heart are the net result of the combined effects of the determinants of $M\dot{V}O_2$. In the normal heart, coronary blood flow is thus ultimately dependent on and directly responsive to changes in these hemodynamic variables as they affect $M\dot{V}O_2$. Increase in $M\dot{V}O_2$ is precisely balanced by elevation of coronary blood flow, which is effected through reduction of coronary vascular resistance.

Regulation of Coronary Blood Flow

The factors influencing coronary blood flow are multiple, may be of systemic or local myocardial origin and may act directly or indirectly on the coronary circulation. They may be generally categorized as mechanical or hydraulic, neural and humoral, and metabolic.[7] The autoregulatory mechanisms referred to previously act chiefly through local metabolic factors to alter coronary vascular resistance to maintain appropriate myocardial blood supply.

Mechanical Factors—There are a number of important mechanical factors that have differing influences on coronary blood flow.[8] The latter varies directly with aortic perfusion pressure and is inversely related to coronary vascular resistance. Further, since left ventricular systolic intramyocardial pressure exceeds left ventricular intracavitary and aortic pressures, left ventricular coronary blood flow, as opposed to that of the right ventricle, occurs primarily during diastole. Diastolic pressure and duration of diastole are therefore of prime importance to left ventricular myocardial blood flow, and pathologic conditions that significantly alter these mechanical variables can adversely affect coronary flow. Thus prolongation of systole (as occurs in significant obstruction to left ventricular outflow) and tachycardia may impinge on diastolic time; and rapid runoff of systemic blood flow during diastole (a complication of aortic regurgitation, arteriovenous fistula, and other circulatory disturbances) is associated with reduced aortic diastolic pressure. In addition, the diastolic perfusion gradient is determined by both aortic and left ventricular pressure during diastole. Factors which elevate the latter, such as cardiac failure, will reduce the perfusion gradient for left ventricular coronary flow and, conversely, this gradient can be enhanced by lowering of left ventricular diastolic pressure.

Alteration of coronary vascular resistance is normally a function of the arterioles. However, in the presence of significant obstructive disease compromising 70% or more of the lumen of large coronary arteries, the latter assume an important resistance function. The arterial obstruction presents a fixed mechanical resistance that both impairs coronary blood flow and is unresponsive to factors that modulate vascular caliber in the normal resistance vessels, thus preventing normal circulatory-metabolic relationships in the involved segment of myocardium. A common accompaniment of severe coronary artery disease is the presence of coronary collateral arteries, which potentially may modify regional coronary vascular resistance in the presence of obstructive narrowing in the native circulation. However, the functional significance of these collateral vessels, which will be discussed below, has not been clarified.

Neurohumoral Factors—Both the sympathetic and parasympathetic nervous systems innervate the coronary arteries, as well as the myocardium and sinoatrial and atrioventricular nodes. This close relation of both divisions of the autonomic nervous system to the structures, and thereby the functions, of the heart has been a major source of the difficulty in elucidating their complex actions on the coronary circulation, which are the result of both direct and indirect effects on the coronary arteries. Thus both sympathetic and parasympathetic stimulation produce significant cardiac chronotropic, inotropic and metabolic alterations, which in themselves affect coronary blood flow and can obscure the direct action of these stimuli on the coronary vasculature.

Clarification of the effects of neurohumoral mechanisms on the coronary circulation has been achieved through investigations on intact organisms and isolated vascular tissues and the application of adrenergic receptor stimulating and blocking drugs. These studies have produced a number of conclusions.[9] It has been established that there are α- and β-adrenergic receptors in the coronary arteries, with evidence of predominance of the latter in the small arteries and presence of both in the large vessels. The α receptors, which mediate constrictor effects via adrenergic stimuli, appear to have a more important physiologic role than the β receptors, the significance of which in the coronary circulation remains uncertain. Sympathetic nerve stimulation produces direct coronary vasoconstriction through its effect on α-adrenergic receptors and indirect vasodilation by its enhancement of myocardial mechanical function and consequent augmentation of $M\dot{V}O_2$. The latter effect is predominant, and the net result of these simultaneous influences is a reduction of coronary vascular resistance and increase in coronary blood flow. In a similar manner the catecholamines, norepinephrine and epinephrine, which cause direct coronary vasoconstriction through α-adrenergic stimulation, increase coronary blood flow by the indirect coronary vasodilating effect of their positive inotropic action. The primacy, in the regulation of coronary vascular resistance, of indirect metabolic effects on the myocardium over direct vascular actions, is a general characteristic of the coronary circulation. However, it is now apparent that the latter play a more important role in the regulation of coronary vascular resistance than previously appreciated.

The direct effect of parasympathetic stimulation is cholinergic coronary vasodilation. However, this may be complicated by the indirect effects of the vagus nerves, which tend to indirectly increase coronary vascular resistance by a negative inotropic action and to reduce extravascular coronary resistance through diminished systolic myocardial compression.[9]

Metabolic Factors—Although it is likely that no single factor is responsible for coronary blood flow regulation under all circumstances, the metabolic requirements of the myocardium appear to be dominant in this process. Coronary vascular resistance is inversely related to $M\dot{V}O_2$, which thereby correlates directly with coronary blood flow. As proposed by Berne,[7] these relationships appear to be primarily mediated by the potent vasodilator, adenosine. Berne and coworkers have provided evidence that through the breakdown of intracellular adenine nucleotides, myocardial cells release adenosine continuously into the surrounding interstitial fluid. This process is directly responsive to myocardial cellular oxygen tension and is enhanced by inadequate oxygen supply and inhibited when oxygen delivery exceeds requirements, providing a feedback system for coronary flow regulation. Recent demonstration of adenosine release from the human heart during angina supports these studies.[10]

Other metabolic factors and vasoactive substances that have received consideration regarding the regulation of coronary blood flow are potassium ion, phosphate ion, plasma osmolarity and prostaglandins. Evidence regarding these factors is inconsistent and their role, if any, appears to be subordinate to that of the oxygen tension–adenine nucleotide system.[7]

Pathophysiology of Myocardial Oxygen Deprivation

As a result of its dependence on a continuous, abundant supply of oxygen, the myocardium is extremely sensitive to deprivation of this vital substrate. Inadequate myocardial oxygenation is associated with rapid deterioration of function and a complex of pathophysiologic events including impaired metabolic activity, deranged mechanical performance, abnormal electrophysiology, altered structural and physical properties, and clinical signs and symptoms. These abnormalities can culminate in irreversible structural and functional impairment within minutes if cellular hypoxia is sufficiently severe. However, even after marked deterioration there is a limited period during which myocardial structural and functional integrity can be restored by restitution of adequate oxygen delivery.

Experimental Studies—Although considerable caution must be exercised in relating experimental findings to clinical problems, laboratory studies have provided a systematic means, not feasible clinically, of analyzing the pathophysiologic consequences of myocardial oxygen deprivation. Experimental investigation of inadequate myocardial oxygen supply has involved studies of

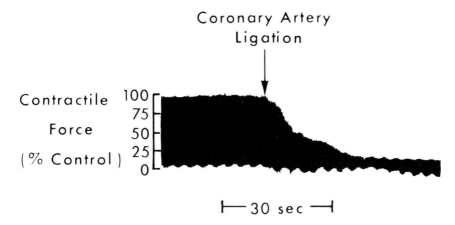

Figure 3. Left ventricular contractile force measured by an isometric strain gauge arch sutured to the myocardium of a dog. Note the rapid decline in force after ligation of the left anterior descending coronary artery.

both myocardial ischemia and hypoxia. Ischemia is defined as inadequate oxygen supply due to diminished coronary blood flow and is analogous to the clinical situation of coronary artery disease. It is studied in the intact heart and coronary circulation. Hypoxia applied experimentally refers to reduced oxygen concentration in the perfusate or supporting medium in which cardiac tissue is immersed. Studies of hypoxia have been carried out in the isolated whole heart or isolated cardiac tissue. Both ischemia and hypoxia produce inadequate myocardial cellular oxygen delivery. However, since ischemia is related to hypoperfusion, it produces a deficiency of, in addition to oxygen, substrates for energy production and it also results in an accumulation of metabolic end products and other substances from damaged cells which, in themselves, may be deleterious to cardiac processes.

In the laboratory animal resting coronary blood flow falls only when stenosis of a coronary artery exceeds 80%,[11] indicating the degree of reserve in the coronary circulation. However, when severe coronary stenosis is induced, interrupting coronary flow and oxygen supply, deterioration of myocardial function is abrupt and profound, as indicated in Figure 3. Of interest is the demonstration of adequate levels of high-energy phosphate compounds in the early phase of myocardial ischemia when marked reduction in function has already ensued, suggesting that inadequate energy production is not the critical factor in the initial phase of this process.[12]

Experimental coronary artery ligation results in diminution of contraction of the ischemic myocardial segment within 10 seconds and, within 1 minute, passive, systolic expansion of this area is produced by the intraventricular pressure generated by the unaffected, normally contracting myocardium which distends the ischemic zone.[13] If a sufficient quantity of myocardium is involved, the impairment of mechanical function is accompanied by alterations in cardiac

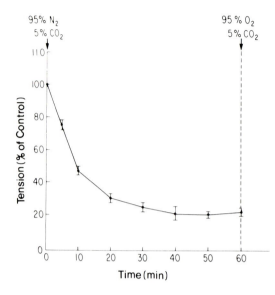

95% N_2
5% CO_2

95% O_2
5% CO_2

Figure 4. Effect of hypoxia on tension (mean ± standard error) developed by isolated cat papillary muscle supported in a Krebs bath. The bath is initially perfused with 95% oxygen and 5% carbon dioxide. Tension decreases abruptly after substitution of 95% nitrogen (N_2) for oxygen.

pump performance, electrical activity, and metabolism.[14, 15] These alterations include reduction in cardiac output, stroke volume and blood pressure and increase in left atrial and left ventricular diastolic pressures, as well as electrocardiographic ST-segment depression, lactate production, enhanced glucose extraction and decreased free fatty acid extraction by the myocardium. Typical ST changes and myocardial lactate production correlate closely as indicators of myocardial ischemia. Although the major consequence of interruption of coronary blood flow is cessation of myocardial oxygen supply, excessive accumulation of products of cellular metabolism and breakdown such as potassium, hydrogen ion and lysosomal enzymes, can depress myocardial metabolic, electrical and functional processes.[12, 14, 16, 17]

The effects of hypoxia on the mechanics of myocardial contraction, as demonstrated in the isolated, supported cat right ventricular papillary muscle, consist of rapid and severe loss of contractile performance (Figure 4). This involves decrease in both tension development and the period during which tension generation occurs.[18, 19] Anoxia, studied in the isolated, perfused heart, produces marked impairment of myocardial mechanical performance, abnormal electrical activity and structural disruption.[20] With the onset of anoxia, pulse pressure and maximal rate of rise of left ventricular pressure are reduced, ventricular end-diastolic pressure increases sharply, and alterations occur in myocardial subcellular architecture.

Clinical Coronary Artery Disease

Clinical-Pathophysiologic Correlations—Coronary heart disease may be manifested by a spectrum of clinical syndromes, including angina pectoris, in-

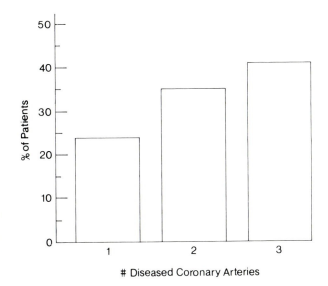

Figure 5. Proportion of coronary patients with one (1), two (2) and three (3) vessel coronary artery disease. Based on coronary angiography of 382 patients at the School of Medicine, University of California, Davis.

termediate coronary syndrome (preinfarction angina, coronary insufficiency), myocardial infarction and sudden death. Cardiac arrhythmias, congestive heart failure and cardiogenic shock may also result from myocardial ischemia and injury due to coronary artery disease.

The advent of coronary angiography has elucidated the relation between coronary artery anatomy and clinical manifestations of coronary heart disease and its prognosis. It is now established that a majority of patients with clinical coronary heart disease, such as angina pectoris, myocardial infarction or sudden death have severe and extensive obstruction of the coronary arteries. Approximately three-fourths of these patients have major stenoses in two or three coronary arteries.[21, 22] Patients with clinical coronary heart disease and involvement of only one coronary artery are more unusual, comprising less than 30% of the coronary population. Data from our laboratories, shown in Figure 4, exemplify these findings. Angiographic studies have further demonstrated that clinically manifest myocardial ischemia is usually associated with compromise of more than 70% of the lumen of one or more coronary arteries.[21, 22] This finding is in accord with experimental data which have shown that constriction of a coronary artery does not reduce flow in the vessel until the stenosis exceeds 80%.[11] Abnormalities of myocardial function in coronary artery disease, whether transient or permanent, are characteristically segmental in location,[23] as described below. These defects are distributed according to the perfusion deficits in the myocardium, the regions of which are determined by the sites of coronary obstruction.

Although the basis of restricted coronary blood flow is typically atherosclerotic coronary artery narrowing, it is now also appreciated that coronary spasm may compromise flow and produce myocardial ischemia. Coronary arterial spasm has been considered chiefly in relation to Prinzmetal or variant angina pectoris, and has been documented in this entity in the presence of both normal [24, 25] and diseased coronary arteries [26] in which it is associated with myocardial ischemic pain, electrocardiographic ST elevation, hemodynamic dysfunction and ventricular arrhythmias. The extent to which this phenomenon may be involved in the clinical manifestations of myocardial ischemia, *ie*, angina, infarction and sudden death, is currently unknown.

Although clinical symptoms are characteristically the initial indication of coronary artery disease, these do not occur, as previously noted, until coronary obstruction is severe. However, the atherosclerotic process is a chronic, progressive one and begins at least several decades prior to its reaching the critical degree productive of clinical manifestations, as indicated by postmortem evidence of considerable coronary atherosclerosis in asymptomatic American men in the third decade of life.[27] Since a group of major risk factors related to development of coronary heart disease have been identified (see Chapter 1), this prolonged incubation process has major implications for both preventive cardiology and identification and management of individuals with preclinical coronary artery atherosclerosis.[28]

The clinical presentation of coronary heart disease is well demonstrated by the Framingham Study, a classic epidemiological investigation of over 5,000 persons followed for more than 20 years.[28] In the male population that developed clinical coronary heart disease, the most common initial presentation was myocardial infarction (45%). Angina pectoris was next in frequency (32%) and sudden death was not rare, occurring as the initial manifestation in 9% of cases. Angina was frequently preceded by myocardial infarction in men. Findings in women differed, angina accounting for 56% of the presenting manifestations of coronary heart disease and occurring chiefly as a new event.

Coronary heart disease is a highly lethal process in which immediate mortality is substantial and long-term survival is generally impaired. However, the latter varies within the coronary population according to the presence of a number of factors. The Framingham experience demonstrated that in 20% of coronary episodes (exclusive of angina), sudden death was the initial event and more than half of the deaths due to coronary heart disease were sudden and unexpected, occurring away from hospital and medical care.[29] Overall immediate mortality related to onset of clinical coronary disease was 33%.

Meaningful analysis of long-term prognosis in coronary heart disease is predicated on appreciation of the heterogeneity of this population with respect to those variables influencing survival. Although the annual mortality rate is 4 to 8% in patients with clinical evidence of coronary heart disease without angiographic confirmation,[28, 30] recent studies based on coronary angiography demonstrated significant differences in survival relating to the extent of coronary artery involvement. These investigations have consistently shown that annual mortality is directly proportional to the number of significantly diseased coronary arteries. In two surveys of a total of 1,295 patients, annual mortality related to angiographically documented coronary artery disease was similar: one-vessel disease—2 to 3%; two-vessel disease—6 to 8%; three-vessel disease—10 to 12%.[31, 32] Other factors, in addition to the number of diseased coronary vessels, contribute to mortality in this group of patients. With any degree of coronary artery disease, mortality is increased by the presence at cardiac catheterization of impaired ventricular function and left main coronary artery disease, and by clinical factors such as prior myocardial infarction, cardiac failure, atrial fibrillation and hypertension.[33]

Angina Pectoris—Myocardial ischemia may be transient and reversible in terms of symptoms and associated cardiac functional alterations, as in the syndrome of angina pectoris. Ischemia of sufficient severity and duration results in irreversible loss of structure and function, usually manifested clinically as myocardial infarction. Circulatory dynamics and patterns of ventricular function during ischemia have been clarified to a considerable extent by the recent application of hemodynamic and angiographic techniques to this problem.

Although the symptom of ischemic cardiac pain is the most apparent manifestation of angina, the imbalance between myocardial oxygen supply and demand productive of this syndrome results in fundamental derangements of cardiac function that also characterize this clinical entity. Coronary blood flow and myocardial oxygen delivery are typically normal and symptoms are absent in angina patients in the resting state. However, myocardial ischemia and angina are usually provoked by augmentation of cardiac oxygen demand, through its aforementioned determinants (Table I), beyond the capacity of the restricted coronary circulation to respond. This commonly occurs with physical or emotional stress. Whereas in normal coronary arteries, flow can increase by fivefold or more,[5] coronary obstructive disease commonly limits this increase in flow to less than double the resting level.[34]

Among the most consistent findings during myocardial ischemia is the usually striking evidence of depressed left ventricular function. The hemodynamic impairment is directly related to the presence of myocardial ischemia, and the extent of functional loss is dependent on the quantity of myocardial muscle involved. With subsidence of ischemia, as occurs in angina, ventricular function returns to its preischemic level. However, after myocardial infarction there is usually permanent reduction in cardiac functional capacity. Consistent with the concept that angina is a result of myocardial ischemia is evidence of increased myocardial oxygen requirements, together with inability to commensurately augment coronary blood flow, during angina, whether provoked or spontaneous. Indeed, in the clinical evaluation of patients, angina is induced or alleviated by manipulation of those hemodynamic variables that determine myocardial oxygen needs [22, 35] (Table I). The basis of restricted coronary blood flow is, in all but unusual instances, coronary artery atherosclerosis.

Although clinical studies have evaluated angina induced by a variety of stresses (catecholamine infusion, pacing tachycardia, exercise) or occurring spontaneously, the hemodynamic response has been consistent. Thus, as in the

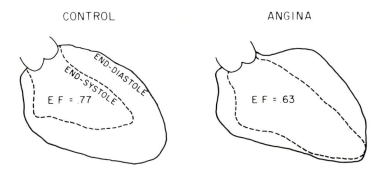

Figure 6. Diagrams of left ventricular angiograms from a patient with coronary artery disease. Control angiogram demonstrates a normal contraction pattern. With the onset of angina produced by atrial pacing, there is impairment of myocardial contraction manifested by hypokinesis of the apical-inferior area of the left ventricle which is associated with a fall in ejection fraction (EF).

experimental studies previously discussed, abnormal cardiac performance indicative of left ventricular failure has been repeatedly demonstrated at the time of angina pectoris.[22, 35] Left ventricular end-diastolic pressure is increased in association with reduced cardiac output, stroke volume and stroke work, and the left ventricular function curve is thereby depressed. That this evidence of depressed myocardial contractile function during ischemic pain is intrinsic to the angina state is indicated by lack of these findings in patients with coronary artery disease who do not manifest angina under identical conditions. A further alteration during acute ischemia that contributes to elevation in end-diastolic pressure is reduction of myocardial compliance.[36]

The deterioration of cardiac performance accompanying angina is associated with abnormal ventricular wall motion, which has now been documented in man by angiographic studies during angina. This abnormality of muscle function consists of failure of adequate shortening, which is associated with diminished force development in one or more areas of ventricular myocardium. During acute ischemia the contractile pattern of the ventricle may deteriorate from normal to include one or more areas of inadequate or abnormal motion, or when the latter is already present it may become quantitatively greater in the affected area or involve additional regions of myocardium [14, 36] (Figure 6). Loss of actively contracting muscle deprives the ventricle, for the duration of this defect, of the contribution of involved myocardium to overall cardiac pump function, resulting in decreased stroke volume, cardiac output and ejection fraction, with consequent increase in residual ventricular volume and end-diastolic pressure—hemodynamic findings indicative of ventricular failure.

The impaired ventricular muscle performance in ischemic heart disease is characteristically segmental, as determined by the distribution of coronary artery atherosclerosis. Abnormal ventricular wall motion resulting from coronary disease has been categorized into several descriptive patterns under the general term "asynergy." [23] The degree of hemodynamic impairment is directly related to the quantity of cardiac muscle involved in the asynergic process. Thus, in the presence of inadequate function of 20 to 25% of left ventricular myocardium, as defined by left ventriculography, compensation by the remaining uninvolved myocardium is inadequate, resulting in depression of overall ventricular function leading to cardiac pump failure.[37] Although it is related to coronary artery disease, asynergy is most consistently the result of ischemic myocardial damage. We have found that in patients with acute or remote myocardial infarction, as indicated by the electrocardiogram, abnormal ventricular motion is almost a constant finding, whereas even in severe coronary artery disease without electrocardiographic evidence of infarction, left ventricular asynergy is much less common in the unstressed ventricle.[14] However, with the onset of acute myocardial ischemia, as in angina, frank asynergy can develop in a previously normally contracting ventricle (Figure 6). In angina pectoris this is a transient, reversible phenomenon, whereas in the infarcted ventricle the abnormality of wall motion is a permanent manifestation of necrosis and subsequent scarring. As in experimental myocardial ischemia, alterations in myocardial electrical and metabolic processes accompany the functional defects, as indicated by lactate production, enhanced glucose extraction and ST-segment depression.[22, 35, 38-40]

The reversible nature of angina is emphasized. The acute myocardial ischemia characteristic of this syndrome is transient, and thus the entire spectrum of physiological abnormalities is short-lived, reversion to previous status generally occurring within minutes. Support for the absence of myocardial damage during angina is provided by metabolic studies that document myocardial ischemia during acute episodes of pain and simultaneously reveal no evidence of necrosis, as indicated by coronary sinus sampling for cardiac enzymes.[41]

Myocardial Infarction—Myocardial infarction is the result of irreversible ischemic injury to myocardial cells (Figure 7). Cellular metabolic and electrical activity cease, necrosis of cardiac muscle ensues, and electrocardiographic evidence of transmural loss of myocardium appears and is generally permanent. The consequent loss of functioning cardiac tissue is the primary cause of sustained cardiac failure in patients with coronary artery disease. Diminution or disappearance of abnormal Q waves may occur, especially in inferior infarction, within months or years.[14] When infarction is not transmural, the electrocardiographic changes are less specific.

The functional derangements observed in the acute transient ischemia of the anginal syndrome are usually present to an equal or greater degree in myocardial infarction, and they are usually permanent. However, there is some capacity for recovery, as indicated by experimental studies demonstrating improved hemodynamic function in the early postinfarction period as compared to the acute stage.[42]

Although there is some evidence of impaired cardiac performance in most

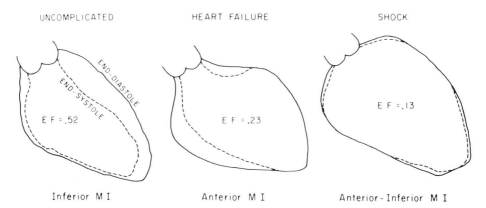

Figure 7. Diagrams of left ventricular angiograms of patients with acute myocardial infarction (MI). The inferior infarction is associated with inferior wall hypokinesis and is clinically uncomplicated. Heart failure is associated with extensive anterior wall akinesis in the anterior infarction. The anterior-inferior infarction is complicated by shock resulting from the severe diffuse impairment of contractile function. Ejection fraction (EF) is progressively decreased with increasing involvement of left ventricular myocardium.

patients with acute myocardial infarction, virtually the entire functional spectrum is present in the group as a whole (Figure 7). Hemodynamic evaluation has revealed myocardial function ranging from normal to the shock state in this syndrome. However, significant depression of ventricular performance is common, as indicated by a 40 to 50% prevalence of congestive cardiac failure and a 10 to 15% prevalence of cardiogenic shock.[43, 44] Depression of ventricular function is more common in anterior than in inferior infarction because, as we have found, the former usually involves a greater quantity of myocardium than does the latter.[45]

Congestive Heart Failure—Although transient episodes of myocardial ischemia can clearly produce temporary depression of left ventricular function, coronary artery disease in the absence of permanent damage to myocardial muscle is uncommonly associated with significant sustained impairment of cardiac performance. In the great majority of patients with coronary artery disease without previous myocardial infarction, indices of ventricular performance such as cardiac output, left ventricular end-diastolic pressure and synergy of contraction are unimpaired.[46] This finding is consistent with the clinical observation that cardiac failure is not usually a significant feature in the patient with angina who has not had a previous myocardial infarction.[47]

Of clinical interest is the relatively consistent relation between the electrocardiogram and ventricular function. Electrocardiographic pathologic Q waves correlate closely with the presence and location of left ventricular asynergy.[48] Q waves of anterior or combined anterior-inferior location are usually associated with hemodynamic dysfunction, whereas inferior Q waves alone are seldom indicative of abnormal function. Further, utilized in this manner the electrocardiogram bears a closer relation to ventricular functional status than does associated coronary artery disease, as indicated by coronary arteriography.[46]

Cardiogenic Shock—The chief cause of mortality in patients hospitalized with myocardial infarction is cardiogenic shock, which is associated with a fatality rate of 80% or greater.[43, 44] This syndrome results from severe depression of myocardial function consequent to loss of cardiac muscle. Impairment of ventricular performance in myocardial infarction is quantitatively related to degree of cardiac damage. Whereas uncomplicated infarction is usually associated with relatively small areas of injury, myocardial destruction in shock involves 40% or more of the ventricle, as indicated by postmortem evaluation.[44, 49] Our angiographic studies in patients with acute infarction have provided *in vivo* confirmation of these findings [50] (Figure 7). Although extent of myocardial damage is the primary factor in the pathogenesis of myocardial infarction shock, associated mechanical complications involving the heart and extracardiac factors such as hypovolemia and impairment of systemic vasoconstriction contribute in some patients.[43, 44]

Sudden Death—As previously noted, sudden death accounts for the majority of mortality from coronary heart disease and in some studies it is the initial and terminal coronary event in as many as 25% of victims.[51] Sudden coronary death chiefly results from the lethal arrhythmias, ventricular tachycardia and fibrillation, which are attributed to electrical instability of the myocardium due to ischemia.[52]

Myocardial ischemia predisposes to ventricular fibrillation by alteration and inhomogeneity of cardiac electrical properties. These consist of disparities in conduction velocity and duration of refractory periods in adjoining fibers which produce multiple reentry circuits and consequent disorganized electrical activity. The net result is ventricular fibrillation. The pathologic basis of this problem is severe coronary artery disease, as indicated by postmortem studies demonstrating multivessel involvement in approximately 75% of individuals dying suddenly.[53] It is of interest that in only a minority of patients is myocardial infarction associated with sudden death. This is reflected by a study of 239 patients resuscitated from ventricular fibrillation, of whom only 16% had associated transmural myocardial infarction.[54]

The major approach to management of this problem has been an attempt to identify those individuals in the coronary population who are at high risk for sudden death.[55] Much interest is currently centered on the chronic presence of ventricular ectopic beats as harbingers of ventricular fibrillation in ambulatory coronary patients. Recent studies have shown a close correlation between sudden death and the prior presence of ventricular ectopic beats detected by standard electrocardiography [56] or portable electrocardiographic monitoring.[57] The incidence of sudden death was 6 to 10 times as high in the group with frequent ventricular ectopic beats as in patients without this finding. We have found that ventricular arrhythmias are closely correlated with the presence of coronary artery disease, as shown in Table II. Further, prolonged portable electro-

TABLE II

Prevalence of Ventricular Ectopic Beats in 139 Patients
(12-Hour Portable Electrocardiographic Monitoring)

	Coronary Artery Disease (n = 102)	Normal (n = 37)
Ventricular Ectopic Beats	85.3% (n = 87)	37.8% (n = 14)

TABLE III

Detection of Ventricular Ectopic Beats in 22 Patients with Coronary Artery Disease
(Angiographically Documented)

	Electrocardiogram	Exercise Test	Portable ECG
Ventricular Ectopic Beats	23% (n = 5)	59% (n = 13)	82% (n = 18)

cardiographic monitoring, when compared to standard electrocardiography and exercise testing, has been the most sensitive means of detecting ventricular arrhythmias in stable coronary patients (Table III). However, exercise testing has also been a convenient, useful method for this purpose and has allowed certain conclusions. Thus, ventricular arrhythmias provoked by exertion are more frequent in coronary patients than in normals; ventricular ectopic beats which are of high frequency, multifocal, paired or occur at low exercise heart rates are particularly suggestive of coronary disease; and abolition during exercise of ventricular ectopic beats present at rest does not exclude coronary artery disease.[58]

We have evaluated the implications of ventricular ectopic beats in patients with recent myocardial infarction, a population of generally high prognostic risk. Interestingly, the frequency of ventricular arrhythmias was similar during the acute and late hospital phases of myocardial infarction.[59] Further, a prospective study of 64 postinfarction patients demonstrated that all 12 patients with subsequent sudden death during a two-year observation period had ventricular arrhythmias on portable monitoring prior to hospital discharge.[60] Serious ventricular ectopic beats (defined as >5/min, multifocal, R on T and ≥ 2 consecutive discharges) were particularly related to subsequent sudden death. In addition, the extent of ST-segment alteration on standard electrocardiography was greater in the sudden death group than in survivors, suggesting a relation of ventricular arrhythmias to persistent ischemia or segmental myocardial dysfunction.

Current findings suggest that the clinical implications of ventricular ectopic beats are related to their pattern and the clinical setting in which they occur. These arrhythmias appear to have serious prognostic significance when they occur in patients with documented coronary heart disease and are of the serious type, as defined above.[55] Associated factors, such as evidence of persistent myocardial ischemia and dysfunction, also affect the course of patients with coronary disease, either in relation to or independently of ventricular arrhythmias.[61]

Angiographically demonstrable coronary collateral vessels are consistently associated with severe obstructive coronary disease, and the coronary collateral circulation has been classically considered to play an important protective role in the ischemic myocardium. However, the results of recent investigations on the functional significance of coronary collaterals in man have generally been at variance with this view. There has been no consistent clinical evidence for a beneficial effect of coronary collaterals on symptoms, resting or exercise electrocardiogram, hemodynamic performance, or segmental myocardial function.[62, 63] Further, isotope studies of regional myocardial perfusion have shown that in zones of hypoperfusion collateral vessels provide minimal augmentation of coronary flow at rest [64] and confer no protective effect during exercise stress.[65]

Consistent with these findings and directly related to the issue of a protective effect of collaterals are postmortem studies demonstrating a lack of relation between them and the presence and extent of myocardial infarction.[66] However, earlier pathologic data support a protective effect of collaterals against infarction [67] and in patients with infarction who underwent acute angiography, we correlated the presence of collateral vessels with reduced complications.[68]

Many aspects of the function of coronary collaterals remain uncertain, including their flow potential. However, their documented ability to augment human regional myocardial perfusion [64] suggests a potential for support of cell viability in ischemic myocardium that may be of importance in the presence of marginal perfusion. Conclusions concerning this important subject must await further investigation by more advanced techniques.

Summary

The fundamental physiologic defect in coronary heart disease is inadequate oxygen delivery to the myocardium. This results in derangement of metabolic and functional processes and clinical signs and symptoms, which occur rapidly when oxygen deprivation is acute. Clinical manifestations of myocardial ischemia typically occur when coronary artery obstruction compromises more than 70% of the arterial lumen and are usually associated with multivessel coronary disease. Reversible derangements of function are characteristic of angina and permanent loss of myocardium and function result from infarction. Cardiac failure from coronary heart disease occurs when more than 25% of left ventricular myocardium is permanently damaged and cardiogenic shock is associated with loss of 40% or more of myocardium. Sudden death is commonly the initial manifestation of coronary heart disease and is usually due to a lethal ventricular arrhythmia caused by myocardial ischemia. Studies of the coronary collateral circulation have not yet provided clinical evidence that it has a protective effect by them in coronary heart disease, although further studies of this problem are needed.

Parts of this chapter were adapted with permission from Amsterdam EA, Miller RR, Foley DH, et al: "Pathophysiology and Treatment of Coronary Artery Disease," in Zelis R (Ed): *The Peripheral Circulations*, pp 363-394, New York: Grune & Stratton, 1975.

This study was supported by Research Program Project Grant HL-14780 from the National Institutes of Health, Bethesda, Maryland.

References

1. James TN: *Anatomy of the Coronary Arteries*, New York: Hoeber Medical Division, Harper & Row, 1961.
2. Opie LH: The glucose hypothesis: relation to acute myocardial ischaemia (editorial). *J Molec Cell Cardiol* 1:107, 1970.
3. Gorlin R: Physiologic studies in coronary atherosclerosis. *Fed Proc* 21:93-97, 1962.
4. Wade OL, Bishop JM: "The Distribution of the Cardiac Output in Normal Subjects at Rest," in Jones RB, Doc JP (Eds): *Cardiac Output and Regional Blood Flow*, pp 86-94, Oxford: Blackwell Scientific, 1962.
5. Mellander S, Johansson B: Control of resistance, exchange and capacitance functions in the peripheral circulation. *Pharmacol Rev* 20:117-196, 1968.
6. Sonnenblick EH, Skelton CL: Oxygen consumption of the heart: physiological principles and clinical implications. *Mod Conc Cardiovasc Dis* 40:9-16, 1971.
7. Berne RM: "The Coronary Circulation," in Langer G, Brady A (Eds): *The Mammalian Myocardium*, pp 251-281, New York: John Wiley & Sons, 1974.
8. Gorlin R: "Physiology of the Coronary Circulation," in Hurst JW, Logue RB, Schlant RC, et al (Eds): *The Heart*, pp 109-115, New York: McGraw-Hill, 1974.
9. Mark AL, Abboud FM: "Myocardial Blood Flow—Neurohumoral Determinants," in Zelis R (Ed): *The Peripheral Circulations*, pp 95-115, New York: Grune & Stratton, 1975.
10. Fox AC, Reed GE, Glassman E, et al: Release of adenosine from human hearts during angina induced by rapid atrial pacing. *J Clin Invest* 53:1447-1457, 1974.
11. Gould KL, Lipscomb K, Hamilton GW: Physiologic basis for assessing critical coronary stenosis. *Amer J Cardiol* 33:87-94, 1974.
12. Katz AM: Effects of ischemia on the contractile processes of heart muscle. *Amer J Cardiol* 32:456-460, 1973.
13. Tennant R, Wiggers CJ: Effect of coronary occlusion on myocardial contraction. *Amer J Physiol* 112:351-361, 1935.
14. Amsterdam EA: Function of the hypoxic myocardium. *Amer J Cardiol* 32:461-471, 1973.
15. Scheuer J, Brachfeld N: Coronary insufficiency: relations between hemodynamic, electrical and biochemical parameters. *Circ Res* 18:178-189, 1966.
16. Katz AM: "Effects of Ischemia and Hypoxia Upon the Myocardium," in Russek HI, Zohman BL (Eds): *Coronary Heart Disease*, pp 45-56, Philadelphia: J. B. Lippincott, 1971.
17. Sommers HM, Jennings RB: Experimental acute myocardial infarction. *Lab Invest* 13:1491-1503, 1964.
18. Amsterdam EA, Foley D, Massumi RA, et al: Enhancement of myocardial function during hypoxia by increased glucose availability (abstract). *Amer J Cardiol* 29:251, 1972.
19. Tyberg JV, Yeatman LA, Parmley WW, et al: Effects of hypoxia on mechanics of cardiac contraction. *Amer J Physiol* 218:1780-1788, 1970.
20. Weissler AM, Kruger FA, Baba N, et al: Role of anaerobic metabolism in the preservation of functional capacity and structure of anoxic myocardium. *J Clin Invest* 47:403-416, 1968.
21. Proudfit WL, Shirey EK, Sones FM: Distribution of arterial lesions demonstrated by selective cinecoronary arteriography. *Circulation* 36:54-62, 1967.

22. Amsterdam EA, Miller RR, Hughes JL, et al: "Pathophysiology of Angina Pectoris," in Kikoff W, Segal BL, Insull W, et al (Eds): *Atherosclerosis and Coronary Heart Disease*, pp 178-189, New York: Grune & Stratton, 1972.
23. Herman MV, Heinle RA, Klein MD, et al: Localized disorders in myocardial contraction. Asynergy and its role in congestive heart failure. *New Eng J Med* 277:222-232, 1967.
24. Oliva PB, Potts DE, Pluss RG: Coronary arterial spasm in Prinzmetal angina. Documentation by coronary arteriography. *New Eng J Med* 288:788-789, 1973.
25. Endo M, Hirosawa K, Kaneko N, et al: Prinzmetal's variant angina. Coronary arteriogram and left ventriculogram during angina attack induced by Methacholine. *New Eng J Med* 294:252-255, 1976.
26. Maseri R, Mimmo R, Chierchia S, et al: Coronary artery spasm as a cause of acute myocardial ischemia in man. *Chest* 68:625-633, 1975.
27. Enos WF Jr, Beyer JC, Holmes RH: Pathogenesis of coronary disease in American soldiers killed in Korea. *JAMA* 158:912-914, 1955.
28. Kannel WB: Some lessons in cardiovascular epidemiology from Framingham. *Amer J Cardiol* 37:269-282, 1976.
29. Gordon T, Kannel WB: Premature mortality from coronary heart disease. The Framingham Study. *JAMA* 215:1617-1625, 1971.
30. Block WJ Jr, Crumpacker EL, Dry TJ, et al: Prognosis of angina pectoris. Observations in 6,882 cases. *JAMA* 150:259-264, 1952.
31. Reeves TJ, Oberman R, Jones WB, et al: Natural history of angina pectoris. *Amer J Cardiol* 33:423-430, 1974.
32. Bruschke AVG, Proudfit WL, Sones FM: Progress study of 590 consecutive nonsurgical cases of coronary disease followed 5-9 years. I: Arteriographic correlations. *Circulation* 47:1147-1153, 1973.
33. Amsterdam EA, DeMaria AN, Lee G, et al: Long-term prognosis after acute myocardial infarction: influence of infarction location and hemodynamic function (abstract). *Clin Res* 25:87, 1977.
34. Parker JO, West RO, DiGiorgi S: The effect of nitroglycerin on coronary blood flow and the hemodynamic response to exercise in coronary artery disease. *Amer J Cardiol* 27:59-65, 1971.
35. Parker JO, Chiong MA, West RO, et al: Sequential alterations in myocardial lactate metabolism, S-T segments, and left ventricular function during angina induced by atrial pacing. *Circulation* 40:113-131, 1969.
36. Dwyer EM Jr: Left ventricular pressure-volume alterations and regional disorders of contraction during myocardial ischemia induced by atrial pacing. *Circulation* 42:1111-1122, 1970.
37. Klein MD, Herman MV, Gorlin R: A hemodynamic study of left ventricular aneurysm. *Circulation* 35:614-630, 1967.
38. Amsterdam EA, Manchester JH, Kemp HG, et al: Spontaneous angina pectoris (SAP): hemodynamic and metabolic changes (abstract). *Clin Res* 17:225, 1969.
39. Most AS, Gorlin R, Soeldner JS: Glucose extraction by the human myocardium during pacing stress. *Circulation* 45:92-96, 1972.
40. Amsterdam EA, Zelis R, Mason DT: "Chemical Assessment of Cardiovascular Function," in Ray CD (Ed): *Medical Engineering*, pp 298-304, Chicago: Year Book Medical Publishers, 1974.
41. Amsterdam EA, Zelis R, Bonanno JA, et al: Relation of cardiac ischemia and necrosis during angina pectoris: comparison of lactate metabolism and enzyme release by the human myocardium (abstract). *Circulation* 43, 44:130, 1971.
42. Kumar R, Hood WB Jr, Joison J, et al: Experimental myocardial infarction. II: Acute depression and subsequent recovery of left ventricular function: serial measurements in intact conscious dogs. *J Clin Invest* 49:55-62, 1970.
43. Amsterdam EA, Hughes JL, Iben A, et al: "Surgery for Acute Myocardial Infarction," in Gunnar RM, Loeb HS, Rahimtoola SH (Eds): *Shock in Myocardial Infarction*, pp 257-283, New York: Grune & Stratton, 1974.
44. Amsterdam EA, DeMaria AN, Hughes JL, et al: "Myocardial Infarction Shock: Mechanisms and Management," in Mason D (Ed): *Congestive Heart Failure*, pp 365-396, New York: Yorke Medical Books, 1976.
45. Miller RR, Olson HG, Vismara LA, et al: Pump dysfunction after myocardial infarction: importance of location extent and pattern of abnormal left ventricular segmental contraction. *Amer J Cardiol* 37:340-344, 1976.
46. Miller RR, Bonanno J, Massumi RA, et al: Usefulness of the electrocardiogram in assessment of

ventricular performance and comparison with coronary arteriography. *Amer J Cardiol* 29:281, 1972.

47. Roberts WC, Buja LM, Bulkley BH, et al: Congestive heart failure and angina pectoris. Opposite ends of the spectrum of symptomatic ischemic heart disease. *Amer J Cardiol* 34:870-872, 1974.

48. Miller RR, Amsterdam EA, Bogren HG, et al: Electrocardiographic and cineangiographic correlations in assessment of the location, nature and extent of abnormal left ventricular segmental contraction in coronary artery disease. *Circulation* 49:447-454, 1974.

49. Page DL, Caulfield JB, Kastor JA, et al: Myocardial changes associated with cardiogenic shock. *New Eng J Med* 285:133-137, 1971.

50. Amsterdam EA, Choquet Y, Bonanno JA, et al: Correlative hemodynamic and angiographic studies in acute coronary syndromes (abstract). *Clin Res* 21:232, 1973.

51. Kuller L: Sudden and unexpected non-traumatic deaths in adults: a review of epidemiological and clinical studies. *J Chronic Dis* 19:1165-1192, 1966.

52. Wit AL, Bigger T Jr: Possible electrophysiological mechanisms for lethal arrhythmias accompanying myocardial ischemia and infarction. *Circulation* 52 (suppl 3):96-115, 1975.

53. Perper JA, Kuller LH, Cooper M: Arteriosclerosis of coronary arteries in sudden, unexpected deaths. *Circulation* 52 (suppl 3):27-33, 1975.

54. Cobb LA, Baum RS, Alvarez H III, et al: Resuscitation from out-of-hospital ventricular fibrillation: 4 years follow-up. *Circulation* 52 (suppl 3):223-235, 1975.

55. Amsterdam EA, Vismara L, DeMaria AN, et al: "Lethal Arrhythmias in the Pathogenesis of Prehospital Sudden Death," in Gensini GG (Ed): *Concepts on the Mechanisms and Treatment of Arrhythmias*, pp 29-37, Mt. Kisco, New York: Futura, 1974.

56. Chiang BN, Perlman LV, Ostrander LD Jr, et al: Relationship of premature systoles to coronary heart disease and sudden death in the Tecumseh epidemiologic study. *Ann Intern Med* 70:1159-1166, 1969.

57. Hinkle LE Jr, Carver ST, Stevens M: The frequency of asymptomatic disturbances of cardiac rhythm and conduction in middle-aged men. *Amer J Cardiol* 24:629-650, 1969.

58. DeMaria AN, Vera Z, Amsterdam EA, et al: Disturbances of cardiac rhythm and conduction induced by exercise: diagnostic, prognostic, and therapeutic implications. *Amer J Cardiol* 33:732-736, 1974.

59. Vismara LA, DeMaria AN, Hughes JL, et al: Evaluation of arrhythmias in the late hospital phase of acute myocardial infarction compared to coronary care unit ectopy. *Brit Heart J* 37:598-603, 1975.

60. Vismara LA, Amsterdam EA, Mason DT: Relation of ventricular arrhythmias in the late hospital phase of acute myocardial infarction to sudden death after hospital discharge. *Amer J Med* 59:6-12, 1975.

61. Vismara LA, Vera Z, Foerster JM, et al: Identification of sudden death risk factors in acute and chronic coronary artery disease. *Amer J Cardiol* 39:821-828, 1977.

62. Helfant RH, Vokonas PS, Gorlin R: Functional importance of the human coronary collateral circulation. *New Eng J Med* 284:1277-1281, 1971.

63. Miller RR, Amsterdam EA, Zelis R, et al: "Determinants and Functional Significance of the Coronary Collateral Circulation in Ischemic Heart Disease," in Russek HI (Ed): *Cardiovascular Disease*, pp 75-83, Baltimore, Maryland: University Park Press, 1974.

64. Smith SC, Gorlin R, Herman NV, et al: Myocardial blood flow in man: effects of coronary collateral circulation and coronary artery bypass surgery. *J Clin Invest* 51:2556-2565, 1972.

65. Berman DS, Salel AF, DeNardo GL, et al: Comparison of Rubidium-81 and Thallium-201 rest and exercise myocardial scintigraphy in the noninvasive detection of regional myocardial ischemia (abstract). *Clin Res* 25:87, 1977.

66. Snow PJD, Jones AM, Daper KS: Coronary disease: a pathological study. *Brit Heart J* 17:503-510, 1955.

67. Zoll TM, Wessler S, Schlesinger MJ: Interarterial coronary anastomoses in the human heart, with particular reference to anemia and relative cardiac anoxia. *Circulation* 4:797-806, 1951.

68. Williams DO, Amsterdam EA, Miller RR, et al: Functional significance of coronary collateral vessels in patients with acute myocardial infarction: relation to pump performance, cardiogenic shock and survival. *Amer J Cardiol* 37:345-351, 1976.

3

Physical Activity and Fatal Heart Attack: Protection or Selection?

Ralph S. Paffenbarger, Jr, MD

Controversy continues to surround interpretation of the relationship between physical activity and reduced incidence of coronary heart disease. Most data demonstrating an association between physical activity and reduced coronary mortality fail to distinguish between any protective effect afforded by vigorous exertion and any selective effect gained from a strong cardiovascular endowment. Thus, in previous studies, one wonders whether the London bus conductors enjoyed a favored coronary experience because of increased energy expenditure or because their companion drivers were more obese, hypertensive and hypercholesterolemic?[1-3] Did the North Dakota, California and Georgia farmers experience a lowered coronary risk because of an added work load, or had they so selected themselves because of a rugged constitution?[4-6] Did postal carriers in Great Britain and the United States experience lower coronary mortality than postal clerks because letter carrying exerted a protective effect or because mail clerking selected those with an incipient cardiovascular weakness?[7,8] We can ask similar questions of "protection or selection" about American and Italian railway switchmen and clerks,[9,10] more and less active American Cancer Society volunteers,[11] New York Health Insurance Plan subscribers,[12] British civil servants,[13] Israeli kibbutz residents,[14] college athletes and their classmates,[15] and even about cross-cultural studies of vigorously active Eskimos, Bushmen and Masai, as compared with Western societies.[16-18]

In the United States a population of 3,686 San Francisco longshoremen offered certain advantages and opportunities for study of the role of energy expenditure in cardiovascular health.[19,20] Work on the waterfront involved a high level of energy output under conditions rather well governed and documented by the rules and records of the International Longshoremen's and Warehousemen's

Union. The longshoremen tended to be a stable workforce who entered the industry in youth and remained active in it for many years. Their history present-ed here covers a 22-year follow-up from 1951 through 1972, and totals 59,401 man years of energy expenditure on the job; one-third of this experience was classified as high energy output and the rest as low energy output.

The energy output ratings of various jobs performed by longshoremen were established by measurements conducted at the quay.[21] High energy output jobs required 5.2 to 7.5 kcal/min or about 1,876 kcal over basal energy expenditure per 8-hour day. Low energy output jobs rated 1.5 to 5.0 kcal/min, or 1,066 kcal over basal energy expenditure per day. By union rules, the longshoremen rou-tinely began their career in heavy work and continued such for an average of 13 years before transferring to less strenuous assignments. Even men who experi-enced clinical heart disease were expected to return to the same heavy job after their convalescence, and may be presumed to have done so.

A multiphasic screening examination in 1951 [22] recorded various personal traits and characteristics such as obesity, smoking habits, blood pressure levels and prior history of heart disease. Cholesterol measurements were added to this information in 1961. These recognized risk factors commonly associated with fatal heart attack could be adjusted for in assessing the influence of energy expenditure or change in level of physical activity.

It could be expected that study of these longshoremen would reaffirm tenden-cies noted in other studies of energy expenditure and heart attack. Since cardio-vascular fitness is readily lost after physical activity is reduced,[23] especially in older men, note was taken of change in job assignment that altered energy output requirements. An annual accounting was taken of job transfers to refine the data on energy expenditure which were to be assessed in relation to occurrence of fatal heart attack among these workers. Deaths from heart attack were assigned to the category in which the decedent had been employed at the last pay period of the June before death (on average six months before death), to avoid selective bias from last-minute transfers to less active jobs. We hoped to be able to quantify key distinctions by resolving effects of job shifts and other variables. To further reduce possible bias of job transfers related to premonitory symptoms of heart disease, we classified fatal heart attacks as sudden and delayed deaths, on the assumption that sudden deaths would be less likely to have involved a pre-monitory transfer to lighter work.

To a limited extent the 22-year follow-up interval afforded consideration of temporal or technological changes in the longshoring industry from manual work to mechanized assistance, to nearly automated containerization methods of cargo handling. Despite these trends, the levels of energy expenditure in the various jobs represented in this study continued to cover a wide range from extremely high output down to fairly sedentary activity, and the energy specifi-cations of jobs were not changed. Examination of the histories of four birth cohorts of dock workers provided some information on the persistence of physi-cal activity in different periods of experience.

TABLE I

Age-adjusted Frequencies (%) of Personal Characteristics Among Longshoremen,
by Energy Expenditure of Work at Multiphasic Screening in 1951

Characteristic	Energy Expenditure of Work*	
	High (n = 2,511)	Low (n = 1,454)
Cigarette smoking		
One or more pack/day	34.2	39.1***
Systolic blood pressure		
Equal to or greater than mean	45.3	44.3
Diastolic blood pressure		
Equal to or greater than mean	48.7	47.2
Diagnosed heart disease	18.2	17.0
Body weight-for-height		
Equal to or greater than mean	45.9	48.0***
Abnormal glucose metabolism	4.0	4.1
Blood cholesterol		
Equal to or greater than mean**	42.8	48.4

*High energy output averaged about 1,876 kcal over basal energy expenditure per 8-hour day; low energy output, about 1,066 kcal
**As measured on 853 high and 1,148 low energy output workers in 1961
***Significantly different from figure for high energy output workers at P < .05

In a number of ways, the San Francisco longshoremen afforded an exceptional opportunity to investigate in detail some of the protective or potentially interventional relationships of physical activity to risk of fatal heart attack.

Methods

Descriptions and explanations of the basic organization and plan of the longshoremen study have been presented elsewhere.[19, 20] Initially, 49 tasks of longshoremen were classified as high, intermediate or light in energy requirements: high, 5.2 to 7.5 kcal/min; intermediate, 2.4 to 5.0 kcal/min; light, 1.5 to 2.0 kcal/min. As the intermediate and light categories differed little in risk of fatal heart attack, they were combined into a single "low" category, above which an apparent "threshold" effect at 5.2 kcal/min provided an empirical breakpoint for definition of energy expenditure levels (Table I, Figure 1 and 2).

Longshoring tasks in cargo handling and related work at the bulkhead ranged from the relatively low level of energy output (2.3 kcal/min or 9.1 BTU/min) required by light machine work to the high energy output (9.7 kcal/min, 38.5 BTU/min) of heavy shoveling and lumbering. Lifting, toting, shoving, stacking, *etc*, comprised a mix of isometric and isotonic movements that would further

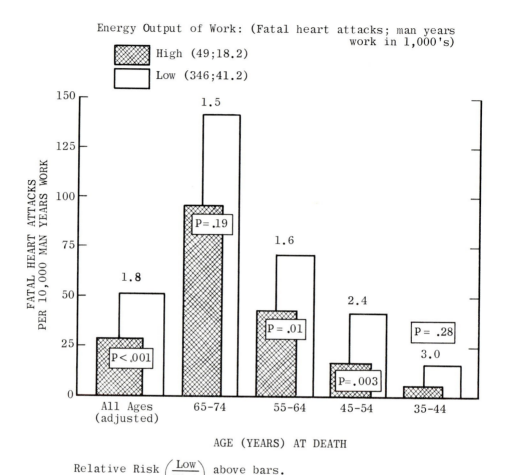

Figure 1. Rates and relative risks of fatal heart attack in longshoremen, 1951-1972, by energy expenditure of work and age at death.

characterize energy output in cargo handling. Systems of work/rest relationships for hold gangs of eight men varied considerably (eg, all men working for 45 minutes and then resting for 15 minutes each hour, or six men working for an hour while two rest for a half hour), but each called for rather sustained bursts of heavy exertion by the workers in the high energy output jobs.

The detailed information available on these study subjects from the multiphasic health examination in 1951 permitted adjustment for other variables such as age, personal habits or characteristics, cohort status, *etc*. Energy expenditure and personal characteristics were examined separately as risk factors of fatal heart attack, and multivariate analysis permitted assessment of their independent

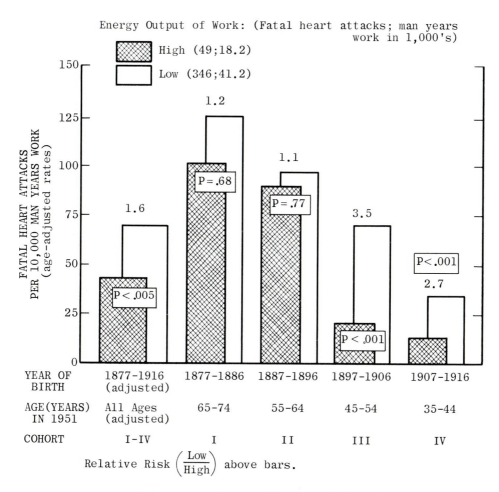

Figure 2. Rates and relative risks of fatal heart attack in cohorts
of longshoremen, 1951-1972, by energy expenditure of work.

contributions. In fact, the data showed that longshoremen in high energy output
jobs differed little from their less active associates in personal characteristics at
the time of multiphasic screening. Moreover, the role of physical exertion remained dominant whether or not added risk was present from some unfavorable
trait such as heavy cigarette smoking or above average blood pressure.

Age and cohort-adjusted death rates from heart attack were computed according to level of energy expenditure and presence of personal characteristics. High
and low levels of six personal characteristics were established at arbitrary cut-
points: cigarette smoking, one or more packs a day vs. less or none; systolic blood
pressure at or above mean for five-year age group vs. lower; diagnosed heart

disease, yes or no; body weight-for-height, equal to or greater than mean for five-year age group vs. less; glucose metabolism, abnormal (diagnosed diabetes mellitus or a blood-sugar level of 205 mg% or more one hour after a 50 gm glucose load) vs. normal; and blood cholesterol equal to or greater than mean for five-year age group vs. less. Adjustments were made by the direct method using the population of California men in 1960 as standard. Differences in death rates by levels of energy expenditure or personal characteristics were expressed as relative risks, taking the lower risk as unity.

Potential reductions in fatal heart attacks associated with major risk factors in this study were estimated by conversion of one or more factors from high to low level. Theoretical results corresponding to conversion of these high risk levels to lower risk levels will be expressed as percent reduction in the overall rate of fatal heart attack for the study population.

Findings

Some key trends in the investigation have been mentioned in the introductory sections of this chapter. Table I, II and III and Figure 1, 2 and 3 present more detailed results in compact form. Relationships observed in these findings will be discussed and their implications noted.

Table I shows the age-adjusted frequencies (percent) of personal characteristics among longshoremen by energy expenditure level of work at the time of multiphasic screening in 1951. These prevalence data describe the study population at the beginning of the 22-year follow-up period.

The Table shows that the initial distribution of the longshoremen was nearly two to one in high energy as compared with low energy output jobs (2,511 vs. 1,454 men). The proportion of workers in high energy output jobs declined from 40% in 1951-1960, to 15% in 1961-1970, to 5% in 1971-1972, reflecting progress of the industry from manual labor to mechanization to containerization in cargo handling. Overall, as has been mentioned, about one-third of the man years of work performed during the 22-year follow-up represented high energy output activity. The total number of longshoremen in Table I is slightly more than 3,686 because a few outside the age range of 35 to 74 years were included in that summation of the screening examination. The basic design of the study is limited to men aged 35 to 74 years, as will be seen in the later analyses.

Little difference in prevalence of characteristics is seen between the two groups of longshoremen defined by job energy categories (high and low) in Table I. The observed difference in cigarette smoking habits is ascribed partly to the fact that high energy output workers tended to be cargo handlers who were not allowed to smoke on the job except in certain designated rest areas. Also, the high energy output workers tended to be slightly more wiry than the longshoremen engaged in less energetic jobs. Further analyses will make clear, however, that these differences, although statistically significant, do not nearly account for the spread between the two groups in risk of fatal heart attack. The

TABLE II

Relative Risks of Fatal Heart Attack in Longshoremen, 1951 to 1972, by Interval
From Onset of Symptoms to Death and Three Characteristics of High Risk

Fatal Heart Attack	Characteristic of High Risk*		
	Low Work Energy Output	Cigarettes, One or More Pack/Day	Systolic Blood Pressure Equal to or Greater Than Mean
Total	2.0 (<.001)	2.1 (<.001)	2.1 (<.001)
Sudden	3.3 (<.001)	1.6 (.008)	2.7 (<.001)
Delayed	1.6 (.006)	2.1 (<.001)	1.4 (.005)
Unspecified	1.7 (.034)	2.5 (<.001)	2.2 (<.001)

*Adjusted for differences in age and each of the other two characteristics of high risk
P values in parentheses

TABLE III

Potential Reduction in Rates of Fatal Heart Attack (a Theoretical Effect
of Intervention) with the Elimination of Specific Combinations of Low Work
Energy Output, Heavy Cigarette Smoking and Higher Levels of Blood Pressure

Characteristic Eliminated	Man Years Work with the Characteristic	Observed Fatal Heart Attacks/10,000 Man Years with Characteristic*	Potential Reduction in percent (95% Confidence Limits)**
1. Low energy output	41,199	69.7	48.8 (30.6-67.0)
2. Heavy cigarette smoking	21,479	94.3	27.9 (20.1-35.7)
3. Higher systolic blood pressure	23,455	89.1	28.8 (20.6-37.0)
1 and 2 above	15,110	95.7	64.7 (44.5-84.9)
1 and 3 above	15,938	91.5	73.5 (56.9-90.1)
2 and 3 above	8,157	161.6	50.3 (39.7-60.9)
1, 2, and 3 above	5,493	151.9	88.2 (70.2-100)

*Cohort and age-adjusted
**Observed-Expected   (see methods)
     Observed

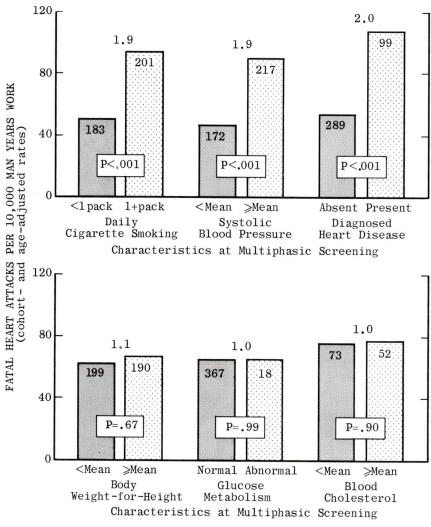

Figure 3. Rates and relative risks of fatal heart attack in long-shoremen, 1951-1972, by selected personal characteristics.

differences in energy expenditure will be seen as far more influential in the relative risk of fatal heart attack.

Some readers may be surprised that blood cholesterol levels are not significantly different in this tabulation and make little or no contribution to fatal heart attack risk in the longshoremen's experience (Figure 3). This observation may reflect the still energetic work background of the longshoremen in 1961, the date of measurement, and their age range (45 to 74 years) at that time. Similar findings have been noted for Italian railway workers.[10]

It is rather striking that Table I shows that 18% of the high energy output workers had had previously diagnosed heart disease, yet were continuing to work in the high energy output category. They even slightly outnumbered the heart disease cases in the low energy output group. Such a history of heart disease did increase risk of fatal heart attack, but this influence was reduced by high as contrasted with low energy output status.[24] A protective intervention effect of vigorous exertion seems evident here.

Figure 1 shows fatal heart attack rates per 10,000 man years of work among the 3,686 longshoremen by energy output category and age at death. Also given is the age-adjusted composite comparison for the total group. For this analysis, long-shoremen 35 to 74 years old upon entry were followed for 22 years or to death or to age 75. Less than 1% were lost to follow-up observation. The low energy output workers had an 80% increased risk of fatal heart attack as compared with the high energy output job holders, shown by the relative risk of 1.8. In Figure 1 the difference in fatal heart attack risk for high energy output and low energy output workers is evident at all ages. Thus, if high energy output is a protective factor, it is influential throughout the 40-year work span covered in the figure. The differential ascribed to high energy output activity remains evident in the oldest age group, though to a somewhat diminished degree. The rate differences are significant in the middle age brackets, but marginal in the two extremes. The increased risk of fatal heart attack in sedentary workers as compared with those more active was continuous throughout developmental stages and technological changes in the industry.[20] The decades in the 22-year follow-up included periods of manual work (1951-1960), mechanization (1961-1970), and the beginning of containerization (1971-1972).

To further compare the alternative hypotheses of protection vs. selection accounting for the reduced risk among high energy output workers, we examined the data with and without allowance for job transfer during the 22-year follow-up period.[20] With unity as base, the relative risk for less active longshoremen was 1.6 when job shifts were not considered, only slightly less than 1.8 when they were.

Figure 2 presents the same information as Figure 1, except that the data are arranged by birth cohort rather than by age at death. Within cohorts adjustments were made for differences between high and low energy workers in age at death. A pattern is seen similar to that in Figure 1, but the significant gaps between high energy output and low energy output risks are concentrated in the two younger cohorts. It appears that the effect of energy expenditure is more active in staving off fatal heart attacks there, while the two older cohorts experience little difference as expressed by relative risk. This may signify that the high energy output workers in the older cohorts did not actually work as hard as represented by job assignment records. Or, the older low energy output dockers may have worked slightly harder, by habit or choice, than their job assignment actually required of them. Or the younger decedents in the older cohorts had died before the study began. By any of these means, relative risk of fatal heart attack would appear to be lower in the earlier generations of workers.

The above analyses were restricted to fatal heart attack identified from official death certificates as the underlying cause of death. Comparison of death certificates of high and low energy output workers for secondary and associated causes of death showed similar proportions of each group to have experienced prior evidence of coronary heart disease (25 vs. 19%), hypertensive disease (2 vs. 6%), and general arteriosclerosis (12 vs. 10%). Or stated differently, 65% of vigorous workers and 67% of those more sedentary were not stated to have had prior evidence of hypertensive-arteriosclerotic abnormalities. This fits the idea of there having been little downward shift in job assignments as a result of cardiovascular symptomatology; it argues against the hypothesis of selective bias.

Although the high and low energy output levels have been defined on the basis of an empirically chosen threshold or breakpoint, as described earlier, the consistency of their relationship to risk of fatal heart attack offers a fairly strong support for the hypothesis of a protective level of vigorous exertion. Figure 1 and 2 and Table II and III, taken all together, provide this same answer from a diversity of analyses based on various approaches to the work situation of the longshoremen. Interpretations of this observation will be discussed later.

To test the specificity of the relationship between physical activity and fatal heart attack, we looked for associations between high energy output and other causes of death. An inverse relationship was found with fatal stroke, but none with site-specific cancers, other natural causes of death, accidental death or suicide. These findings were consistent whether or not account was taken of job shifts during the 22-year follow-up. Specificity of the relationship thus would seem to exist for hypertensive-arteriosclerotic diseases.

While vigorous work energy output was common to all longshoremen, varying rather widely with time and age, their risk of fatal heart attack was affected also by several personal characteristics measured at multiphasic screening in 1951 (blood cholesterol in 1961). Cohort and age-adjusted rates of fatal heart attack, together with relative risks, are shown for high and low levels of each of these personal characteristics (Figure 3). On the high or abnormal side of the two-level scale depicted for each characteristic, the percentages of man years of work contributed were: heavy cigarette smokers, 38%; higher systolic blood pressure, 40%; diagnosed heart disease, 14%; overweight, 46%; abnormal glucose metabolism, 4%; and higher blood cholesterol, 43%.

Relative risks of fatal heart attack were 1.9 for heavy cigarette smoking, 1.9 for systolic blood pressure equal to or greater than mean and 2.0 for diagnosed heart disease—all significantly greater than unity. Cohort and age-adjusted death rates from heart attack for high and low levels of any of the three remaining characteristics were not significantly different.

The strong univariate association with fatal heart attack demonstrated for heavy smoking and higher blood pressure, both prevalent characteristics during the 22-year follow-up, invites multivariate analysis to assess their predictive power relative to that of physical inactivity. Table II gives relative risks of fatal heart attack, by interval from onset of symptoms to death, for each of three characteristics: low work energy output, cigarette smoking of one or more packs a day and systolic blood pressure level equal to or greater than average for men in the same group.[25] The relative risk estimates were derived by a summary chi-square procedure. Each set of relative risks for any one of the characteristics was adjusted for differences in age and the other two characteristics.

The 395 deaths included 115 classified as sudden (within one hour or dead on arrival after an observed attack), 112 delayed (more than one hour) and 168 unspecified. The association between low work energy and fatal heart attack is strongest for sudden death, where the relative risk is 3.3 for low contrasted with high energy workers. The association persists, but at lower estimates of relative risk, for fatal heart attacks with longer or unspecified intervals from onset to death. Similarly, increased relative risks of all three types of fatal heart attack are seen for both heavy smoking and higher levels of blood pressure. It can be concluded that each of these three characteristics contributes independently to risk of fatal heart attack of sudden or delayed finality.

Not shown in the Table are the results of another analysis using a multivariate logistic risk approach to study work energy output where adjustments between high and low energy levels were made for differences in age, race, cigarette smoking, systolic blood pressure, diagnosed heart disease, weight-for-height and glucose metabolism.[26] Relative risks of fatal heart attack for low as compared with high energy workers were 2.0 (P < .001), 3.5 (P < .001), 1.7 (P = .08) and 2.0 (P = .008) for total, sudden, delayed and unspecified deaths, respectively.

It might be anticipated that elimination of the three characteristics of high risk shown in Table II would have lowered appreciably the death rate from fatal heart attack over the 22-year follow-up period. Computations show that if all the long-shoremen had worked only at high energy output levels, the death rate from heart attack would have been reduced 31 to 67%; if all men had smoked less than a pack of cigarettes per day (or not at all), the rate would have been reduced 20 to 36%; and if all had had blood pressure levels below the actual mean, the reduction would have been 21 to 37%. Finally, if none of the three characteristics of high risk had prevailed, rates of fatal heart attack would have been reduced in this population and follow-up period by as much as 70 to 100%.

Discussion

The data and analyses used in this study of San Francisco longshoremen provide an extensive review of work experience and personal characteristics of the study subjects. The rates and relative risks of fatal heart attack are computed in terms of man years of work rather than population at risk, and emphasis is directed to the protective influence of work energy output as opposed to any selective influence of personal characteristics or causal interventions such as job transfers to lighter work. The bulk of evidence from analyses of all these aspects repeatedly points to reduced work energy output level as equally as influential in increasing risk of fatal heart attack as such commonly recognized characteristics as cigarette smoking, prior heart disease and higher blood pressure. And reduced work energy output is more influential than obesity, abnormal glucose metabolism or higher blood cholesterol. This holds true after all adjustments and allowances have been made for the other personal characteristics.

If, as appears here, the protective effect of high energy output is quite pronounced, unanswered questions remain as to the mode and extent of its influence. By most standards the longshoremen as a group were exceptionally energetic workers whose benefit threshold or optimum level of energy output would seem rather high for workers in other industries. However, the apparent threshold (eg, 5+ kcal/min, or perhaps 1,500 kcal over basal output per day) is that of a composite experience over a 22-year span or it is assessed in terms of some average experience, from which the actual experience of any individual could have departed widely. This energy "threshold" is more an indicator than a precise measure; it is a compass rather than a yardstick, and in this sense it is referable to other populations. We may safely expect a relatively high energy output pattern to show a protective influence against risk of fatal heart attack wherever it is studied in a similar manner. This conclusion becomes a strong endorsement of adequate exercise for anyone, not merely for longshoremen.

There is another way of looking at this apparent threshold of energy output. We may consider the high energy workers as protected or we may consider the low energy workers as endangered. The latter are at an 80% greater risk of fatal heart attack than the former, and it is conceivable that some degree of intervention could reduce this difference.

It is encouraging that the inverse association between work energy output and risk of fatal heart attack is consistent in all age classes and cohorts in this study, and persists throughout the 22 years of modernization in the industry, even after adjustments are made for personal characteristics such as smoking or previous coronary heart disease. These findings show that the benefits of energetic activity are widespread and far-ranging in both the population and the life span. Whether the new mechanized technology will have an adverse effect on the life expectancy of the longshoremen is a question beyond the scope of the present investigation in which follow-up ended in 1972.

The interest in looking at sudden death from heart attack stemmed partly from an idea of avoiding or reducing a possible bias from last-minute or premonitory transfers to lighter work because of ill health. It is presumed that sudden deaths were less likely to be forewarned or foreseen. Data were assessed with and without allowance for job transfers. Despite these precautions and others (Table II), sudden death from heart attack emerged as the strongest correlate of low work energy output. There were some indications that this relationship was more pronounced in the younger birth cohorts than in the older work groups, and hence that it especially influenced sudden death at young or middle age [24] among men whose counterparts had failed to survive in the older cohorts before the

study began. Possibly these results could also signify that more energetic workers were less likely candidates for sudden death, having perhaps more stamina to
survive. In several ways the analysis for sudden death proved to be of interest for
the study of fatal heart attack risk in general as related to energy output patterns.

The usual adjustments for age differences were applied in this study, but there
were also investigations of particular age groups such as birth cohorts (Figure 2)
and age at death (Figure 1). In view of union rules including seniority, it might be
assumed that the light energy workers would tend to be the older workers, thus
building an age bias into that category. However, it was observed that many of the
older longshoremen continued in heavy work output jobs. Also, during the 22-
year follow-up period, the proportions of heavy and light jobs available changed
noticeably with increasing mechanization, so that a larger proportion of young
men tended to be doing lighter work than earlier. For these reasons, plus whatever job transfers were taken into account, the work categories were probably
less influenced by age than might be supposed. A birth cohort analysis provided
an opportunity to look at these matters in a different perspective, with helpful
results. The importance of energy output to reduced risk of fatal heart attack was
found to vary somewhat with different situations, but the trend persisted in all
age groups and cohorts studied.

Many questions remain to be answered by further investigations. Perhaps
controlled clinical studies might fully differentiate the roles of physical exercise
and protection against fatal heart attack. Yet, the role of energy output is assessed
in the longshoremen's experience in such a manner and to such an extent that
this study can be placed alongside the studies of other work populations previously mentioned and add contributions of its own to the total picture as it is
presently understood.

Summary

A strong inverse association between vigorous energy expenditure and fatal
heart attack is evident in the longshoring industry. Although we are unable to
determine to what extent high energy output decreases the risk, and low energy
output increases the risk, the association should be considered primarily protective rather than selective in nature. It is protective (a *cause* of reduced fatal heart
attack), not selective (an *effect* of coronary heart disease symptomatology or
specific longshoring practices), as based on the following evidence:

(1) Men engaged in heavy work in 1951 were similar to less active longshoremen relative to selected risk factors of coronary heart disease. There were
no differences in the prevalence of higher blood pressure, higher blood cholesterol, abnormal glucose metabolism or diagnosed heart disease; but heavy workers
were less apt to be heavy smokers and weighed less than the less active. Neither
smoking nor excess weight could account, however, for the 80% excess risk of
fatal heart attack among the lighter workers. (2) Risk was reduced for vigorous
workers even though decedents were charged against the job category held an

average of six months earlier, to offset selective bias from any health related transfers to less active jobs. (3) The reduced risk persisted for longshoremen registered in the industry in 1951 and followed forward for 22 years, whether or not account was taken of job transfers that occurred. This strongly implies that few longshoremen shifted downward in physical activity categories due to health reasons related to coronary heart disease. (4) The reduced risk for vigorous workers was consistent in all age classes and cohorts, and persisted throughout the 22 years of modernization in the industry. Also, the reduced risk was maintained when account was taken of race, cigarette smoking, systolic blood pressure, diagnosed heart disease, weight-for-height and glucose metabolism. (5) The reduced risk seemed to involve a threshold effect in that a fairly well-defined critical level of energy output was required to achieve the protection. The threshold level perhaps signified strenuous bursts of peaked energy output rather than sustained lesser effort. (6) Similar proportions of high and low energy output workers who died from heart attack were reported to have had prior coronary heart disease, hypertensive disease and general arteriosclerosis as secondary or associated causes listed on their respective death certificates. Their longshoring job assignments would seem not to have been influenced by any symptoms from these chronic conditions. (7) Specificity of the findings was indicated by the absence of any association between energy expenditure and such other causes of death, as cancer of specific sites, other natural causes and violence. (8) The reduced risk for high energy output was stronger for sudden death as compared with delayed or unspecified death from heart attack. Yet the sudden death, as more unexpected and unforeseen, usually would not be related to premonitory job transfer.

References

1. Morris JN, Heady JA, Raffle PA, et al: Coronary heart disease and physical activity of work. *Lancet* II: 1053-1057, 1111-1120, 1953.
2. Morris JN, Heady JA, Raffle PA: Physique of London busmen. *Lancet* II:569-570, 1956.
3. Morris JN, Kagan A, Pattison DC, et al: Incidence and prediction of ischaemic heart-disease in London busmen. *Lancet* II:553-559, 1966.
4. Zukel WJ, Lewis RH, Enterline PE, et al: A short-term community study of the epidemiology of coronary heart disease: a preliminary report on the North Dakota study. *Amer J Public Health* 49:1630-1639, 1959.
5. Breslow L, Buell P: Mortality from coronary heart disease and physical activity of work in California. *J Chronic Dis* 11:421-444, 1960.
6. Cassel J, Heyden S, Bartel AG, et al: Occupation and physical activity and coronary heart disease. *Arch Intern Med* 128:920-928, 1971.
7. Morris JN: Occupation and coronary heart disease. *Arch Intern Med* 104:903-907, 1959.
8. Kahn HA: The relationship of reported coronary heart disease mortality to physical activity of work. *Amer J Public Health* 53:1058-1067, 1963.
9. Taylor HL, Klepetar E, Keys A, et al: Death rates among physically active and sedentary employees of the railroad industry. *Amer J Public Health* 52:1697-1707, 1962.
10. Menotti A, Puddu V, Monti M, et al: Habitual physical activity and myocardial infarction. *Cardiologia* 54:119-128, 1969.
11. Hammond EC, Garfinkel L: Coronary heart disease, stroke, and aneurysm: factors in the etiology. *Arch Environ Health* 19:167-182, 1969.
12. Shapiro S, Weinblatt E, Frank CW, et al: Incidence of coronary heart disease in a population

insured for medical care (HIP): myocardial infarction, angina pectoris, and possible myocardial infarction. *Amer J Public Health* 59:1-101, 1969.

13. Morris JN, Chave SPW, Adam C, et al: Vigorous exercise in leisure-time and the incidence of coronary heart disease. *Lancet* I:333-339, 1973.

14. Brunner D, Manelis G, Modan M, et al: Physical activity at work and the incidence of myocardial infarction, angina pectoris and death due to ischemic heart disease: an epidemiological study in Israeli collective settlements (Kibbutzim). *J Chronic Dis* 27:217-233, 1974.

15. Paffenbarger RS, Wolf PA, Notkin J, et al: Chronic disease in former college students. I: Early precursors of fatal coronary heart disease. *Amer J Epidemiol* 83:314-328, 1966.

16. Mann GV, Shaffer RD, Anderson RS, et al: Cardiovascular disease in the Masai. *J Atheroscler Res* 4:289-312, 1964.

17. Biss K, Ho K-J, Mikkelson B, et al: Some unique biologic characteristics of the Masai of East Africa. *New Eng J Med* 284:694-699, 1971.

18. Schaefer O: Vigorous exercise and coronary heart-disease. *Lancet* I:840, 1973.

19. Paffenbarger RS Jr, Laughlin ME, Gima AS, et al: Work activity of longshoremen as related to death from coronary heart disease and stroke. *New Eng J Med* 282:1109-1114, 1970.

20. Paffenbarger RS Jr, Hale WE: Work activity and coronary heart mortality. *New Eng J Med* 292:545-550, 1975.

21. Hale RC, O'Hara JJ: An Engineering Analysis of Cargo Handling. X: Energy Expenditure of Longshoremen (Report 59-20). Los Angeles: Department of Engineering, University of California, June 1959.

22. Weinerman ER, Breslow L, Belloc NB, et al: Multiphasic screening of longshoremen with organized medical follow-up. *Amer J Public Health* 42:1552-1567, 1952.

23. Cooper KH: *Aerobics*, New York: Bantam Books, 1968.

24. Paffenbarger RS Jr, Hale WE, Brand RJ, et al: Work-energy level, personal characteristics, and fatal heart attack: a birth-cohort effect. *Amer J Epidemiol* 105:200-213, 1977.

25. Paffenbarger RS Jr, Brand RJ, Sholtz RI, et al: Work-energy level, host characteristics and specific causes of death. Unpublished data, 1976.

26. Brand RJ, Paffenbarger RS Jr, Sholtz RI, et al: Job activity and fatal heart attacks studied by multiple logistic risk analysis (abstract). *Circulation* 54 (suppl 2): 51, 1976.

PART II

Physiological Aspects of Exercise

4

Acute and Chronic Physiological Responses to Exercise

Jack H. Wilmore, PhD

"Man is a remarkable animal. He can sprint 100 yards in 9.0 seconds, run a sub-four-minute mile, and complete a 26.2-mile marathon at an average rate of less than 5 minutes per mile. He can swim for both distance and speed, jump over 29 feet horizontally, over 7 feet vertically, and perform many other tasks requiring high levels of skill and dexterity."[1]

Man is able to accomplish these feats only through a series of complex interactions within the body involving nearly all of the body's systems. While the muscles perform the work, the heart and blood vessels deliver the nutrients and, with the help of the lungs, provide oxygen to and remove carbon dioxide from the tissues. The nervous and endocrine systems integrate all of this activity into a meaningful performance. Practically no tissue or organ escapes involvement in even the simplest movement. At the cellular level, the mitochondria and numerous enzymes are activated and energy generated to enable the muscle to contract. The skin becomes a critical part of the body's heating and cooling system as activity is prolonged. The kidneys assist in maintaining fluid balance. While textbooks could be, and have been, written on each of the involved systems individually, this chapter attempts to focus briefly, and in rather general terms, on the major or most significant physiological aspects of human performance. This chapter is concerned with the cardiovascular, respiratory and metabolic adaptations to exercise.

Historical Perspective

It wasn't until the early twentieth century that efforts were made to gain insight into man's ability to functionally adapt to the stress of exercise. With the establishment of the Harvard Fatigue Laboratory in 1927,[2] and the work of A. V. Hill [3] in England in the 1920's, a group of dedicated scientists began a concerted effort to push back the frontiers in the area of exercise and sport physiology. While isolated research laboratories and individual research experiments had investigated specific aspects of man's physical performance as early as the mid-to-late 1800's, these early efforts in the 1920's marked the start of a new era with scientists dedicated to the sequential study of how man adapts to the unique condition of exercise. Since this time in history, considerable knowledge has accumulated, but this area of investigation is still in the stage of infancy. With the availability of new techniques and instrumentation and the efforts of current investigators, the period of rapid growth is quickly approaching.

Assessing Man's Response to Exercise

How does one go about determining the various physiological responses to exercise? The individual exercising in his natural environment or the athlete performing his sport do not present the researcher with the most desirable situations from which to gather this basic information. With the development of radiotelemetry, limited information can be obtained during natural exercise or actual competitive experiences. A small transmitter, less than two inches cubed, can be attached to the body of an athlete and with the appropriate attachments data relative to heart rate, body temperature and additional physiological parameters can be transmitted to a receiver stationed alongside the field, court or pool. While this information is of considerable interest and importance, it provides only limited insight into the total body's response to exercise.

The limitations of field testing have forced the researcher and his subject into the research laboratory. In the laboratory, the subject can be studied in much greater depth and detail and within a controlled environment. While the situation is artificial, relative to a truly natural performance situation, a great deal of information can be obtained that provides a better understanding of the individual in his natural environment.

One of the goals of studying exercise in the laboratory is to be able to produce a level of exercise which can be quantified and is reproducible. In order to determine the functional relationship between exercise as a stimulus and the resulting adaptations of the different body systems, one must be able to quantify both the level of exercise and the specific response to that exercise. There are a number of ways the individual can be exercised within the confines of the laboratory. The simplest form of exercise is bench stepping, where the individual steps up and down on a bench of standard height (12 to 18 inches), at a fixed rate of stepping established by a metronome, eg, 24 ascensions per minute. This is the least expensive and most portable of the various testing devices, but it has several disadvantages. First, the total amount of work that is performed in a set period of time is totally dependent on the individual's body weight, *ie*, the heavier individual must lift more weight each step. Secondly, the athlete makes considerable movement during a stepping test, making it difficult to obtain certain physiological measurements.

A second device that is used for producing an exercise response in the laboratory is the bicycle ergometer, which can be used in either the normal upright or supine position. In addition, the bicycle ergometer can be used for arm cycling. Ergometers work on the basis of one of two principles, mechanical friction or electromagnetic resistance. With the mechanical friction devices, a belt surrounding the fly wheel of the bicycle can be tightened or loosened, adjusting the resistance against which the individual pedals. The pedal rate must be accurately maintained to provide a constant work output. With electromagnetic resistance, the fly wheel moves through an electromagnetic field, and the strength of the field determines the resistance to pedalling. With electromagnetic devices, a constant level of work is maintained independent of the pedalling rate, as a feedback loop increases the resistance when the rate slows, and decreases the resistance as the rate increases. Advantages to using the bicycle ergometer include the following: it is relatively inexpensive and portable, the work level or power output can be accurately defined and the task is weight-independent, ie, the work level can be set independent of the individual's body weight. It does have the distinct disadvantage, however, that the individual is restricted or limited more by local muscle fatigue than by general, overall cardiovascular, respiratory and metabolic fatigue. In addition, and closely related to the problem of local fatigue, the peak or maximum physiological parameters obtained on the bicycle ergometer are frequently lower than those obtained from the other forms of laboratory exercise.

Probably the most widely used laboratory exercise device is the motor-driven treadmill. This device appears to provide the highest maximum physiological responses to exercise, and the work rate is constant, ie, the subject either keeps up with the rate of work or is thrown off of the back of the treadmill. The treadmill is an expensive device, however, and lacks portability. In addition, it can be somewhat dangerous if the individual loses his balance.

Two unique laboratory work devices have been recently developed, the rowing ergometer [4] and the swimming flume.[5] The rowing ergometer was devised to test competitive oarsmen in an activity that more closely approximated their competitive task. The swimming flume was developed for the same purpose. Valuable research data had been obtained by instrumenting swimmers in a swimming pool. The problem of turns and of not having a stationary swimmer led to the use of tethered swimming. The subject was placed in a harness, which was connected to a rope and a series of pulleys, with attached weights, and he would swim in a stationary position against different resistances. While these initial attempts provided useful data, they did not accurately duplicate the true environment of the swimmer. The swimming flume, while very expensive, has resolved this problem and has created many new opportunities to investigate almost all aspects of swimming.

Each of these laboratory modes of exercise makes it possible to exercise the individual from low to exhaustive levels, while maintaining his body in a relatively stable position. This allows the individual to be instrumented to measure a variety of physiological parameters. Expired air can be collected for the determination of the volume and rate of respiration as well as the amount of oxygen or energy used during exercise; electrodes placed on the chest allow the monitoring of the electrocardiogram to determine the normality and rate of the heart; blood pressure can be monitored either directly (arterial catheter) or indirectly (sphygmomanometer); arterial and venous blood samples can be drawn and analyzed for various components; body and skin temperatures can be monitored; and many other specific parameters can be either recorded or observed. Advances in technology have made it possible to define man's response to exercise quite explicitly, but even with these advances, there are still many areas that cannot be accurately assessed or described. Only as technology pushes ahead will the total picture start to come more clearly into focus. Bruce discusses additional aspects of exercise testing methodology in Chapter 10.

Physiological Adaptations to Acute Exercise

Physiological adaptations to exercise fall into two major categories: acute and chronic. Acute adaptations are those that occur during a single bout of work. Chronic adaptations are those that result after a period of physical training, *ie*, changes that result from conditioning. Chronic adaptations will only be briefly discussed in this chapter but are covered in depth by Adams et al in Chapter 24. Also, histological, biochemical and hematological alterations with acute and chronic exercise are presented in separate chapters.

Cardiovascular Adaptations—The major function of the cardiovascular system during exercise is to deliver blood to the active tissues, and thereby supply oxygen and nutrients and remove metabolic waste products. If the exercise bout is prolonged, the cardiovascular system also assists in maintaining body temperature, so the individual doesn't overheat. A series of cardiovascular adaptations results when the individual goes from the resting to the exercise state.

The resting heart rate is influenced by age, body position, level of cardiorespiratory fitness and various environmental factors. It becomes progressively lower with increasing age and better physical fitness, and is higher with increases in temperature and altitude.[6] It is not uncommon to find resting heart rates varying from the extremes of 30 beats/min or lower in the highly trained endurance athlete, to over 100 beats/min in the sedentary, deconditioned adult.[1] Before the start of exercise the pre-exercise heart rate may be increased above normal resting levels. This is due to an anticipatory response which probably reflects a sympathetic neurohumoral effect. Thus, reliable estimates of resting heart rate should only be made under conditions which are conducive to the individual's total rest and relaxation.

As exercise begins, the heart rate increases. During low levels of exercise at a constant workload, the heart rate will usually attain a plateau or steady-state

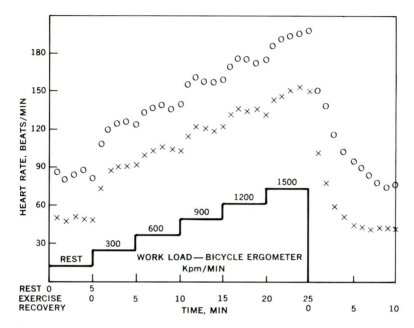

Figure 1. Relationship of heart rate to work intensity, illustrating the difference in response between the trained (X) and untrained (O) individual. Reproduced with permission from Wilmore JH, Norton AC: *The Heart and Lungs at Work*, p 3, Beckman Instruments, 1974.

within several minutes.[6] As the workload is progressively increased, the heart rate will also increase, ie, a roughly linear relationship exists between the heart rate and workload (Figure 1). At higher workloads, it takes progressively longer to attain a steady-state rate.[7] For the same workload, the more fit individual will have a lower steady-state value (Figure 1). The older individual of comparable fitness will also have a lower submaximal heart rate for the same workload. But since he will also have a lower maximum heart rate, his relative rate (submaximal steady-state rate/maximum rate) will be similar to that for the younger individual.[8]

At progressively higher workloads, there eventually will be a level which totally exhausts the individual. Prior to this, however, the heart rate will have reached a plateau at its maximum. Each individual has a definable maximum heart rate (HRmax) which is highly reproducible from test to test. Maximum heart rates are quite variable between individuals, but do decrease linearly with age (Figure 2).[9] The equation, HRmax = 220 – age, provides an approximation of the mean maximal heart rate for any one age category. However, the variance for any one age category is high, ie, the standard deviation is approximately ±10 beats/min;[9] thus, the predicted HRmax for any one individual can be in error by a considerable amount. For this reason, submaximal testing with end points determined on the basis of a predicted HRmax, is not considered to be desirable.

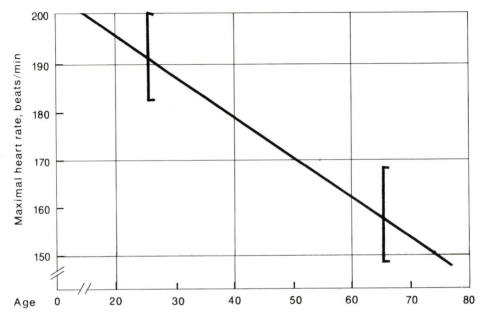

Figure 2. Decrease in maximal heart rate with age. Reproduced with permission from Andersen KL et al: *Fundamentals of Exercise Testing*, p 78, Geneva: World Health Organization, 1971.

The stroke volume response to exercise is highly dependent on hydrostatic pressure effects. When sitting or standing, without exercising, stroke volume is reduced relative to the supine position due to blood pooling in the extremities. The maximum stroke volume attained during exercise, however, in the supine, sitting or erect position is nearly identical [6] or slightly higher [10] than the value attained during supine rest. Stroke volume changes very little during supine exercise up to maximum, and the increase in stroke volume from rest to maximum exercise in the sitting or erect posture is sufficient to overcome the effect of venous pooling in the lower extremities.[10]

Stroke volume at rest in the erect position varies among adults between 50 and 80 ml, while maximum stroke volume will approach 200 ml or higher in highly trained athletes.[6] It appears that when exercising in the erect position stroke volume will increase linearly with the workload until it reaches its maximum value at approximately 50% of the individual's capacity for exercise. It has been suggested that stroke volume starts to decrease at the higher heart rates due to a shortened diastolic filling time, but there is little research available to support this theory.[6, 11] For example, at a heart rate of 180 beats/min the complete filling and emptying of the heart takes only 1/3 second. This suggestion, however, is not unequivocally supported by the available data.

The cardiac output at rest is 4 to 6 liters per minute. It increases linearly with increases in work level up to the point of exhaustion, although there is some evidence that it reaches a maximum and then decreases with prolonged exhaustive work. At exercise levels up to 40 to 60% of the individual's maximal capacity, the increase in cardiac output is accomplished through increases both in heart rate and in stroke volume. At higher exercise levels, the increase results solely from the continued increase in heart rate.[6] Maximal values of cardiac output during exercise are dependent upon many factors, the two most prominent being body size and degree of fitness. The maximal cardiac output for a small deconditioned man may well be under 20 liters per minute while a large, well-conditioned athlete may have values in excess of 40 liters per minute.[6]

The flow of blood from the heart is not constant through all tissues, but varies with the tissue needs. During exercise, blood will be shunted from areas of little or no metabolic activity (such as the gut) to those areas of active tissue involved in the exercise.[6] The absolute amount of blood flowing to the heart is increased in proportion to the increased metabolic activity of the heart during exercise, while that to the kidneys, stomach and intestines appears to be diminished. The skin and muscles receive a substantially greater proportion of the cardiac output as the body engages in exercise of increasing intensity.[6]

The amount of blood going to the working muscles is referred to as the effective blood volume, and this may decrease from a maximum with prolonged work, particularly in hot environments. This is due to the increased flow to the periphery to promote both metabolic and environmental heat loss.

Blood pressure is one of the more difficult variables to measure during exercise. Direct measurement of blood pressure by inserting a catheter into an artery is not justifiable for most tests due to the inherent risks and expense. Most available information on blood pressure responses to exercise has been obtained by indirect methods. From the data that have been reported to date, there is a linear increase in the systolic pressure with increasing levels of work, the peak values reaching 200 mm Hg or higher.[6] Diastolic pressure changes little from rest to maximum exercise in the normal, healthy individual. Thus, both pulse pressure and mean pressure increase with increasing work. In the pulmonary circulation, the systolic pressure can double from 20 to 40 mm Hg with maximal exercise, while diastolic pressure remains unchanged.[6]

The composition of blood changes as the individual goes from a resting to an exercising state. The red blood cell may actually undergo a decrease in size as the body is exposed to prolonged exercise where there is a substantial fluid loss.[12] Proteins may also be lost from the plasma volume, although data at the present time are conflicting.

With substantial fluid loss in prolonged exercise due to sweating, there is a reduction in plasma volume which results in a hemoconcentration of the red blood cells and the plasma proteins, ie, since the fluid portion is reduced, the cellular and protein portion of the blood volume represents a larger fraction of the total blood volume. This hemoconcentration results in a substantial rise in the red blood cell count by 20 to 25%. Whereas at one time it was thought that red blood cells were added to the circulation to facilitate oxygen transport, it is now recognized that plasma volume is reduced, producing a rise in only the relative but not absolute number of red blood cells. Plasma volume loss results from a shift of fluid from the plasma to the interstitial fluid.

At rest, the blood pH remains constant at a value slightly below 7.4.[6] Thus, normal blood at rest is slightly alkaline. There is little change in blood pH up to about 50% intensity of exercise. As the intensity of exercise increases above 50%, the pH will start to drop, becoming more acidic. This drop is gradual at first, but becomes more rapid as the individual approaches exhaustion. Values of 7.0 or lower have been reported following maximal exercise, and tissue pH reaches levels even lower than 7.0.[13] The lowering of the blood pH is primarily the result of increased anaerobic muscle metabolism and corresponds to the increase observed in blood lactate. Blood lactate levels range from an average of 10 mg/100 ml of blood (1.1 millimoles per liter of blood) at rest to 200 mg/100 ml of blood (22 millimoles per liter of blood) or higher within five minutes following exercise,[6] (lactate values reach their maximum in the blood during the initial five minutes of recovery from exhaustive exercise). Large concentrations of blood lactate do not appear in the blood until the workload reaches or exceeds 50% of the individual's capacity.

Respiratory Adaptations—The pulmonary ventilation or minute volume increases from a resting value of approximately 6 liters per minute to values above 100 liters per minute during the end stages of exhaustive exercise in men, and can reach values in excess of 200 liters per minute in large, well-conditioned male athletes.[14] This is accomplished by an increase in both the tidal volume and in the respiratory frequency. Tidal volume may increase from a resting average of 0.5 liters per minute up to 2.5 to 3.0 liters per minute during maximal exercise. This would correspond to an increase from 10% of the vital capacity at rest to 50% during exercise. The respiratory frequency can increase from 12 to 16 breaths per minute at rest, to 40 to 50 breaths per minute during maximal exercise. There is a direct, linear relationship between the increase in pulmonary ventilation and the increase in work level up to about 60 to 90% of the individual's capacity.[15] At this point, the ventilation increases at a much faster rate through the end of maximal exercise, which may be related to the onset of anaerobic metabolism, ie, anaerobic threshold.[15, 16]

Two practical respiratory phenomena, which are poorly understood and almost impossible to duplicate in the research laboratory, periodically occur during exercise. These are the phenomena of "second wind" and "stitch in the side," both brought on through running. The stitch in the side is usually felt as a sharp, severe pain in the lower thoracic or upper abdominal area. Many theories exist to explain this phenomenon, but to date none have any conclusive scientific support. The two most logical explanations are ischemia of the diaphragm and gastrointestinal gas or ischemia of the large intestine.[17] Whatever the cause, there is no simple remedy that works equally well for all people. Some can continue, and run right on through their pain, while others find it necessary to slow down or stop. Specific dietary modifications have been suggested as a preventive meas-

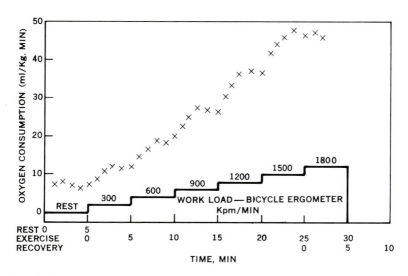

Figure 3. Oxygen consumption in relationship to work intensity. The peak oxygen consumption would be the $\dot{V}O_2$ max. Reproduced with permission from Wilmore JH, Norton AC: *The Heart and Lungs at Work*, p 10, Schiller Park, Illinois: Beckman Instruments, 1974.

ure, but sufficient evidence is not available to demonstrate their effectiveness.

Second wind is an equally confusing phenomenon.[17] During a workout at a constant pace, the effort seems labored, or the individual isn't "in the groove." Suddenly, the individual feels a sense of freedom, the distress of labored breathing is gone and he has experienced second wind. The feeling of second wind does relate to a more comfortable pattern of breathing, but this appears to be the result of a more basic physiological alteration which has yet to be defined. It is possibly a result of more efficient circulation to the active tissues or to a more efficient metabolic process. The answer will have to await better understanding of how respiration is controlled during exercise.[12]

Metabolism—As the body shifts from rest to exercise there is an increase in total body metabolism. While this has been documented through direct calorimetry, much more data is available using indirect calorimetry, primarily through the assessment of oxygen consumption levels. Oxygen consumption ($\dot{V}O_2$) varies in direct proportion to the level of work being performed (Figure 3), up to a peak or maximum value ($\dot{V}O_2$ max). $\dot{V}O_2$ max is a well-defined and reproducible physiological endpoint which dictates to a large extent the individual's physical working capacity.[6] It is widely accepted as the best criterion of cardiorespiratory endurance capacity or "physical fitness." $\dot{V}O_2$ max is used synonymously with the terms "physical working capacity" and "aerobic power."

To increase oxygen delivery to the exercising muscles, the cardiac output is increased, which is a result of both an increase in heart rate (HR) and stroke volume (SV). Heart rate can increase from 2.5 to 4 times its resting value and stroke volume (sitting or erect posture) can nearly double its pre-exercise resting value. The difference in arterial and venous oxygen content (a-v̄ O$_2$ diff) can also increase approximately 2.5 to 3.0 times its resting value, ie, from 5 to 15 ml of oxygen/100 ml of blood. Since oxygen uptake is the product of cardiac output (Q̇) and a-v̄ O$_2$ diff, or more specifically, V̇O$_2$ = HR·SV·a-v̄ O$_2$ diff; the V̇O$_2$ max is approximately 12.5 times greater than V̇O$_2$ at rest, ie, V̇O$_2$ max = (HR rest · 2.5) (SV rest · 2) (a-v̄ O$_2$ diff rest · 2.5). These basic relationships, however, will vary considerably with the state of conditioning of the subject (Table I).

V̇O$_2$ max values are influenced greatly by size, age and level of fitness.[6] To account for individual differences in size, V̇O$_2$ max is frequently expressed relative to body weight (ml of oxygen/kg of body weight · min) or to lean body weight. This allows a meaningful comparison between individuals of different size. V̇O$_2$ max decreases with age beyond the age of 15 to 20 years.[19] This is probably due to a combination of true biological aging and a sedentary life style. In addition, girls beyond the age of 10 to 12 years have V̇O$_2$ max values considerably below those of boys of the same age.[20] It is questionable as to whether these represent true differences between the sexes, or whether the female is a victim of her culture which imposes on her a sedentary life style once she reaches menarche.

V̇O$_2$ max values vary from high levels of 80 to 84 ml/kg · min in long distance runners and cross-country skiers, to values in the mid 20's or lower for poorly conditioned sedentary adults.[17] The highest V̇O$_2$ max recorded was 94 ml/kg · min for a champion Norwegian cross-country skier.[21] The highest value recorded for a woman was 74 ml/kg · min, in a Russian cross-country skier.[22] Values for athletes in various sports are illustrated in Table I.

Oxygen debt refers to the volume of oxygen consumed during the recovery period following exercise which is in excess of that normally consumed at rest. There is an oxygen debt associated with even low levels of exercise. This is due to the fact that oxygen consumption requires several minutes to reach the required or steady-state level, even though the requirement to perform the exercise is constant from the very start of the exercise.[6] This initial period, where the oxygen consumption is below the steady state or required level, is referred to as the period of oxygen deficit, and the deficit is simply calculated as the difference between that which is required and that which is actually consumed.

While V̇O$_2$ max is regarded as the best physiological criterion of endurance capacity, it does have certain limitations. With a group of endurance athletes, it is not possible to accurately predict the order of finish in an endurance race using only the V̇O$_2$ max values. Likewise, correlations of endurance running performance tests, ie, Cooper's 12 minute run, the Balke 1.5 mile run, the 2 mile run, etc, with V̇O$_2$ max are variable (r = 0.40 to r = 0.89), indicating that there is more to endurance performance than just V̇O$_2$ max. It is also well documented that V̇O$_2$ max will increase with physical training for only 12 to 18 months,[23] at which time it plateaus, even with continued, higher intensity training. The individual can still improve his times for the various distances after this period where the V̇O$_2$ max stops increasing. Thus, performance can improve even

TABLE I

Range of Maximal Oxygen Consumption Values for Athletes in Various Sports

Sport	Maximal Oxygen Consumption ml/kg · min
Men	
Cross-Country Skiers	70-94
Long Distance Runners	65-85
Rowers	58-75
Bicyclists	55-70
Long Distance Swimmers	48-68
Gymnasts	48-64
Speed Skaters	50-75
Ice Hockey Players	50-60
Football Players	45-64
Baseball Players	45-55
Tennis Players	42-56
Women	
Cross-Country Skiers	56-74
Long Distance Runners	55-72
Rowers	41-58
Distance Swimmers	45-60
Speed Skaters	40-52
Sprinters	38-52
Basketball Players	35-45

Reproduced with permission from Wilmore JH: Athletic Training and Physical Fitness: Physiological Principles and Practices of the Conditioning Process, Boston: Allyn and Bacon, 1977.

though $\dot{V}O_2$ max has reached its peak.

Figure 4 illustrates one possible explanation for this apparent inconsistency. The athlete is able to improve his performance even after he reaches an upper limit or ceiling for his $\dot{V}O_2$ max, by developing the ability to work at a higher percentage of his capacity for prolonged periods of time. Costill [24] found most marathon runners complete the 26.2 miles averaging a pace which corresponds to 65 to 80% of their $\dot{V}O_2$ max. Derek Clayton, holder of the best time in the world for the marathon (2 hours, 8 minutes, 33 seconds), had a measured $\dot{V}O_2$ max below that which would normally be expected on the basis of his world record performance (69.7 ml/kg · min). Costill, however, found that Clayton was able to work at 86% of his $\dot{V}O_2$ max when running on the treadmill at his racing pace, a value considerably higher than the average world class marathoner, and a value that probably accounts for his world record running ability. Similar results were found for Frank Shorter, 1972 Olympic gold medal winner in the marathon.[25] It would appear that both $\dot{V}O_2$ max and the percentage of $\dot{V}O_2$ max the athlete can maintain for a prolonged period of time are the determining factors in perform-

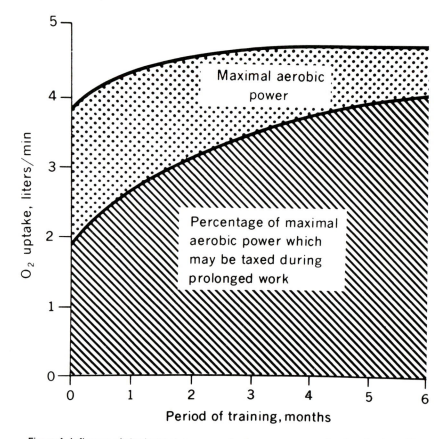

Figure 4. Influence of physical training on maximal oxygen consumption (maximal aerobic power) as well as on the fraction of maximal oxygen consumption that one can maintain during prolonged work. Reproduced with permission from Åstrand P-O, Rodahl K: *Textbook of Work Physiology*, p 381, Copyright 1970, McGraw-Hill Book Company.

ance. This could explain the lower than expected correlations between $\dot{V}O_2$ max and endurance performance tests, and the ability of the athlete to improve performance while $\dot{V}O_2$ max plateaus.

Carbon dioxide production ($\dot{V}_{CO_2}$) increases in approximate proportion to increases in oxygen consumption. The amount of carbon dioxide produced divided by the oxygen consumed is the respiratory exchange ratio, $R = \dot{V}_{CO_2}/\dot{V}_{O_2}$. Values for R vary from lows of 0.65 to 0.80 at rest, to more than 1.5 during recovery following short-term exhaustive exercise. This ratio is an extremely helpful guide to the investigator, alerting him to the ensuing attainment of exhaustion. When the R value reaches a level of 1.0, the individual will not be able to continue exercising for longer than from several seconds to several minutes. Under these conditions, metabolism becomes increasingly dependent on anaerobic processes.[6] Some patients with pulmonary disorders reach exhaustion at R values below 1. The R value has also been used to approximate the proportion of energy derived from carbohydrate, fat and protein sources during rest and steady-state submaximal exercise.[20]

Chronic Adaptations to Exercise

The physiological alterations which occur with physical training programs will be discussed in detail in Chapter 24. The purpose of this section is to provide a brief summary of those chronic adaptations that result from physical training relative to the acute changes presented in the previous section.

Assuming a previously sedentary individual is involved in a 3-day-a-week, 20-minutes-a-day jogging program, exercising at 75% of his endurance capacity, his resting heart rate will be reduced by 1 beat/min for each week of participation in the program. Resting heart rates of 40 beats/min are not uncommon in highly trained endurance athletes. Maximal heart rate is changed very little with training, although Pollock[26] suggested that there is a tendency for maximal heart rate to decrease with training if it is initially above 180 beats/min. In any case, maximal heart rate is more closely related to age than state of conditioning.[27] During standardized, submaximal bouts of exercise, the heart rate will be considerably lower following training. Likewise, postexercise recovery heart rates will be considerably lower following both standardized submaximal as well as maximal bouts of exercise.

Associated with the changes in exercise and recovery heart rates are changes of similar magnitude in stroke volume. The stroke volume at rest, during standardized, submaximal exercise and at maximal exercise is increased as a result of training. The combined effects on stroke volume and heart rate result in little or no change in $\dot{Q}$ at rest or during a standardized submaximal exercise, but a considerable increase in $\dot{Q}$ max. Pretraining $\dot{Q}$ max values of 18 to 20 liters per minute can be increased to 23 to 25 liters per minute following training. Values as high as 42 liters per minute have been reported in highly trained endurance athletes.[6]

Heart volume and weight also undergo a slight increase with training. The cardiac hypertrophy, once considered to be of pathological origin, ie, "athlete's heart," is now recognized as a normal response to the continued stress of exercise.[28] Blood volume is also increased, in addition to total hemoglobin, although the hematocrit will remain unchanged or will be slightly lowered.

Arterial blood pressure is probably influenced little by training in the normal individual, but will probably decrease in the hypertensive.[26] Peripheral blood flow is influenced by training due to an apparently higher density of capillaries in the active muscles,[6] thus providing better muscle perfusion and a greater total blood supply during maximal levels of exercise.

Pulmonary ventilation is lowered at standardized submaximal levels of exercise, but is greatly increased during maximal levels of work following training.[26] Pulmonary diffusion is unaltered at rest or during submaximal exercise, but is increased during maximal exercise. This could be the result of an increased perfusion of the lung due to greater pulmonary blood flow in the upper regions of the lung.[1]

Changes in a-$\bar{v}$ O$_2$ diff are somewhat controversial. It appears that following training there is little change in submaximal exercise values. During maximal exercise, there is a modest increase.

$\dot{V}O_2$ at rest and at standardized submaximal levels of exercise is either unchanged or slightly reduced following training. $\dot{V}O_2$ max is substantially increased following endurance training. Increases of from 4 to 93% have been reported, but most studies have reported increases of from 15 to 30%.[26]

The factors responsible for this increase in $\dot{V}O_2$ max have been identified but there is presently a great deal of controversy regarding the relative importance of these factors. Logical arguments have been raised to support the concept that a substantial portion of the change in $\dot{V}O_2$ max is the result of changes in size, number and content of the muscle mitochondria, ie, $\dot{V}O_2$ max is limited by the oxidative capacity of the muscle cell as opposed to the concept that it is the inadequate supply of oxygen to the mitochondria that is the limiting factor.[29]

Others support the more traditional approach that $\dot{V}O_2$ max is limited by $\dot{Q}$ max and local tissue perfusion, ie, there is an inadequate supply of oxygen being delivered to the active tissue. Several recent studies have given support to this latter theory. Pirnay et al[30] had their subjects breathe a mixture of CO in air that would effectively block 15% of the circulating hemoglobin. This resulted in a 15.1% reduction in $\dot{V}O_2$ max. Eckblom et al[31] removed 800 and 1,200 ml of whole blood from two groups of subjects and noted a 13 and 18% reduction in both Hb and $\dot{V}O_2$ max in both groups and a 30% reduction in both groups' total working capacity (time to exhaustion). Upon reinfusion of the red cell mass, following the restoration of total blood volume and Hb to normal levels, Hb levels increased 13% and $\dot{V}O_2$ max increased 9%.

Kaijser[32] felt this problem could be resolved by assessing changes in working capacity with alterations in arterial oxygen content. He postulated that if the cardiovascular system limits working capacity, work performance should vary with induced changes in arterial oxygen content. He had his subjects breathe oxygen at 3 atmospheres in comparison to normal breathing. He found no differences in the performance times between the two conditions, and that under maximal exercise conditions the subjects didn't utilize $\dot{Q}$ max while breathing oxygen at 3 atmospheres. This led him to support the first concept that the oxidative capacity of the muscle is the major limiting factor, not inadequate oxygen transport by the circulatory system. A recent review on the efficacy of oxygen as a work facilitating agent,[33] however, demonstrated just the opposite effect, ie, oxygen breathing increased maximal work performance by approximately the same percentage as the increase in the partial pressure of oxygen. Thus, this area remains one of open debate and controversy.

There is apparently a limit as to what levels $\dot{V}O_2$ max can reach with training, and this is undoubtedly set by heredity.[6] However, it does appear that one's

TABLE II

Hypothetical Physiological and Body Composition Changes in a Sedentary Normal Individual Resulting from an Endurance Training Program,* Compared to the Values of a World Class Endurance Runner of the Same Age

Variables	Sedentary Normal		World Class
	Pretraining	Post-training	Endurance Runner
Cardiovascular			
HR_{rest}, beats/min	71	59	36
HR_{max}, beats/min	185	183	174
SV_{rest}, ml†	65	80	125
SV_{max}, ml†	120	140	200
$\dot{Q}_{rest}$, liters/min	4.6	4.7	4.5
$\dot{Q}_{max}$, liters/min	22.2	25.6	34.8
Heart volume, ml	750	820	1,200
Blood Volume, liters	4.7	5.1	6.0
Systolic BP_{rest}, mmHg	135	130	120
Systolic BP_{max}, mmHg	210	205	210
Diastolic BP_{rest}, mmHg	78	76	65
Diastolic BP_{max}, mmHg	82	80	65
Respiratory			
$\dot{V}_{E\ rest}$, liters/min (BTPS)	7	6	6
$\dot{V}_{E\ max}$, liters/min (BTPS)	110	135	195
f_{rest}, breaths/min	14	12	12
f_{max}, breaths/min	40	45	55
TV_{rest}, liters	0.5	0.5	0.5
TV_{max}, liters	2.75	3.0	3.5
VC, liters	5.8	6.0	6.2
RV, liters	1.4	1.2	1.2
Metabolic			
a-v̄ O_2 $diff_{rest}$, ml/100 ml	6.0	6.0	6.0
a-v̄ O_2 $diff_{max}$, ml/100 ml	14.5	15.0	16.0
$\dot{V}O_{2\ rest}$, ml/kg · min	3.5	3.7	4.0
$\dot{V}O_{2\ max}$, ml/kg · min	40.5	49.8	76.7
Blood $lactate_{rest}$, mg/100 ml	10	10	10
Blood $lactate_{max}$, mg/100 ml	110	125	185
Body Composition			
Weight, lbs	175	170	150
Fat weight, lbs	28	21.3	11.3
Lean weight, lbs	147	148.7	138.7
Relative fat, %	16.0	12.5	7.5

*6-month training program, jogging 3 to 4 times/week, 30 min/day, at 75% of his $\dot{V}O_2$ max
†Upright position

Reproduced with permission from Wilmore JH, Norton AC: The Heart and Lungs at Work: A Primer of Exercise Physiology, Schiller Park, Illinois: Beckman Instruments, 1974.

performance can continue to improve by developing the ability to maintain a working pace that represents a higher percentage of $\dot{V}O_2$ max. This is a relatively new area of research in which a great deal of information is lacking.

Summary

As a result of endurance training, important physiological changes take place which facilitate the delivery of oxygen to the active muscles during submaximal and maximal exercise. Table II lists typical values before and after a training program for a number of physiological and body composition parameters. In addition, the values for a world class endurance runner are listed for comparative purposes. This illustrates the tremendous adaptability of man, as well as the great spread in values between a trained normal and a highly trained and skilled athlete. The latter phenomenon is due to basic genetic differences between individuals and illustrates that endurance athletic performance is an innate capacity, and that training can only take one to the limit of his or her genetic potential.

Adapted in part with permission from Wilmore JH: *Athletic Training and Physical Fitness: Physiological Principles and Practices of the Conditioning Process*, Boston: Allyn and Bacon, 1977.

References

1. Wilmore JH, Norton AC: *The Heart and Lungs at Work: A Primer of Exercise Physiology*, Schiller Park, Illinois: Beckman Instruments, 1974.
2. Horvath SM, Horvath EC: *The Harvard Fatigue Laboratory: Its History and Contributions*, Englewood Cliffs, New Jersey: Prentice-Hall, 1973.
3. Hill AV: *Muscular Movement in Man*, New York: McGraw-Hill, 1927.
4. Hagerman FC, Lee WD: Measurement of oxygen consumption, heart rate, and work output during rowing, *Med Sci Sports* 3:155-160, 1971.
5. Åstrand P-O, Englesson S: A swimming flume. *J Appl Physiol* 33:514, 1972.
6. Åstrand P-O, Rodahl K: *Textbook of Work Physiology*, New York: McGraw-Hill, 1971.
7. Maksud MG, Coutts KD, Hamilton LH: Time course of heart rate, ventilation and $\dot{V}O_2$ during laboratory and field exercise. *J Appl Physiol* 30:536-539, 1971.
8. Becklake MR, Frank H, Dagenais GR, et al: Influence of age and sex on exercise cardiac output. *J Appl Physiol* 20:938-947, 1965.
9. Taylor HL, Haskell W, Fox SM III, et al: "Exercise Tests: a Summary of Procedures and Concepts of Stress Testing for Cardiovascular Diagnosis and Function Evaluation." in Blackburn H (Ed): *Measurement in Exercise Electrocardiography*, Springfield, Illinois: Charles C Thomas, 1969.
10. Stenberg J, Åstrand P-O, Ekblom B, et al: Hemodynamic response to work with different muscle groups, sitting and supine. *J Appl Physiol* 22:61-70, 1967.
11. Carlsten A, Grimby G: *The Circulatory Response to Muscular Exercise in Man*, Springfield, Illinois: Charles C Thomas, 1966.
12. Costill DL, Fink WJ: Plasma volume changes following exercise and thermal dehydration. *J Appl Physiol* 37:521-525, 1974.
13. Hermansen L, Osness J-B: Blood and muscle pH after maximal exercise in man. *J Appl Physiol* 32:304-308, 1972.
14. Wilmore JH, Haskell WL: Body composition and endurance capacity of professional football players. *J Appl Physiol* 33:564-567, 1972.
15. Davis JA, Vodak P, Wilmore JH, et al: Anaerobic threshold and maximal aerobic power for

three modes of exercise, *J Appl Physiol* 41:544-550, 1976.

16. Wasserman K, McIlroy MB: Detecting the threshold of anaerobic metabolism in cardiac patients during exercise. *Amer J Cardiol* 14:844-852, 1964.
17. Wilmore JH: *Athletic Training and Physical Fitness: Physiological Principles and Practices of the Conditioning Process*, Boston: Allyn and Bacon, 1977.
18. Shephard RJ: What causes second wind. *Physician and Sportsmedicine* 2:37-40, 1974.
19. Robinson S: Experimental studies of physical fitness in relation to age. *Arbeitsphysiol* 10:251-323, 1938.
20. Wilmore JH: Inferiority of female athletes: myth or reality. *J Sports Med* 3:1-6, 1975.
21. Åstrand P-O: Innovations in Athletic Conditioning and Sports Medicine, First Annual Symposium. University of California, Berkeley, December, 1973.
22. Saltin B, Åstrand P-O: Maximal oxygen uptake in athletes. *J Appl Physiol* 20:425-431, 1965.
23. Bergstrand CG: Physical training in normal boys in adolescence. *Acta Paediat Scand* 217:60-61, 1971.
24. Costill DL: Physiology of marathon running. *JAMA* 221:1024-1029, 1972.
25. Costill DL, Fink WJ, Pollock ML: Muscle fiber composition and enzyme activities of elite distance runners. *Med Sci Sports* 8:96-100, 1976.
26. Pollock ML: "The Quantification of Endurance Training Programs," in Wilmore JH (Ed): *Exercise and Sport Sciences Reviews*, vol 1, pp 155-188, New York: Academic Press, 1973.
27. Fox SM, Haskell WL: "The Exercise Stress Test: Needs for Standardization," in: *Cardiology—Current Topics and Progress*, p 149, New York: Academic Press, 1970.
28. Barnard RJ: "Long-term Effects of Exercise on Cardiac Function," in Wilmore JH (Ed): *Exercise and Sport Sciences Reviews*, vol 3, pp 113-133, New York: Academic Press, 1975.
29. Holloszy JO: "Biochemical Adaptations to Exercise: Aerobic Metabolism," in Wilmore JH (Ed): *Exercise and Sport Sciences Reviews*, vol 1, pp 45-71, New York: Academic Press, 1973.
30. Pirnay F, Dujardin J, Derdanne R, et al: Muscular exercise during intoxication by carbon monoxide. *J Appl Physiol* 31:573-575, 1971.
31. Ekblom BJ, Goldbarg AN, Gullbring B: Response to exercise after blood loss and reinfusion. *J Appl Physiol* 33:175-180, 1972.
32. Kaijser L: "On the Limiting Factors for Heavy Exercise in Normal Man," in Larsen OA, Malmborg RO (Eds): *Coronary Heart Disease and Physical Fitness*, p 41, Baltimore: University Park Press, 1971.
33. Wilmore JH: "Oxygen," in Morgan WP (Ed): *Ergogenic Aids and Muscular Performance*, pp 321-343, New York: Academic Press, 1972.

Editors' Note—$\dot{V}O_2$ is expressed in some chapters in this book as ml/kg · min and in other chapters as ml/kg per min.

5

Adaptations in Human Skeletal Muscle as a Result of Training

Philip D. Gollnick
Walter L. Sembrowich

Collectively, skeletal muscle constitutes the single largest tissue mass of the body. This tissue mass is distributed over the skeleton as individual specialized muscles controlled by the nervous system in a manner that produces an effective and intricate system for controlling bodily movement. These movements, in addition to being essential for survival, are used by man for physical labor and for participation in sports and games. By viewing the different developmental patterns of the muscles of athletes it is clear that skeletal muscle possesses a remarkable ability to adapt to patterns of use. Thus, endurance athletes have muscles of normal size but with a capacity for prolonged, high intensity activity. In contrast, individuals engaged in activities requiring a large power output have enlarged muscles that are usually low in endurance capacity. The purpose of this chapter is to examine the spectrum of developmental patterns in human skeletal muscle from disuse to highly trained state.

The topic of adaptation in skeletal muscle is important since this tissue, in addition to constituting the body's largest tissue mass, possesses the greatest capacity for increasing its metabolic rate and thereby stressing the circulatory system.

Skeletal Muscle Composition

Skeletal muscle is composed of fibers that can be differentiated into distinct types on the basis of their contractile and metabolic properties.[1-3] Fibers of similar type are innervated by motor nerves to form motor units.[4] Since the performance characteristics and adaptability of muscle are related to its motor unit (fiber) composition,[5] a brief description of the major fiber types of human skeletal muscle will be given here.

Muscle fibers are most frequently characterized by histochemical methods. With these methods, fibers in serial cross sections are stained for characteristics such as myofibrillar adenosinetriphosphatase (ATPase) and enzymes that reflect aerobic and anaerobic potentials. These techniques have been applied to entire human muscles obtained at autopsy and from muscle samples taken via either the open or needle biopsy techniques. From these studies a significant body of knowledge has developed concerning the skeletal muscle of sedentary individuals and athletes, as well as adaptations to physical training.

It is generally accepted that two major fiber types (motor units) exist in man.[6] One fiber type stains darkly for myofibrillar ATPase after alkaline preincubation, whereas the other stains lightly. It is well documented from animal studies that dark staining fibers possess high myosin ATPase activity and have fast twitch characteristics.[4, 7, 8] Conversely, light staining fibers have low myosin ATPase activity and slow twitch properties. Although direct correlations between contractile speed and myosin ATPase activity have not been made for human skeletal muscle, indirect evidence supports this concept. First, it is well established that human muscle possesses motor units that can be divided into a clear dichotomy on the basis of contractile speed.[9-13] The percentage of the fast and slow motor units in a given muscle is closely related to the overall identification of fibers that stain dark and light for myofibrillar ATPase.[9, 14]

Second, Taylor et al [15] have prepared myosin from human muscle and related its ATPase activity to the percentage of the two fiber types as identified by histochemical methods. Extrapolation of these data to represent muscles with a theoretical 100% light or dark staining fibers resulted in estimated myosin ATPase activities of .16 and .49 μmol Pi/mg myosin/min, respectively. These values are similar to those reported in slow and fast twitch muscles of other mammalian species.[16] On the basis of these relationships, we have adopted the nomenclature of slow twitch (ST) and fast twitch (FT) to identify the fiber types of human skeletal muscle. Perhaps the most frequently used system for identifying fibers from the histochemical staining for myofibrillar ATPase uses the terms type I and type II for the low and high ATPase fibers, respectively.[6, 17] It should also be emphasized that through appropriate manipulation of the pH of the preincubation medium a subspecies of the FT fibers can be identified.[4] Although it has been reported that the fiber types of animal skeletal muscle can be identified from ultrastructural features,[18] this approach has not been used extensively with human muscle to date.[19]

Generally ST fibers stain more intensely than FT fibers for oxidative capacity (mitochondrial density) by reactions such as succinate dehydrogenase (SDH), cytochrome oxidase, NADH diaphorase or sudan black.[4, 7-9, 20, 21] It is clear from such staining procedures that a continuum of staining intensities for oxidative capacity exists within each major fiber classification.[4, 22] In fact, some overlap of oxidative staining probably exists for low oxidative ST fibers and the FT fibers

TABLE I

Some Histochemically and Biochemically Determined Features
of the Two Major Fiber Types of Human Skeletal Muscle

Property		ST Fibers (Type I)	FT Fibers (Type II)	Reference
Myofibrillar ATPase (alkaline preincubation)	(H)	Light	Dark	6, 7, 17
Oxidative Activity				
NADH-diaphorase	(H)	Dark	Light	15
SDH	(H)	Dark	Light	14, 22, 26, 27, 34-36, 47, 93
	(B)	High	Low	21, 29
HOADH	(B)	High	Low	96
Anaerobic Activity				
Phosphorylase	(H)	Light	Dark	20
LDH (total)	(H)	Light	Dark	23
	(B)	Low	High	50, 97
LDH-1	(H)	Dark	Light	23
	(B)	High	Low	50, 97
LDH-5	(H)	Light	Dark	23
	(B)	Low	High	50, 97
a-GPDH	(H)	Light	Dark	14, 22, 26, 27, 34-36, 47, 93
PFK	(B)	Low	High	96
Glycogen Content	(H)	Dark	Dark	14, 22, 26, 27, 34-36, 47, 93
	(B)	High	High	28

NADH-diaphorase = reduced nicotinamide adenine dinucleotide

SDH = succinate dehydrogenase

HOADH = beta-hydroxyacyl-CoA-dehydrogenase

LDH = lactate dehydrogenase

a-GPDH = alpha glycerophosphate dehydrogenase

PFK = phosphofructokinase

H = histochemically determined

B = biochemically determined

References are a representative sampling and not an inclusive list

that have the highest oxidative activity of this subgroup. Fast twitch fibers stain more intensely than ST fibers for anaerobic enzymes such as phosphorylase, alpha glycerophosphate dehydrogenase and total lactate dehydrogenase (LDH). A sharp dichotomy exists in anaerobic staining intensity with no apparent overlap between the major fiber types. Differential staining for LDH isozymes has revealed that FT fibers possess primarily the muscle type (LDH-5) LDH whereas the heart type (LDH-1) LDH predominates in ST fibers.[23]

Electrical stimulation of high oxidative motor units in animal preparations has demonstrated that they possess a high resistance to fatigue.[1, 3, 4] Conversely, low oxidative motor units have low endurance capacity. A general summary of the

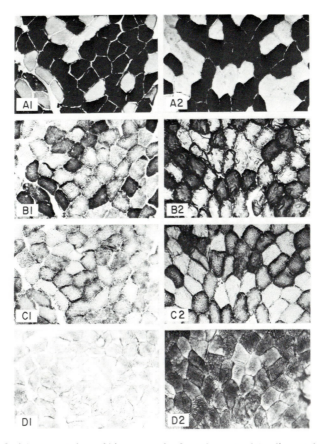

Figure 1. Serial cross sections of biopsy samples from the vastus lateralis muscle of man strained for myofibrillar ATPase (series A) to show ST (light) and FT (dark) fibers. Series B is stained for NADH-diaphorase activity to show oxidative enzymes, series C is an alpha-glycerophosphate stain for anaerobic activity, and series D is the periodic acid Schiff's reaction for glycogen. Series 1 is from a subject before training whereas series 2 is the same subject after a 5-month endurance training program. Reproduced with permission from Gollnick PD, Armstrong RB, Saubert CW IV, et al: Enzyme activity and fiber composition in skeletal muscle of untrained and trained men. *J Appl Physiol* 33:312-319, 1972.

characteristics of human skeletal muscle fibers is presented in Table I and illustrated in Figure 1.

Historically, human muscle fibers have been identified as red and white on the basis of oxidative staining properties. However, the overlap in staining intensity for this property and the fact that it can be shifted as a result of changes in physical activity make such an identification scheme obsolete.

The glycogen content of skeletal muscle of normal male subjects is approximately 80 mM of glucose units $\times$ kg^{-1} wet weight.[22, 24, 25] Histochemical localization of glycogen in muscle samples from such individuals produces a uniform staining intensity. This suggests an equal concentration of glycogen in all fi-

TABLE II

Comparison of the Diameter and the Area of Human Skeletal Muscle Fibers

| | ST Fibers | | FT Fibers | | |
| | Diameter | Area | Diameter | Area | |
Muscle	μM	μM^2 $\times$ 10^{-2}	μM	μM^2 $\times$ 10^{-2}	Reference
VL		54.95		66.38	42
VL	72.2	42.83	80.4	52.18	41
D	63.6	32.34	67.3	35.94	41
VL		50.60		55.00	96
VL		45.56		48.92	27
BB		40.58		61.38	27
VL		45.60		50.70	26
RF	57.5		55.9		64
BB	48.2		52.4		64
Mean	60.4	44.64	64.0	52.93	

VL = vastus lateralis; BB = biceps brachii; RF = rectus femoris; D = deltoid

bers.[14, 22] Reports of a higher glycogen staining in FT (Type II) fibers of human skeletal muscle do exist in the literature.[20] Observations by Gollnick et al [26, 27] have shown that such a differential staining pattern occurs only when the total muscle glycogen is below about 60 mM of glucose units per kg wet weight. The isolation of individual muscle fibers and estimation of their glycogen content has verified the histochemical observation that both fiber types of man normally have about the same glycogen concentration.[28]

Fiber Size

A compilation of data from normal man [21, 22, 29] and from autopsy material [30, 31] reveals that the diameter of FT fibers is approximately 10% greater than that of ST fibers whereas the area of FT fibers is about 20% larger. Therefore, the size of the two major fibers of human muscle is roughly equal (Table II). This near equivalence of size makes it possible to predict with reasonable accuracy the relative area that a given fiber type occupies in a muscle from its percent composition (Figure 2).[21, 22] This similarity in the fiber size of man is in marked contrast to that of animals where the anaerobic fibers are two to threefold larger than the oxidative fibers.[32, 33] Thus, in animals it is not possible to use the simple percentage of a given fiber type as an estimate of the area it occupies in the muscle.

Fiber Types in Muscular Activity

The contractile and metabolic properties of the two major motor unit types of human skeletal muscle suggest that each may be engaged preferentially to meet

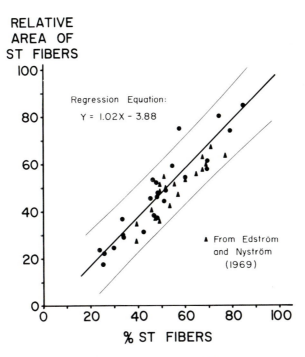

RELATIVE
AREA OF
ST FIBERS

Regression Equation:
Y = 1.02X − 3.88

▲ From Edström
and Nyström
(1969)

% ST FIBERS

Figure 2. The relationship between the percent of ST fibers in a muscle and the relative area occupied.[22] Reproduced with permission from Gollnick PD, Armstrong RB, Saubert CW IV, et al: Enzyme activity and fiber composition in skeletal muscles of untrained and trained men. *J Appl Physiol* 33:312-319, 1972.

the varying demands of different types of work.[5] Slow twitch fibers are well suited for prolonged submaximal exercise where full advantage can be made of their aerobic capacity. Conversely, FT fibers perform best during short, high intensity contractions where energy demands are met by anaerobic metabolism. Gollnick et al [26, 27, 34-36] have attempted to gain some insight into the patterns of muscle fiber involvement in different types of exercise through glycogen depletion patterns as identified histochemically. Initial studies were performed with subjects working on bicycle ergometers under standardized conditions. Muscle samples were obtained at selected intervals from the vastus lateralis muscle with the needle biopsy method. These studies demonstrated that at loads requiring oxygen uptake ($\dot{V}O_2$) below maximal ($\dot{V}O_2$ max) an initial glycogen depletion occurred in the ST fibers. During the course of a 3-hour exercise session at a load requiring about 70% of $\dot{V}O_2$ max a progressive depletion of glycogen occurred in ST fibers. After the ST fibers were depleted of glycogen, a rapid glycogen loss then occurred in FT fibers (Figure 3). It was of interest that when all fibers were depleted of glycogen the subjects were unable to continue the work at the initial level. Thus a loss of muscle glycogen may be related to fatigue. At low work intensities (30% $\dot{V}O_2$ for 3 hours) only a small percentage of ST fibers were

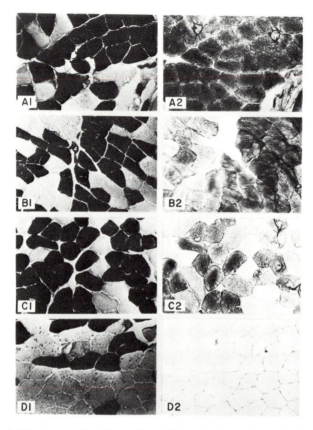

Figure 3. The glycogen depletion pattern in the vastus lateralis muscle of a subject during 3 hours of bicycle exercise at a load requiring about 70% of $\dot{V}O_2$ max (60 rpm). Series 1 is a stain for myofibrillar ATPase showing ST (light) and FT (dark) fibers. Series 2 is the PAS stain for glycogen. A, B, C and D are samples at rest and after 60, 120 and 180 minutes of exercise respectively. Reproduced with permission from Gollnick PD, Armstrong RB, Saubert CW IV, et al: Glycogen depletion patterns in human skeletal muscle fibers during prolonged work. *Pflueger Arch* 344:1-12, 1973.

depleted of glycogen whereas at very high submaximal loads (90% $\dot{V}O_2$ max for 1 hour) all ST fibers were depleted of glycogen. In these latter studies no glycogen loss could be detected via histochemical methods from FT fibers. It should be emphasized that the exercise load of 90% of $\dot{V}O_2$ max was performed by well trained, highly motivated young men and it would not be anticipated that untrained individuals would be capable of a similar effort.

All of the studies described above were conducted at a pedal speed of 60 rpm. When pedal speed was adjusted between 30 and 120 rpm with the power output held constant, the glycogen depletion did not change from that observed at 60 rpm.[36] Thus, the work rate (pedal speed) did not exert any effect on the pattern of motor unit involvement at the submaximal work loads. A rapid glycogen deple-

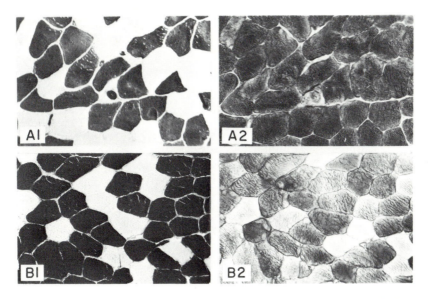

Figure 4. Serial sections showing the glycogen depletion in the vastus lateralis muscle of a man after the 6th bout of one minute of bicycle exercise at a load equal to 150% of $\dot{V}O_2$ max. Ten-minute rest pauses were given between exercise bouts. Series 1 shows ST and FT fibers with the myofibrillar ATPase stain and series 2 is the PAS stain for glycogen. Reproduced with permission from Gollnick PD, Armstrong RB, Sembrowich WL, et al: Glycogen depletion pattern in human skeletal muscle fibers after heavy exercise. *J Appl Physiol* 34:615-618, 1973.

tion occurred in FT fibers when the exercise intensity was increased to loads above $\dot{V}O_2$ max (Figure 4). This suggests a significant contribution of FT motor units at high work loads. It should not be construed, however, as an indication that ST fibers were not utilized under these conditions since a large amount of oxygen is still taken up during such exercise. Subsequent studies of endurance running have confirmed the glycogen depletion patterns observed in the laboratory experiments.[37, 38] Studies where individual muscle fibers were isolated and their glycogen content estimated chemically have also shown that a differential glycogen depletion occurs during exercise.[28] At very high exercise intensities lactate accumulation is greatest in FT fibers [39] suggesting primary reliance of these fibers on anaerobic metabolism.

Factors in Motor Unit Recruitment

The studies with glycogen depletion during exercise strongly suggest a differential recruitment of motor units depending upon the intensity of the work. The underlying factor(s) that cause the shift in fiber recruitment are unknown. Measurement of the force exerted on the pedal of a bicycle during work has demonstrated that only 20 to 35% of the maximal voluntary contractile force of the leg muscles is exerted during loads that elicit $\dot{V}O_2$ max.[36, 40] It seems unlikely that at this relatively low force output a massive recruitment of FT motor units would be required to generate the tension needed for the work. The enhanced involvement of FT fibers is more closely related to the oxygen requirement of the work than to the development of tension. Thus, the development of tension and the need for different types of motor units may be governed by the state of the metabolism and perhaps the blood flow through the muscle.

The physiological basis for the differential recruitment of motor units is probably based upon differences in the size of the motor nerves supplying the muscle fibers and their ease of activation.[41] It has been demonstrated in animals that the smallest motor nerves are the most easily activated [42, 43] and that these innervate the oxidative fibers.[41] Undoubtedly a continuum of activation ease for motor units exists with muscles (both for the ST and FT motor units) and it is this physiological characteristic that forms the basis for motor control.[41] For example, it has been shown that the most easily activated motor nerves supply the most oxidative fibers of a given fiber type.[4] This ease of activation and the constant use of a motor unit that would result may be the factor that leads to the well developed oxidative metabolism of such fibers.

Fiber Composition of Muscles

A considerable body of literature exists concerning the fiber composition of human skeletal muscles.[9, 21, 22, 29-31, 44-46] From these studies it is apparent that most human muscles contain both ST and FT fibers distributed throughout in a mosaic pattern. The percentage of ST and FT fibers is approximately equal for the majority of the population. However, some muscles contain a majority of one or the other fiber type. Notable examples are the postural muscles, such as the soleus, which contains a high percentage (in some cases nearly 100%) of ST fibers.[31, 47] In direct contrast, the orbicularis oculi muscle has a predominance of FT fibers (up to 99%).[31, 48]

Since the properties of skeletal muscle fibers endow them for use in either endurance (ST) or power (FT) activity, the question remains as to whether athletes possess a predominance of either fiber type depending upon the activity in which they excell. Gollnick et al [14, 22] used both cross-sectional and longitudinal approaches to study this problem. In their cross-sectional study both untrained and trained men were examined. The trained men encompassed a variety of activities and training methods and included individuals of average ability as well as Olympic and world champions. These studies revealed that athletes who were successful in endurance activities (long distance running and bicycling) possessed a higher average percentage of ST fibers in their muscles than did sedentary and nonendurance trained individuals. However, a wide variation existed and it was impossible to state that only individuals with a high percentage of ST fibers were capable of endurance work. The means and ranges of ST fiber distribution of these groups are presented in Figure 5. Subsequent studies with international caliber skiers [49] and runners [44-46] confirmed these findings.

In a group of ten highly trained young men it was also observed that the time of

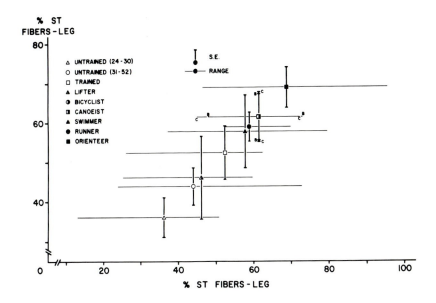

% ST
FIBERS – LEG

△ UNTRAINED (24-30)
○ UNTRAINED (31-52)
□ TRAINED
▲ LIFTER
◑ BICYCLIST
▣ CANOEIST
⬥ SWIMMER
● RUNNER
■ ORIENTEER

S.E.
RANGE

% ST FIBERS – LEG

Figure 5. The percentage of ST fibers in the vastus lateralis muscle of subjects engaged in a wide variety of athletic events. Values of means with the
SE given in the vertical direction and the range in the horizontal direction.[22]

completing a 30 km cross-country race was directly related to the percentage of
ST fibers in the vastus lateralis muscle.[38] However, great caution must be used
not to extrapolate these observations to the general population since this was a
highly select group.

The results of these cross-sectional studies raise the question as to whether the
variation in fiber composition seen in athletes was the result of training or was
from natural endowment. The answer to this question can only come from longitudinal studies. In an attempt to answer this question Gollnick et al [14] studied six
sedentary subjects before and after 5 months of endurance training. Training
consisted of pedaling a bicycle 4 days per week at a load requiring between 65
and 75% of the subject's $\dot{V}O_2$ max. Determination of the fiber composition of the
vastus lateralis muscle from biopsy samples taken before and after the training
revealed that there was no change in the percentage of ST fibers. This was true
even though as a group the initial percentage of ST fibers was low. Although the
number of subjects was small and the training program rather short, the general
conclusion reached was that endurance training did not result in the conversion
of FT to ST fibers. Whether such a conclusion will hold for those who perform
endurance work for many years (as with world caliber distance runners) is not
settled.

Athletes engaged in activities such as weight lifting and sprint events appear
to have an equal percentage of both fiber types with a slight tendency towards a
greater percent of FT fibers in their muscles.[21, 22] Consequently they are well

suited for power activities. Karlsson et al [50] could not find any change in the fiber composition of subjects before and after a strength training program. Similarly, Saltin et al [51] observed no difference in the fiber composition of subjects after either an endurance or sprint training program on the cycle ergometer.

Some earlier studies have reported an increase in "red" fibers after training.[52-55] Unfortunately these studies classified fibers on the basis of oxidative staining intensity. Associated with endurance training there is an increase in the staining intensity for NADH diaphorase and SDH activity as determined biochemically. If this is the only criterion for fiber identification, these changes could be taken as a change in fibers from "white to red."[2] In highly trained endurance athletes the FT fibers that stain lightly for oxidative capacity are often as dark as the darkest staining ST fibers in the muscles from sedentary individuals. These observations point to the problems of relying upon stains for oxidative capacity to identify fibers. Thus, we have used the myofibrillar ATPase as a method of fiber identification because it is not readily influenced by the activity pattern of the muscle.

The general conclusion reached from these data is that the fiber composition of skeletal muscle as established by myofibrillar ATPase staining is not changed by normal physical training. Persons who are successful in endurance activities were probably born with a high percentage of ST fibers in their muscles and through trial and error find their way into activities for which they are physiologically well suited. The finding of Taylor et al [15] that the ATPase of myosin isolated from the muscle of well trained athletes does not differ from that of untrained individuals also supports this conclusion. Similar findings have been made in rats.[56]

Muscle Strength and Fiber Size and Number Relations

It is well established that the cross-sectional area of a muscle is directly related to its strength. This has been demonstrated over a wide range of ages and maximal strengths through both cross-sectional and longitudinal studies.[57, 58] Thus, the strength of a particular muscle can be considered to be governed by the size and number of fibers contained within it. Women's muscles have the same strength per unit of cross-sectional area as those of men. The only factor that can account for a difference in total strength between the sexes is the smaller total muscle mass of women.[57, 59] Contributing to this smaller muscle mass is the overall small size of the fibers in the muscle of women.[60] Whether there is also a smaller total number of fibers is unknown. Increases in strength in response to training also occur at the same relative rate in men and women irrespective of age.[60]

The range of fiber areas that exists within a single species attests to the remarkable adaptability of skeletal muscle. For example, the average fiber area in the biceps brachii of a small dog (Chihuahua) is only about one-tenth (290 as compared to 2,080 u^2) that of a large dog (St. Bernard).[61] Comparative studies of human muscle have also been made with autopsy material. Etemadi and Hosseini [62] reported that mean fiber diameter of the biceps brachii muscle of normal individuals to be only 50% that of a lumberjack. The muscle of the lumberjack also contained 40% more fibers than that from normal subjects. Similarly, Jennekens et al [30] found that the muscle fibers in the biceps brachii from a male laborer were 36% (ST) and 57% (FT) larger than those in the same muscle from a slender girl.

Effect of Training on Muscle Fiber Size and Number

One of the earliest reports of changes in muscle fibers as a result of training was that of Morpurgo.[48] He observed an increase in fiber size but not number in the dog sartorius muscle after training. Subsequent studies on animals seemed to confirm the fact that total fiber number did not change during enlargement produced by functional overloads. However, Morpurgo studied the sartorius muscle and this muscle may not be used extensively in running. In fact this muscle does not exist in some quadrupedal animals.

The muscle fibers of individuals doing heavy resistance work (weight lifters) are larger than those of sedentary persons and of endurance athletes.[22, 29] In one study this difference was 50 and 70% for FT and ST fibers, respectively. Edström and Ekblom [29] reported that the FT fibers of weight lifters were 45% larger than endurance athletes and sedentary individuals. In these subjects there were no differences in ST fibers. It should be pointed out that fiber areas vary considerably in a single muscle sample and considerable overlap exists between subjects.

Gollnick et al [14] observed a significant increase in the size of ST but not FT fibers after 5 months of endurance training. This may suggest that in previously sedentary individuals a change in muscle fiber size can occur even from endurance exercise.

In an electron-microscopic study of human skeletal muscle MacDougall et al [63] found a 30 and 36% increase in the areas of the fibers and myofibrills after strength training. They also noted a fivefold increase in the incidence of myofibrillar splitting. No change was noted in filament packing density. Histochemical data suggested that these changes occurred primarily in the FT fibers.

The early studies of Morpurgo [48] and others have suggested that the total fiber population of a muscle was fixed and could not be increased by training. However, the difference in fiber number of a subject described above would suggest that this issue is not completely settled. Furthermore, fiber splitting has been reported in extreme overload studies in rats.[64, 65] Ianuzzo et al [66] observed a 30% increase in the total number of muscle fibers in the rat plantaris after prolonged overload produced by tenotomy of a synergist. Sola et al [67] also suggested that an increase in muscle fibers occurs during work-induced muscle enlargement. One of the major problems in studying this problem has been that most animal models do not lead to the massive hypertrophy that can be produced in man by weight training. Gonyea et al [68, 69] described an exercise procedure for cats that

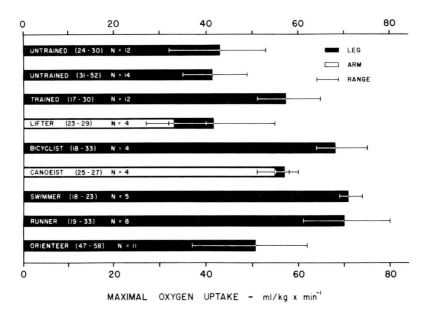

Figure 6. The $\dot{V}O_2$ max of subjects grouped according to the athletic events in which they participate. The age range and number of subjects is given in the bar along with the identification of the group. The black bar represents $\dot{V}O_2$ max during leg exercise and the open bar, $\dot{V}O_2$ max during arm exercise.[22]

produces enlargement and fiber splitting in the front limb muscles. This model shows promise of producing muscle enlargement similar to that which occurs in man. With technical developments such as this it may be possible to settle the question of whether indeed muscle fiber number is fixed or if it can be altered by exercise.

Metabolic Adaptations to Training

Endurance Training—Skeletal muscle from endurance trained individuals possesses oxidative enzyme activities and mitochondrial concentrations higher than those of untrained individuals and nonendurance athletes. This general conclusion is supported by results from cross-sectional and longitudinal studies of man. For example, in the studies described above on fiber distribution in untrained and trained men, Gollnick et al [22] also determined SDH and phosphofructokinase (PFK) activities in muscle samples from the various experimental groups. A total of 78 subjects were studied. Differences in $\dot{V}O_2$ max (Figure 6) clearly differentiated the endurance athletes from the remaining groups. In most of the subjects, muscle samples were obtained from the vastus lateralis and deltoid muscles. SDH activities for the various groups are presented in Figure 7. These data illustrate a greater aerobic potential in the muscles of the endurance

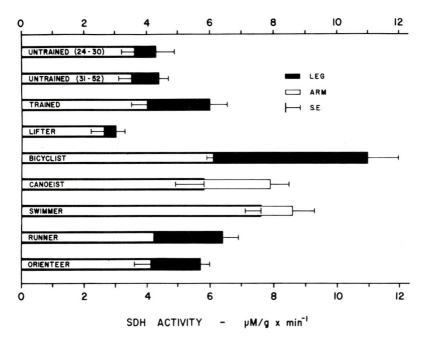

Figure 7. Succinate dehydrogenase activities of the vastus lateralis and deltoid muscles of groups of untrained and trained men.[22]

trained subjects. They also demonstrate that this adaptation is localized to those muscles engaged in the training. For example, bicycle exercise makes extensive use of the thigh muscle and in the highly trained bicyclists SDH activity exceeded that of all other groups including the distance runners who on the basis of their $\dot{V}O_2$ max data, excel at endurance work. Similarly, swimmers and canoeists had highest SDH activities in their deltoid muscles. This specificity of training explains the observation that people who change from one sport activity to another experience the sensation of being essentially untrained for the new activity. It also emphasizes the importance of securing measurements on the muscles that have been trained when an evaluation of a training procedure is being done.

Several cross-sectional studies have confirmed the differences in aerobic enzymes as described above.[29, 44-46, 70-74] Enzymes examined include SDH, cytochrome oxidase, malic dehydrogenase and citrate synthase. The activity of beta hydroxyacyl-CoA-dehydrogenase, an enzyme in fatty acid breakdown, is also elevated in skeletal muscles of trained individuals. This latter observation suggests an increased ability of trained muscle to use fatty acids as energy sources. Observations on women are similar to those on men [45, 46, 75] (Figure 8). A higher capillary density was reported in the muscle of training individuals.[76]

Observations from longitudinal studies of endurance training have clearly

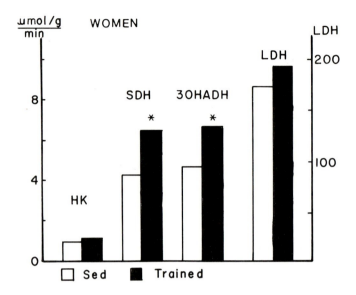

Figure 8. Hexokinase (HK), succinate dehydrogenase (SDH), beta hydroxy-acyl-CoA dehydrogenase (3OHADH) and lactate dehydrogenase (LDH) activities in the vastus lateralis muscle of a group of untrained and endurance trained women. Unpublished observations from Petersen, Rassmusen, Sembrowich and Gollnick, March 1976.

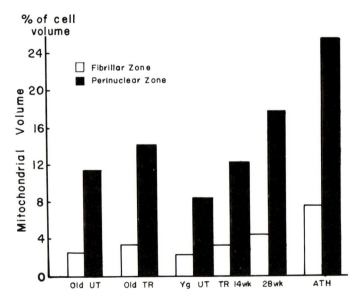

Figure 9. Mitochondrial volumes in the fibrillar and perinuclear zones of untrained and trained old men, young (yg) men before and after 14 and 28 weeks of training and top class athletes (Ath).[72]

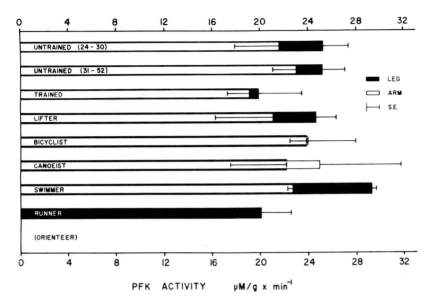

Figure 10. Phosphofructokinase activities in the deltoid and vastus lateralis muscle of groups of untrained and trained men.[22] See Figure 5 for additional information concerning groups.

established that the differences between trained and untrained subjects are due to the exercise.[14, 72, 73, 75, 77, 78] They have also demonstrated that the general findings apply to young as well as mature individuals [79] and to men as well as women.[80]

Electron-microscopic examination of human skeletal muscle has revealed that the increased aerobic potential (elevated enzyme activities) of skeletal muscle of trained subjects is the result of a greater mitochondrial volume.[55, 71, 72, 73] Kiessling et al [72] also examined the muscle of young men after 14 and 28 weeks of training (Figure 9). They found that the mitochondrial volume in both the fibrillar and perinuclear regions of the muscle had increased 48 and 215% respectively. Even after this training program, however, the mitochondrial volumes were less than those of top class endurance athletes. The increase in mitochondrial volume after endurance training is probably the result of increase both in the size and number of mitochondria.

It is unclear whether endurance training influences the enzymes for anaerobic metabolism. Figure 10 contains the results of the PFK from the cross-sectional study with untrained and trained men. There is little difference between groups. Similar data have been reported by others for enzymes such as glycogen phosphorylase, triose phosphate dehydrogenase, hexokinase and LDH.[50, 55, 70, 72, 73, 81] In a longitudinal study Gollnick et al [14] observed an increase in PFK. Taylor et al [82-84] also reported increases in glycogen phosphorylase, synthetase and branching enzyme after endurance training. These changes have not been confirmed and it is too early to accept them and judge their physiological importance.

Strength Training—In cross-sectional studies no major difference in the activities of oxidative enzymes has been found in individuals engaged in weight lifting or sprint running.[22, 29] In fact for weight lifters the SDH activity was lower than that of sedentary individuals. The large muscle bulk without any endurance stimulation may simply result in a growth dilution of the mitochondria. Thorstensson et al [77, 85] also did not observe any change in SDH activity after a program of strength training. Grimby et al [40] observed a significant increase in succinate oxidase activity in the muscle of subjects trained for 6 weeks with a program of isometric contractions. As was true with endurance training, there have been no indications that power training results in a change in the activities of any of the enzymes of glycolytic pathway.

Adaptations in Muscle Glycogen Metabolism

The glycogen content of human skeletal muscle can undergo wide fluctuations, which are greatly influenced by diet and the state of physical training. The concentration of glycogen in muscle is also an important factor in the performance of prolonged, high intensity exercise. This was clearly demonstrated in 1939 by Christensen and Hansen.[80] They exercised subjects to exhaustion after feeding them a mixed diet, a high fat-protein diet, and a high carbohydrate diet. After consumption of a normal diet the subjects exercised for about 120 minutes as compared to about 90 and 240 minutes after the high fat-protein and carbohydrate enriched diets, respectively. The work for these subjects averaged 175 watts per minute. Carbohydrate combustion based on respiratory exchange ratio and $\dot{V}O_2$ was highest after consumption of the carbohydrate diet. Subsequent studies where muscle samples were obtained with the needle technique confirmed the fact that glycogen storage and use were greatest after the consumption of a high carbohydrate diet.[25]

Using a classic experimental design, Bergström and Hultman [24] demonstrated the importance of prior exercise in the adaptive response of glycogen loading in skeletal muscle. They exercised one leg of subjects on a bicycle ergometer with the unexercised leg serving as a control. In these experiments a supercompensation of glycogen occurred only in the muscles of the exercised leg even though a carbohydrate enriched diet was consumed. Subsequently it has been demonstrated that the most effective method for glycogen loading of skeletal muscle is to first deplete the glycogen from the muscles by strenuous exercise. The glycogen content of the muscle is then kept low by a combination of a low carbohydrate diet and light exercise for 3 days. For an additional 3 days a carbohydrate enriched diet (about 60% of total kcal as carbohydrates) is consumed while energy requirements are kept at a low level. Through this regimen the glycogen content of the muscle may be raised in some individuals by as much as three to four times that of normal values. The biochemical mechanism(s) that produce this large accumulation of glycogen in the muscle are unknown. Since 2.7 gm of water are stored in muscle for every gram of glycogen, this glycogen

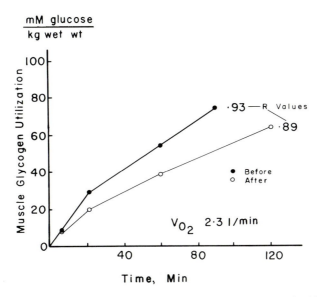

Figure 11. Glycogen utilization rates in the vastus lateralis muscle of subjects doing bicycle exercise at the same power output before and after training.[98]

loading also results in a significant weight gain. Although warnings have been issued about the dangers that may exist through the accumulation of glycogen and water in the heart during such a glycogen loading procedure,[86] there is no evidence that this in fact does occur.

Physical training results in an elevated glycogen in skeletal muscle.[14, 82, 84, 87, 88] This glycogen elevation is associated with an increase in the activity of the enzyme glycogen synthetase which is rate-limiting for glycogen formation.[55, 84] In normal, well fed but sedentary individuals muscle glycogen is usually about 80 mM of glucose units per kg wet weight.[22, 26] Values up to 200 mM of glucose units per kg wet weight and higher [14, 22] have been observed in muscle of highly trained individuals. It has been demonstrated that exercise and the depletion of glycogen associated with it results in an increase in the level of glycogen synthetase I (I is the form of the enzyme active in the absence of glucose-6-P) activity in muscle.[87, 89] This enzyme progressively returns to normal resting values as the glycogen stores of the muscle are returned to normal.

Physical training has a glycogen sparing effect when work is performed at the same absolute work load after as before training (Figure 11). Associated with this is a reduction in the respiratory exchange ratio indicating a greater reliance on fat oxidation. Also the level of lactate in both blood and working muscle is lower in the trained as compared with the untrained state. Whether this is related to the adaptative response in the oxidative systems is uncertain since the oxygen uptake at a given absolute work load and the muscle blood flow [51, 90] are not significantly altered by training.

Specificity of Training

Results from cross-sectional studies suggest that the metabolic adaptations of skeletal muscle are specific both to the muscle involved and the type of training. To further characterize this specificity, Saltin et al [51] used a one-legged training model. Subjects exercised one leg either with an endurance or sprint training program. In some cases both legs were exercised but with a different type of program for each leg. In other subjects one leg served as a sedentary control. Biopsy samples were taken from the vastus lateralis muscle with the needle technique before and after 4 weeks of training. These results demonstrated that no change in fiber composition occurred as a result of the training. SDH activity was unchanged in the untrained leg but was increased 19 and 33% in the sprint and endurance trained legs, respectively. Piehl et al [88] used a similar protocol to demonstrate that the increase in glycogen synthetase activity that occurs with training is limited to the trained leg. From these it is clear that responses are limited to those muscles involved in the exercise used to produce the trained state.

Significance of Adaptations in Skeletal Muscle

The significance of variations in oxidative enzyme activities of skeletal muscle and the changes associated with training are not fully understood. Attempts have been made to correlate the activities of oxidative enzymes with total body $\dot{V}O_2$ max. A correlation coefficient of .61 existed between SDH activity and $\dot{V}O_2$ max for the 78 subjects studied by Gollnick et al.[22] Though statistically significant, its predictive value is limited. Hoppeler et al [71] found r's ranging from .78 to .82 between $\dot{V}O_2$ max and various measures of mitochondrial concentration in the vastus lateralis of 17 subjects. Kiessling et al [72, 73] reported an r of .80 between the cytochrome oxidase activity of the vastus lateralis and $\dot{V}O_2$ max of 18 sedentary, middle-aged subjects. Booth and Narahara [91] reported a similar value in nine subjects. Thus, a positive relationship does exist between $\dot{V}O_2$ max and the oxidative activity of the vastus lateralis muscle. Whether or not this is a cause and effect relationship remains to be determined. In this regard, Gollnick et al [14] found that the SDH activity of the vastus lateralis muscle more than doubled after an endurance training program, whereas the $\dot{V}O_2$ max value increased by an average of only 13%.

The importance of local changes in oxidative activity cannot be discounted however. From glycogen depletion studies it is apparent that only a small number of fibers are activated at any one time. The local increase in oxidative activity may be very important for supporting the metabolism of these motor units. This question will only be settled by further investigation.

Effect of Disuse on Skeletal Muscle

Although the effects of physical training on human skeletal muscle have been fairly extensively studied, less information exists concerning muscular disuse resulting from cessation of training or forced inactivity. Forced inactivity is particularly important from a medical standpoint since many illnesses and surgical treatments result in periods of either total body or isolated limb inactivity. Inactivity of isolated limbs frequently results in a significant reduction in total body activity as well. Saltin et al [92] clearly demonstrated that bed rest for 3 weeks has a severe debilitating effect on the functional capacity of the circulatory system. This was manifest by an average loss of 28% in $\dot{V}O_2$ max, 11% in heart volume, and 26% in maximal cardiac output. Thus, it is obvious that continued activity is essential for maintenance of the functional status of the heart. Loss in work capacity may be greater in the highly trained than sedentary individual following forced inactivity.

Muscular inactivity results in a rapid loss of muscular mass and strength. Studies of bed rest have demonstrated that a strength loss is evident 1 to 2 days after the initiation of inactivity and proceeds at a rate of 1 to 1.5% per day.[60] Müller [60] reported that immobilization of a limb by casting results in a loss of 22% of the initial strength within the first 7 days. After this large initial strength loss little further decline occurred. This plateau effect was attributed to the fact that the subject began to perform isometric contractions within the cast. The smallest decrement in strength during inactivity was observed in subjects who had just completed a training program. Considerable caution must be exercised in interpreting data from most immobilization studies since control data are often inadequate. In spite of this limitation it is clear that inactivity leads to a rapid loss in muscular strength.

Only limited information is available on the effects of inactivity on intracellular components of human skeletal muscle. Gollnick et al [93] studied patients who had one leg immobilized following surgery for the reconstruction of the anterior cruciate ligament. Biopsy samples were obtained from the vastus lateralis muscle of both the operated and control legs before and at selected intervals after surgery. Prior to surgery the injured leg possessed lower "muscle tone" and the SDH activity was lower than the normal leg. This suggested a voluntary reduction in activity as a result of the injury. After a one week bed rest following the surgery, significant reductions in SDH occurred in both legs. Further reductions in SDH activity were evident during the period of recovery while the operated limb was placed in a cast (6 weeks). During this period a 3 cm loss in circumference occurred in the casted leg. These subjects were able to return to normal activity only after 3.75 months. As part of this experiment a group of subjects were fitted with casts that allowed a flexion to 120° and extension to 160°. In these subjects the change in SDH activity was not different from those individuals with the fixed casts. However, the loss in muscle circumference was less (.5 cm) and they were able to return to normal activity sooner (in 1.5 months) than those with fixed casts.

Examination of biopsy samples from these subjects indicated no change in fiber composition. However, the greatest loss in fiber area occurred in the ST fibers. The loss of oxidative activity as indicated by histochemical staining oc-

TABLE III

Effects of Training on Skeletal Muscle

	ST Fibers		FT Fibers	
		Type of Training		
	Strength	Endurance	Strength	Endurance
% Composition	0	0	0	0
Size	+	0	+ +	0
Glycogen content	0	+ +	0	+ +
Contractile property	0	0	0	0
Oxidative capacity	0	+ +	0	+
Fat oxidation	0	+ +	0	+
Anaerobic capacity	0	0	0	0
Capillary density	?	?	?	?
Blood flow during work	?	?	?	?

0 = no change; ? = unknown; + = a moderate increase; + + = a large increase

curred in a uniform manner in all muscle fibers. There was no change in glycolytic activity.

Saltin and Landin [94] examined the properties of muscle of both legs of hemiparetic patients and patients with Parkinson's disease to learn more about the effect of inactivity on these components. They found that the SDH activity of these patients was only 30 to 60% that of normal individuals. In these individuals the activity in the affected leg was only about 65% that of the nonaffected leg. These data further point to the importance of regular physical activity in the maintenance of normal metabolic capacity.

Prolonged immobilization of the limbs of animals has shown that a gradual disintegration of the muscle fibers occurs.[95] This is reversible when activity is restored. The oxidative capacity of muscle is also rapidly lost during inactivation of animal skeletal muscle.[59]

The field of inactivity and its effect on skeletal muscle will be a fruitful and important one for future investigation.

Summary

It is clear from the foregoing discussion that skeletal muscle possesses a remarkable ability to adapt to different patterns of use. Current information suggests that large local adaptations occur to influence the metabolic character of muscle during endurance training. Increases in muscle mass occur during training only when the resistance against the muscle work is high. There is no indication that the basic contractile properties of muscle fibers are altered by training or that the fiber composition changes. These findings clearly illustrate the importance of physical activity in maintaining muscle strength and in the development of the metabolic capacity of the muscle. A summary of training responses of skeletal muscle is presented in Table III.

Note—In this chapter we have intentionally limited our presentation to a description of adaptations in human skeletal muscle to training. In so doing we have eliminated a large body of literature obtained from experiments with animals. For a complete review of studies with animals we recommend the recent review by Drs. John O. Holloszy and Frank W. Booth (*Ann Rev Physiol* 38:273-291, 1976).

References

1. Burke RE, Levine DN, Zajac FE III, et al: Mammalian motor units: physiological-histochemical correlation in three types in cat gastrocnemius. *Science* 174:709-712, 1971.
2. Burke RE, Edgerton VR: "Motor Unit Properties and Selective Involvement in Movement," in Wilmore J (Ed): *Exercise and Sport Sciences Reviews*, pp 31-81, New York: Academic Press, 1975.
3. Edström L, Kugelberg E: Histochemical composition, distribution of fibres and fatiguability of single motor units. *J Neurol Neurosurg Psychiat* 31:415-423, 1968.
4. Kugelberg E: Histochemical composition, contraction speed and fatiguability of rat soleus motor units. *J Neurol Sci* 20:177-198, 1973.
5. Denny-Brown D: On the nature of postural reflexes. *Proc Roy Soc [Biol]* 104:253-301, 1929.
6. Engel WK: The multiplicity of pathological reactions in human skeletal muscle. *Proc Int Congr Neuropathol* 5:613-624, 1966.
7. Barnard RJ, Edgerton VR, Furukawa T, et al: Histochemical, biochemical, and contractile properties of red, white, and intermediate fibers. *Amer J Physiol* 220:410-414, 1971.
8. Peter JB, Barnard RJ, Edgerton VR, et al: Metabolic profiles of three fiber types of skeletal muscle in guinea pigs and rabbits. *Biochemistry* 14:2627-2633, 1972.
9. Buchthal F, Schmalbruch H: Spectrum of contraction times of different fibre bundles in the brachial biceps and triceps muscles of man. *Nature* 221:89, 1969.
10. Buchthal F, Schmalbruch H: Contraction times and fibre types in intact human muscle. *Acta Physiol Scand* 79:435-452, 1970.
11. Buchthal F, Dahl K, Rosenfalck D: Rise time of the spike potential in fast and slowly contracting muscle of man. *Acta Physiol Scand* 87:261-269, 1973.
12. Eberstein D, Goodgold J: Slow and fast twitch fibers in human skeletal muscle. *Amer J Physiol* 215:535-541, 1968.
13. Sica REP, McComas AJ: Fast and slow twitch units in a human muscle. *J Neurol Neurosurg Psychiat* 34:118-120, 1971.
14. Gollnick PD, Armstrong RB, Saltin B, et al: Effect of training an enzyme activity and fiber composition of human skeletal muscle. *J Appl Physiol* 34:107-111, 1973.
15. Taylor AW, Essen B, Saltin B: Myosin ATPase in skeletal muscle of healthy men. *Acta Physiol Scand* 91:568-570, 1974.
16. Bárány M: ATPase activity of myosin correlated with speed of muscle shortening. *J Gen Physiol* 50:197-216, 1967.
17. Engel WK, Brooke NH, Nelson PG: Histochemical studies of denervated or tenotomized cat muscle illustrating difficulties in relating experimental animal conditions to human neuromuscular diseases. *Ann NY Acad Sci* 138:160-185, 1966.
18. Gauthier GF: On the relationships of ultrastructural and cytochemical features to color in mammalian skeletal muscle. *Z Zellforsch* 95:462-482, 1969.
19. Cullen MJ, Weightman D: The ultrastructure of normal human muscle in relation to fiber type. *J Neurol Sci* 25:43-56, 1975.
20. Dubowitz V, Pearse AG: A comparative histochemical study of oxidative enzymes and phosphorylase activity in skeletal muscle. *Histochemie* 2:105-117, 1960.
21. Edström L, Nyström B: Histochemical types and sizes of fibres of normal human muscles. *Acta Neurol Scand* 45:257-269, 1969.

22. Gollnick PD, Armstrong RB, Saubert CW IV, et al: Enzyme activity and fiber composition in skeletal muscle of untrained and trained men. *J Appl Physiol* 33:312-319, 1972.
23. Gollnick PD, Armstrong RB: Histochemical localization of lactate dehydrogenase isozymes in human skeletal muscle fibers. *Life Sci* 18:27-32, 1976.
24. Bergström J, Hultman E: Muscle glycogen synthesis after exercise. An enhancing factor localized to the muscle cells in man. *Nature* 210:309-310, 1966.
25. Bergström J, Hermansen L, Hultman E, et al: Diet, muscle glycogen, and physical performance. *Acta Physiol Scand* 71:140-150, 1967.
26. Gollnick PD, Piehl K, Saubert CW IV, et al: Diet, exercise, and glycogen changes in human muscle fibers. *J Appl Physiol* 33:421-425, 1972.
27. Gollnick PD, Karlsson J, Piehl K, et al: Selective glycogen depletion in skeletal muscle fibres of man following sustained contractions. *J Physiol* 241:59-67, 1974.
28. Essén B, Henriksson J: Glycogen content of individual muscle fibres in man. *Acta Physiol Scand* 90:645-647, 1974.
29. Edström L, Ekblom B: Differences in sizes of red and white muscle fibres in vastus lateralis of musculus quadriceps femoris of normal individuals and athletes, relation to physical performance. *Scand J Clin Lab Invest* 30:175-181, 1972.
30. Jennekens FGI, Tomlinson BE, Walton JN: The sizes of the two main histochemical fibre types in five limb muscles in man. *J Neurol Sci* 13:281-292, 1971.
31. Johnson MA, Polgar J, Weightman D, Appleton D: Data on the distribution of fiber types in thirty-six human muscles: an autopsy study. *J Neurol Sci* 18:111-129, 1973.
32. Armstrong RB, Saubert CW IV, Sembrowich WL, et al: Glycogen depletion in rat skeletal muscle fibers at different intensities and durations of exercise. *Pflueger Arch* 352:243-256, 1974.
33. Lindholm A, Piehl K: Fibre composition, enzyme activity and concentrations of metabolites and electrolytes in muscles of standardbred horses. *Acta Vet Scand* 15:1-23, 1974.
34. Gollnick PD, Armstrong RB, Sembrowich WL, et al: Glycogen depletion pattern in human skeletal muscle fibers after heavy exercise. *J Appl Physiol* 34:615-618, 1973.
35. Gollnick PD, Armstrong RB, Saubert CW IV, et al: Glycogen depletion patterns in human skeletal muscle fibers during prolonged work. *Pflueger Arch* 344:1-12, 1973.
36. Gollnick PD, Piehl K, Saltin B: Selective glycogen depletion pattern in human muscle fibres after exercise of varying intensity and at varying pedalling rates. *J Physiol* 241:45-57, 1974.
37. Costill DL, Jansson E, Gollnick PD, et al: Glycogen utilization in leg muscles of men during level and uphill running. *Acta Physiol Scand* 91:475-481, 1974.
38. Costill DL, Gollnick PD, Jansson ED, et al: Glycogen depletion pattern in human muscle fibres during distance running. *Acta Physiol Scand* 89:374-383, 1973.
39. Essén B, Häggmark T: Lactate concentration in type I and II muscle fibres during muscular contraction in man. *Acta Physiol Scand* 95:344-346, 1975.
40. Grimby G, Björntorp P, Fahlén M, et al: Metabolic effects of isometric training. *Scand J Clin Lab Invest* 31:301-305, 1973.
41. Henneman E, Olson C: Relations between structure and function in the design of skeletal muscle. *J Neurophysiol* 28:481-498, 1965.
42. Hursh JB: Conduction velocity and diameter of nerve fibers. *Amer J Physiol* 127:131-139, 1939.
43. Rushton WAH: A theory of the effects of fiber size in medullated nerve. *J Physiol* 115:101-122, 1951.
44. Costill DL, Fink WJ, Pollock ML: Muscle fiber composition and enzyme activities of elite distance runners. *Med Sci Sports* 8:96-100, 1976.
45. Costill DL, Daniels J, Evans W, et al: Skeletal muscle enzymes and fiber composition in male and female track athletes. *J Appl Physiol* 40:149-154, 1976.
46. Fink WJ, Costill DL, Daniels J, et al: Muscle fiber composition and enzyme activities in male and female athletes (abstract). *Physiologist* 18:213, 1975.
47. Gollnick PD, Sjödin B, Karlsson J, et al: Human soleus muscle: a comparison of fiber composition and enzyme activities with other leg muscles. *Pflueger Arch* 348:247-255, 1974.
48. Morpurgo D: Uber Aktivitäts-Hypertrophie der willkürlichen Muskeln. *Virchow Arch* 150:522-554, 1897.
49. Havu M, Rusko H, Komi PV, et al: Muscle fiber composition, work performance capacity and training in Finnish skiers. *Int Res Comm Sys* 1:10, 1973.
50. Karlsson JB, Sjödin B, Thorstensson A, et al: LDH isozymes in skeletal muscles of endurance and strength trained athletes. *Acta Physiol Scand* 93:150-156, 1975.

51. Saltin B, Nazar K, Costill DL, et al: The nature of the training response; peripheral and central adaptations to one-legged exercise. *Acta Physiol Scand* 96:289-305, 1976.
52. Barnard RJ, Edgerton VR, Peter JB: Effect of exercise on skeletal muscle. I: Biochemical and histological properties. *J Appl Physiol* 28:401-414, 1971.
53. Faulkner JA, Maxwell LC, Brook DA, et al: Adaptation of guinea pig phantaris muscle fibers to endurance training. *Amer J Physiol* 221:291-297, 1971.
54. Faulkner JA, Maxwell LC, Lieberman DA: Histochemical characteristics of muscle fibers from trained and detrained guinea pigs. *Amer J Physiol* 222:836-840, 1972.
55. Morgan TE, Cobb LA, Short FA, et al: "Effects of Long-term Exercise on Human Muscle Mito-chondria," in Pernow B and Saltin B (Eds): *Muscle Metabolism During Exercise*, pp 87-95, New York: Plenum, 1971.
56. Bagby GJ, Sembrowich WL, Gollnick PD: Myosin ATPase and fiber composition from trained and untrained rat skeletal muscle. *Amer J Physiol* 223:1415-1417, 1972.
57. Ikai M, Fukunaga T: Calculation of muscle strength per unit cross-sectional area of human muscle by means of ultrasonic measurement. *Int Z Angew Physiol* 26:26-32, 1968.
58. Ikai M, Fukunaga T: A study on training effect on strength per unit cross-sectional area of muscle by means of ultrasonic measurement. *Int Z Angew Physiol* 28:173-180, 1970.
59. Max SR: Disuse atrophy of skeletal muscle: loss of functional activity of mitochondria. *Biochem Biophys Res Commun* 46:1394-1398, 1972.
60. Müller EA: Influence of training and of inactivity on muscle strength. *Arch Phys Med* 51:449-463, 1970.
61. Julian LM, Cardinet GH III: Fiber sizes of the biceps brachii muscle of dogs which differ greatly in body size. *Anat Rec* 139:243, 1961.
62. Etemadi AA, Hosseini F: Frequency and size of muscle fibers in athletic body build. *Anat Rec* 162:269-274, 1968.
63. MacDougall D, Sale G, Elder G, Sutton JR: Ultrastructural properties of human skeletal muscle following heavy resistance training and immobilization (abstract). *Med Sci Sports* 8:72, 1976.
64. Hall-Craggs ECB: The longitudinal division of fibres in overloaded rat skeletal muscle. *J Anat* 107:459-470, 1970.
65. Reitsma W: Skeletal muscle hypertrophy after heavy exercise in rats with surgically reduced muscle function. *Amer J Phys Med* 48:237-258, 1969.
66. Ianuzzo CD, Gollnick PD, Armstrong RB: Compensatory adaptation of skeletal muscle fiber types to a long-term functional overload. *Life Sci* 9:1517-1524, 1976.
67. Sola OM, Christensen DL, Martin AW: Hypertrophy and hyperplasia of adult chicken anterior latissimus dorsi muscles following stretch with and without denervation. *Exp Neurol* 41:76-100, 1973.
68. Gonyea WJ, Ericson GC: An experimental model for the study of exercise-induced skeletal muscle hypertrophy. *J Appl Physiol* 40:630-633, 1976.
69. Gonyea WJ, Ericson GC, Bonde-Petersen F: Skeletal muscle fibre splitting induced by weight lifting exercise in cats. *Acta Physiol Scand* 99:105-109, 1977.
70. Bass A, Vondra K, Ruth R, et al: Enzyme activity patterns of energy supplying metabolism in the quadriceps femoris muscle (vastus lateralis). *Pflueger Arch* 316:169-173, 1976.
71. Hoppeler H, Luthi P, Claassen H, et al: The ultrastructure of the normal human skeletal muscle. *Pflueger Arch* 344:217-232, 1973.
72. Kiessling KH, Pilström L, Karlsson J, et al: Mitochondrial volume in skeletal muscle from young and old physically untrained and trained healthy men and from alcoholics. *Clin Sci* 44:547-554, 1973.
73. Kiessling KH, Pilström L, Bylund ACH, et al: Enzyme activities and morphometry in skeletal muscle of middle-aged men after training. *Scand J Clin Lab Invest* 33:63-69, 1974.
74. Vihko V, Hirsimaki Y, Rusko H, et al: Adaptation of skeletal muscle to endurance training: succinate dehydrogenase activities in highly trained skiers. *Int Res Comm Sys* 2:1033, 1974.
75. Taylor AW, Lavoic S, Lemiewt G, et al: The effects of endurance training on the number area and enzyme activity of skeletal muscle fibres of French Canadian women (abstract). *Med Sci Sports* 8:54, 1976.
76. Hermansen L, Wachtlova M: Capillary density of skeletal muscle in well-trained and untrained men. *J Appl Physiol* 30:860-863, 1971.
77. Thorstensson A, Sjödin B, Karlsson J: Enzyme activities and muscle strength after "sprint train-ing" in man. *Acta Physiol Scand* 94:313-318, 1975.

78. Varnauskas E, Björntorp P, Fahlén M, et al: Effects of physical training on exercise blood flow and enzymatic activity in skeletal muscle. *Cardiovasc Res* 4:418-422, 1970.
79. Eriksson BO, Gollnick PD, Saltin B: Muscle metabolism and enzyme activities after training in boys 11-13 years old. *Acta Physiol Scand* 87:495-497, 1973.
80. Christensen EH, Hansen O: Arbetisfähigkeit und Ehrährung. *Skand Arch Physiol* 81:160-171, 1939.
81. Sjödin B, Thorstensson A, Frith K, et al: Effect of physical training on LDH activity and LDH isozyme pattern in human skeletal muscle. *Acta Physiol Scand* 97:150-157, 1976.
82. Taylor AW, Stothart J, Booth MA, et al: Human skeletal muscle glycogen branching enzyme activities with exercise and training. *Canad J Physiol Pharmacol* 52:119-122, 1974.
83. Taylor AW, Booth MA, Rao S: Human skeletal muscle phosphorylase activities with exercise and training. *Canad J Physiol Pharmacol* 50:1038-1041, 1972.
84. Taylor AW, Thayer R, Rao S: Human skeletal muscle glycogen synthetase activities with exercise and training. *Canad J Physiol Pharmacol* 50:411-415, 1972.
85. Thorstensson A, Karlsson J: The effect of strength training on muscle enzymes related to high energy phosphate metabolism (abstract). *Acta Physiol Scand* 91:21, 1974.
86. Nelson RA, Gastineau CF: "Exceptional" nutritional needs of the athlete. *The Medical Aspects of Sports* (AMA) 15:19-21, 1974.
87. Piehl K: Time course for refilling of glycogen stores in human muscle fibres following exercise-induced glycogen depletion. *Acta Physiol Scand* 90:297-302, 1974.
88. Piehl K, Adolfsson S, Nazar K: Glycogen storage and glycogen synthetase activity in trained and untrained muscle of man. *Acta Physiol Scand* 90:779-788, 1974.
89. Hultman E, Bergström J, Roch-Norlund AE: "Glycogen Storage in Human Skeletal Muscle," in Pernow B, Saltin B (Eds): *Muscle Metabolism During Exercise*, pp 273-288, New York: Plenum, 1971.
90. Clausen JP, Trap-Jensen J: Effect of training on muscular blood flow during exercise. *Acta Physiol Scand* 94:C18, 1968.
91. Booth FW, Narahara KA: Vastus lateralis cytochrome oxidase activity and its relationship to maximal oxygen consumption in man. *Pflueger Arch* 349:319-324, 1974.
92. Saltin B, Blomqvist G, Mitchell JH, et al: Response to exercise after bed rest and after training. *Circulation* 38(suppl 7):1-78, 1968.
93. Gollnick PD, Eriksson E, Häggmark T, et al: Recovery with a movable or standard cast following intra-articular reconstruction of the anterior cruciate ligament. *The Medical Aspects of Sports* (AMA) 15:56-60, 1974.
94. Saltin B, Landin S: Work capacity, muscle strength and SDH activity in both legs of hemiparetic patients and patients with Parkinson's disease. *Scand J Clin Lab Invest* 35:531-538, 1975.
95. Cooper RG: Alteration during immobilization and regeneration of skeletal muscle in cats. *J Bone Joint Surg* 54:919-953, 1972.
96. Essén B, Jansson E, Henriksson J, et al: Metabolic characteristics of fibre types in human skeletal muscle. *Acta Physiol Scand* 95:153-165, 1975.
97. Karlsson J, Frith K, Sjödin B, et al: Distribution of LDH isozymes in human skeletal muscle. *Scand J Clin Lab Invest* 33:307-312, 1974.
98. Karlsson J, Nordesjö LO, Saltin B: Muscle glycogen utilization during exercise after physical training. *Acta Physiol Scand* 90:210-217, 1974.

6

Myocardial Adaptations to Physical Conditioning

Leigh D. Segel, PhD

The current interest in physical conditioning and the suggestion that regular exercise may prevent or decrease the severity of cardiac disease has stimulated the investigation of the effects of exercise training on the heart. There has been a considerable amount of the literature on this subject during the past six years. However, because of the many variables involved in studies of this nature, a great deal of uncertainty still remains. This review will examine recent advances in areas of cardiac mechanics, microstructure and metabolism affected by long-term physical conditioning.

Much of the difficulty in evaluating results of conditioning experiments is derived from factors involved in the design of the various studies. Among the variables that must be considered are: (1) The age of the animal at the beginning and end of the conditioning; (2) The sex of the animal; (3) The type of exercise and the intensity of the training program; (4) Whether or not the control animals receive the same amount of handling as the conditioned animals; (5) The type of anesthesia used before sacrifice; (6) Whether control animals were fed ad lib or were on a restricted diet to maintain the same growth curve as the exercisers; (7) The influence of the final bout of exercise on the result (ie, the amount of rest the animal had prior to sacrifice); (8) Whether the exercise was spontaneous or enforced; and (9) Whether or not an independent, recognized criterion of conditioning was shown to result from the training program used. Studies which do not consider these factors complicate the analysis and interpretation of the results. This may explain the contradictory nature of much of the data discussed here, relating chronic exercise and myocardial alterations (Table I).

TABLE I

Influence of Exercise Conditioning on Myocardial Function

Enhanced Contractile Performance
    Increased work load at standard heart rate [6]
    Increased tension, $\dot{V}_{max}$, and rate of tension development [7]
    Less impairment of cardiac performance during hypoxia or pressure overload [12, 22]
    Increased isometric tension [20]
    Increased cardiac output and cardiac work [21]

No Improvement in Contractile Performance
    No change in tension or rate of tension development [9]
    No change in length-tension curve [10]
    Depressed tension [14]
    No change in cardiac function measured in situ [16, 22]

Modified Metabolic Activity
    Increased myosin ATPase activity [23-25, 29]
    Increased mitochondrial function or oxidative enzyme activity [33, 34]
    Increased glycolytic enzyme activity [44, 45]
    Increased glycogen concentration [46, 49]
    Increased catecholamine concentration [68, 69]
    Decreased catecholamine concentration [9, 17-19]

No Modification of Metabolic Activity
    No change in ATPase activity [28]
    No change in mitochondrial function or oxidative enzyme activity [11, 15, 30, 31]
    No change in glycogen concentration [41-45]
    No change in catecholamine concentration [70, 71]

Structural and Ultrastructural Changes
    Increased size and/or number of mitochondria [34, 52]
    Decreased size of mitochondria [51]
    Increased extracoronary collaterals or coronary vascularity [8, 64]
    No change in extracoronary collaterals [63]

Cardiac Mechanics

Exercise physiologists have for some time studied the function of the heart during an acute exercise bout and as the result of chronic exercise conditioning.[1] Investigation of the intrinsic contractile properties of the myocardia of experimental animals resulting from exercise and conditioning have recently come under intense investigation. This discussion will focus on work in which the mechanical function of the myocardium (eg, tension, rate of tension development) and hemodynamic function (eg, cardiac output, coronary flow, left ventricular pressure) have been studied in exercise-trained individuals. Well documented effects of conditioning on cardiac tissue include: reduction in resting and intrinsic heart rates,[2-6] and cardiomegaly, which has been reported as increased cardiac mass [5-11] or as an increase in heart weight/body weight ratio.[12-15] While bradycardia appears to be universal and is sometimes used as a criterion of training, cardiomegaly has not been observed consistently.[16-19]

On a mechanical basis hearts from exercise-conditioned experimental animals have generally been reported to have improved intrinsic contractility,[6, 7, 12, 20, 21] although this is not a universal finding.[9, 10, 14, 16, 22] Crews and Aldinger[20] measured myocardial contractile function of swim-conditioned rats with a strain-gauge lever system. Development of right ventricular isometric tension was higher in the exercised rats. Studies by Penpargkul and Scheuer[21] employing the isolated working perfused rat heart suggest that male rats conditioned by swimming have increased cardiac output and cardiac work. The improved pumping performance was shown to persist even during perfusions in which arterial pO_2 was reduced.[12] Wyatt and Mitchell[6] demonstrated an increase in physical work capacity, an increase in left ventricular muscle mass, and a decrease in heart rate at rest and during submaximal exercise in dogs exercised daily for 12 weeks.

Several investigations have utilized isolated papillary muscle preparations as the model for studying the myocardial mechanics of conditioned and non-conditioned rats. Mole and Rabb[7] reported that papillary muscles isolated from exercised-trained, enlarged rat hearts exhibited increased maximum tension, maximum velocity of shortening, and maximum dT/dt, and decreased time to peak tension. These results contrast with those of several other investigators. Amsterdam et al[9] did not find any difference in papillary muscle tension or maximum rate of tension development in normoxic conditions between control and exercise-conditioned rats. Nutter et al[14] reported that a 12-week treadmill training program produced cardiomegaly with depressed myocardial contractility, both of which were reversible with detraining. Peak tension and maximum dT/dt of papillary muscles from trained rats were significantly lower than those of sedentary rats. After a 6-week detraining period these variables returned to control values. Response to hypoxic stress was similar in trained, detrained and control muscles. Grimm et al[10] found no effect of conditioning on length-tension curves studied in papillary muscles. Maximum developed tension per gram wet muscle weight also did not change as a result of conditioning.

In a study by Dowell et al,[16] no difference was evident in control in situ cardiac functional measurements between sedentary and conditioned female rats. Although an 8-week treadmill running program was employed, no independent criterion of conditioning was reported. Body and heart weights and gastrocnemius cytochrome c levels were unchanged as a result of the program. Heart rate, left ventricular systolic and end-diastolic pressures, contractility index, cardiac index and stroke index were uninfluenced by the repetitive exercise. However, after a sustained pressure overload induced by aortic banding for 3 days, contractility index significantly declined in control animals while remaining unchanged in the trained animals, suggesting that conditioned animals have improved ability to withstand the stress of pressure overload.

Carey et al[22] have recently assessed myocardial performance in open-chested conditioned and nonconditioned rats. They recorded no difference in dP/dt_{max} between the two groups in normoxic conditions. However, when the rats were subjected to an hypoxic environment, cardiac performance (dP/dt_{max} and ventricular pressure) was less impaired in the conditioned rats than in the nonconditioned animals.

Morganroth et al [5] analyzed hearts of athletes using echocardiography and reported that athletes participating in isotonic (endurance) exercise (running, swimming) exhibited increased left ventricular mass with cardiac changes similar to those found in chronic volume overloads (increased stroke volume and end-diastolic volume), while athletes participating in heavy resistance exercise (wrestling, shot putting) exhibited increased left ventricular mass with cardiac changes similar to those found in chronic pressure overloads (increased left ventricular wall thickness).

Because of the equivocal nature of the evidence, it would be premature to draw firm conclusions regarding the intrinsic contractility of conditioned hearts at this point. The experiments of Scheuer et al [12, 21] provide the strongest evidence at this time suggesting that cardiac mechanical function is improved in the normal nonstressed heart by conditioning. They suggest that the greater aerobic and mechanical reserve of conditioned hearts is the result of improved mechanisms of oxygen delivery (ie, increased coronary flow). During stress produced either by hypoxia or by pressure overload, the conditioned heart appears to be better able to maintain or increase contractility during the challenge.[12, 16, 22]

Myosin Adenosine Triphosphatase Activity

The suggestion that conditioned hearts have improved contractility raises the possibility that adaptive changes occur in the myofibrillar protein system responsible for contraction. This has been explored by several investigators. Bhan and Scheuer [23] have presented evidence that the enzymatic ATPase activity of cardiac actomyosin increased with an increasing level of conditioning. Rats on a swimming program exhibited the same ATPase activity as controls until after the animals had swum a total of 45 to 60 hours. By 100 hours the activity was approximately 1.7-fold higher than control. At this point, the hearts exhibited significant cardiomegaly, based on heart weight. Earlier in the conditioning regimen when the ATPase activity was increased, heart weight was not significantly increased even though the heart weight/body weight ratio was increased. These data are in agreement with Medugorac et al [24, 25] who found that 100 to 120 hours of swimming by rats resulted in approximately 1.5-fold increased ATPase activity. The authors concluded from their data that an increased proportion of myosin light chain 1 in conditioned hearts is related to the change in enzymatic activity. Bhan and Scheuer,[26] however, reported no change in the number of myosin light chains in hearts from their conditioned rats. Instead, these authors,[27] utilizing a fluorescence probe of the active site of cardiac heavy meromyosin, speculated that an adaptive conformational change occurs at or near the active site of the enzyme in conditioned hearts. They proposed that this uncoiled conformation allows increased accessibility of substrate to the active site and thus results in enhanced activity.

Baldwin et al [28] found no increase in Mg^{++}-ATPase activity of cardiac actomyosin from rats conditioned by a strenuous 18 to 24-week running program. They suggested that the increased ATPase activity, observed by Bhan and Scheuer,[23] is a transient phenomenon that is an adaptation to early training but which decreases with long-term training. This would tend to be refuted by the data of Wilkerson and Evonuk [29] who reported that animals on a mild swimming program (30 minutes every other day for 10 weeks) or on a more rigorous program (swimming to exhaustion every other day for 10 weeks) both exhibited increased cardiac ATPase activities compared to nonconditioned controls. The possibility remains, however, that the rigorous program of Wilkerson and Evonuk was not as strenuous as that of Baldwin et al.[28]

Mitochondrial Function

Myocardial oxidative function has been studied to ascertain whether the heart adapts to the energy requirements of chronic exercise by altering the amount or activity of mitochondria or mitochondrial enzymes. Attempts have also been made in some investigations to correlate changes in mitochondrial function with alterations in fine structure of the myocardium as a result of training.

An early study by Hearn and Wainio [11] using male rats that had undergone a mild conditioning program (1/2 hour daily swimming for 5 to 8 weeks) indicated that enlarged hearts from the conditioned rats exhibited the same succinic dehydrogenase activity as hearts from nonconditioned rats. Later investigators, using conditioned runners and swimmers, reported similar results. Gollnick and Ianuzzo,[30] using rats that had a total running program of approximately 50 hours, found no change in myocardial succinic dehydrogenase activity as a result of training. Oscai et al,[15] examining cardiac cytochrome oxidase and succinic oxidase in runners (approximately 120 hours total conditioning, at a maximum of 2 hours per day) and swimmers (maximum 90 hours training at 30 to 180 min per day), reported no change in the activity levels of those enzymes or in the concentration of cardiac cytochrome c. Dohm et al,[31] studying mitochondrial oxygen consumption in hearts of conditioned runners (approximately 120 total running hours), obtained results in agreement with workers who studied activities of single mitochondrial enzymes: there was no alteration in the oxidative capacity of the mitochondria as a result of conditioning. In a slightly different type of experiment, Sembrowich et al [32] found that there was no difference in *in vitro* swelling of mitochondria from conditioned and nonconditioned hearts. Two groups of investigators, however, have recorded significant increases in parameters related to oxidative metabolism of conditioned hearts. Both groups observed the changes after more strenuous training than that used by the investigators discussed previously. Kraus and Kirsten [33] employed a 16-week swimming program. Rats swam with weights on their tails twice daily, 6 days per week, to the point of exhaustion. The specific activity of succinic dehydrogenase and glycerol phosphate dehydrogenase increased 40 and 100%, respectively, during the conditioning program. These workers, however, did not indicate how long after the final swimming period the rats were allowed to rest before sacrifice and thus the enzyme activities reported may have been influenced by the final bout of exercise if the animals were not allowed a sufficient rest time before sacrifice. In another study, Arcos et al [34] assessed changes in overall mitochondrial function during the course of a conditioning program in which rats swam 6 hours per day, 6 days per week. After 73 total swimming hours, oxygen consumption and respiratory control ratio had increased; this increase persisted in a group of rats that had swum 161 hours. By 410 hours, the mitochondrial activity had returned to control levels. These experiments employed animals having the same weight at sacrifice; no discussion of the age of the animals was presented. Since vigorous conditioning can depress the growth curve of rats, it is possible that the single control group of this study was older than some, if not all, of the swimmers. Age-matched controls were apparently not studied.

These investigations indicate that after a *mild* to *moderate* training program there are no adaptive alterations in mitochondrial function as determined in broken cell preparations. It appears unlikely that a dramatic increase in mitochondrial respiratory capacity, as observed in skeletal muscle in response to endurance training,[35] occurs in cardiac muscle as a result of conditioning. The possibility remains, however, that the myocardium does adapt to a *vigorous* training program by increasing cell oxidative capacity, and this bears further investigation.

Nonoxidative Metabolism

Although the heart is primarily an aerobic organ, deriving most of its energy from oxidative metabolism, during conditions of inadequate oxygen delivery nonoxidative metabolism (glycolysis) becomes predominant.[36] The possibility that hearts from conditioned rats perform better than control hearts in hypoxic conditions [12] and the finding that in a "fit" population the heart exhibits periods of ischemia in a stressful situation [37] have aroused interest in changes that occur in nonoxidative metabolism as a result of conditioning.

It is well established that an acute bout of strenuous exercise by nonconditioned animals diminishes cardiac glycogen stores.[38-43] Upon cessation of exercise there is resynthesis of glycogen and a period of glycogen supercompensation that can last from 4 to 20 hours depending on the severity of the exercise bout.[39, 40, 43] Recent work in our laboratory (L. Segel, unpublished data, February 1975) indicates that the glycogen depletion and supercompensation pattern in hearts of conditioned rats in response to a bout of exercise is different from that observed in nonconditioned rats for the same exercise period. This suggests that adaptive changes occur as a result of conditioning that directly or indirectly influence cardiac glycogen metabolism in response to stress.

There are several other indications in the literature that glycolytic metabolism adapts to conditioning. Simon et al [44] reported a modest increase in cardiac pyruvate kinase activity in rats that had swum for 8 weeks. York et al [45] showed not only a 20% increase in cardiac pyruvate kinase in 16-week swimmers, but also a 32% increase in cardiac lactic dehydrogenase activity and a slight increase in the percentage of LDH "M" isozyme in the conditioned hearts. They did not, however, note any increase based on tissue wet weight of phosphofructokinase activity, an important enzyme in regulating the rate of glycolysis.

Scheuer et al [46] reported that cardiac glycogen stores (resting level) in conditioned animals were increased 20 to 25%. These results were obtained using rats fasted on the day prior to sacrifice which Scheuer et al reported "yielded more consistent differences in glycogen values between sedentary and conditioned animals."[46] Since overnight fasting raises cardiac glycogen 60 to 80% [47] (L. Segel, unpublished data, July 1974), it is possible that the difference Scheuer et al observed in cardiac glycogen between conditioned and nonconditioned rats after fasting involved interactions among factors affected by starvation as well as by conditioning. An early study by Shelley et al [48] showed no difference in cardiac glycogen between rested fed controls and conditioned swimmers but did show a large difference between the two groups when the animals were fasted. These findings must be viewed with caution, however, for two reasons: (1) They did not observe any effect of 24-hour starvation on cardiac glycogen in control rats, and (2) Two groups of essentially identical swimmers were reported to have widely varying mean values of cardiac glycogen (4.65 and 7.23 mg/g heart). Poland and Blount [49] reported results similar to Scheuer et al [46] when hearts from starved conditioned rats were examined. Results from nonstarved rats were not reported. Other investigators [41-45] using fed and fasted animals did not observe any change in cardiac glycogen in resting animals as a result of conditioning. In the study of Lamb et al,[41] the control and conditioned rats were handled similarly by the investigators, thus controlling an important variable.

These provocative observations bear further investigation in light of the possibility that additional cellular energy might be provided by extra glycogen stores in a conditioned heart during ischemic periods.

Ultrastructure

The fine structure of the myocardium has been examined in attempts to detail changes occurring as a result of acute exercise or long-term conditioning. The question as to whether conditioning offers protection against any damage that acute exercise may cause has also been explored. Aldinger and Sohal [50] reported an increase in the number of mitochondria in hearts of rats on a program of swimming conditioning. Arcos et al,[34] who also used swimming rats, reported that there was an apparent increase in the size and number of cardiac mitochondria from female rats conditioned by swimming. Mitochondrial mass, determined as milligrams of mitochondria isolated from one gram of heart tissue, apparently increased with training up to a point, then decreased with excessive training. As the total time in the conditioning program increased, the hearts were less likely to exhibit changes in the number of mitochondria, but were more likely to exhibit signs of exercise-induced damage to the organelles: reduced, swollen, clumped or irregular cristae, and reduction in matrix density. In contrast, a conditioning program of treadmill running was shown to induce a shift toward smaller mitochondria in hearts of male rats examined 24 hours after the last exercise period by Edington and Cosmas,[51] who suggested that this increase in mitochondrial surface-to-volume ratio may imply increased oxidative capacity of these hearts. Another possibility is that the small mitochondria are nonfunctional organelles that could be called upon to respond to a functional overload. Peterson,[52] who examined electron micrographs using a linear analysis technique, agrees with Arcos et al,[34] finding a significant increase in the proportion of the myocardium that is composed of mitochondria. However, he did not evaluate the relative size or volume differences of the mitochondria of the conditioned vs. the nonconditioned hearts.

Several workers have investigated the effects on cardiac ultrastructure of a single bout of exhaustive exercise in conditioned and nonconditioned rats. The work of King and Gollnick [53] suggested that exhaustive exercise causes considerable mitochondrial damage irrespective of prior conditioning. The destruction, including swelling and cristae and membrane disruption, was evident immediately following the exercise bout and was almost completely reversed at 24 hours post exercise. However, more convincing evidence presented by other investigators [54-58] has suggested that there is no damage to cardiac mitochondria or other organelles as a result of the bout of exercise in conditioned or nonconditioned animals. Laguens et al [57, 58] presented evidence from rat and dog hearts that mitochondria enlarge and replicate following an exercise period.

These reports and others [59, 60] emphasize the importance of rapid electron microscopy fixation techniques in instances, such as post exercise, where the fragility of mitochondria and other membranous structures (hence, the possibility of damage during conventional fixation) may be altered. Experiments by Banister et al [61] had indicated that cardiac mitochondria from nonconditioned animals or animals in the early stage of conditioning (up to 3 or 4 weeks of daily treadmill running) exhibited damaged and disrupted inner and outer membranes immediately after an acute bout of running. Later, Cvorkov et al [62] presented evidence that rats fed a high protein diet were protected from myocardial mitochondrial damage from the fourth day of exercise training. Recent work by this group, using perfusion fixation of the hearts for electron microscopy,[56] demonstrated that with this more rapid method of fixation which minimizes postmortem tissue destruction there was no damage to cardiac mitochondria or sarcoplasmic reticulum in nonconditioned rats after exhaustive running. In this study the authors did note dilated vesicles in the intercalated discs of the hearts.

The effect of chronic exercise on the microvasculature of the heart has also been studied by several groups. Bloor and Leon,[8] examining the microstructure of perfusion-fixed hearts from conditioned and nonconditioned rats, found that extracoronary collateral artery areas and the ratio of capillaries to muscle fibers were increased in the ventricles of exercised animals. On the other hand, a study of patients with coronary heart disease by Sim and Neill [63] indicated that an exercise conditioning program did not cause any change in coronary collaterals as evidenced by coronary arteriograms. Stevenson et al,[64] studying vinyl casts of coronary trees of swimmers and runners, found that physical exercise, if not too strenuous or continuous, caused an increase in the relative size of the coronary tree in rats. Whether their positive results with very mildly exercised animals have an application to *in vivo* blood flow (or to species other than rat) remains to be seen.

Cardiac Catecholamine Concentration

Several theories have been advanced to explain the bradycardia exhibited by conditioned animals. Tipton and Taylor [65] suggested that trained animals have more cardiac-bound nonneural acetylcholine (or other cholinergic substance) available than do control animals. Another hypothesis holds that a decrease in sympathetic stimulation of the heart is responsible for the decreased heart rate.[66] This latter possibility was investigated by several researchers who measured catecholamine stores and binding sites in hearts of conditioned animals. The assessment of cardiac catecholamines in conditioned rats requires careful attention to the factors mentioned above. In these studies, handling the control animals, use of the proper anesthesia and the type of training program assume paramount importance. Probably because of these factors, the investigations reported here regarding cardiac catecholamines present a variety of results. DeSchryver et al [17-19] demonstrated in several studies that the cardiac catecholamine content of spontaneously running rats is decreased on a concentration basis and on a whole heart basis. The conditioning program for these rats was mild and did not produce cardiomegaly or a change in body weight. DeSchryver et al [17-19] used decapitation as the method of sacrifice. It also appears that their control animals received the same amount of handling as the exercisers received. Daily handling of animals suppresses the rise in plasma corticosterone that occurs when "unhandled" rats are handled, weighed, etc.[67] It is possible that handling has a similar effect on circulating or tissue catecholamine content and, thus, the controls should be handled by the experimenters in a manner similar to the exercisers.

Ostman et al,[68-70] using a strenuous program of swimming or running, consistently observed only cardiomegaly (increased wet heart weight and heart weight/body weight ratio) as a result of conditioning. They did not obtain consistent results with respect to cardiac catecholamine concentrations or adrenal gland weights in their three studies. The authors did not state whether the controls were handled during their experiments except for weighing once weekly. Their results are also difficult to interpret because different sacrificing methods were used in their three studies. Guinea pigs, conditioned by running for 5 months, exhibited increased cardiac norepinephrine; sacrifice was by a blow to the head. No change in adrenal weight was found. In rats conditioned by running for 15 weeks and sacrificed by decapitation, there was no change in cardiac norepinephrine. Adrenal weight was increased 31%. In a third study, using swim-conditioned rats sacrificed by ether anesthesia and bleeding, cardiac norepinephrine was increased 25% and adrenal weight was increased 10%.

Leon et al [71] recently reported that swim-conditioned rats (1 hour a day for 12 weeks) having enlarged hearts exhibited no change in norepinephrine concentration or total amount of norepinephrine in the heart. Hearts were removed after decapitation of the animals, but remained unfrozen for up to 15 minutes after removal from the animals. The enzymes monoamine oxidase and catechol-O-methyltransferase, both of which metabolize catecholamines, are present in heart tissue [72] and it is possible that during the 15-minute postsacrifice period some of the norepinephrine present was metabolized.

Amsterdam et al [9] studied rats that swam 90 minutes a day for 12 weeks and were sacrificed by a blow to the head followed by rapid excision and freezing of the heart. Controls were not handled daily in this study. Cardiac catecholamine concentration was depressed, although not significantly, in the enlarged conditioned hearts.

In a related study, Salzman et al [73] examined epinephrine uptake in hearts of voluntarily running mice. The ventricles of mice after 9 weeks of running had 26% lower uptake of epinephrine-^{3}H per milligram of tissue than that of controls. Uptake per total ventricle was unchanged, however, as a result of conditioning since heart weight and heart weight/body weight ratio were greater in the conditioned mice. This work suggests that there is a dilution of cardiac binding sites for epinephrine associated with exercise-induced cardiomegaly.

The weight of the evidence from these studies appears to indicate that decreased catecholamine content may be one factor contributing to the bradycardia of conditioned hearts.

Conclusions

Despite the conflicting data surrounding the question of the effect of physical conditioning on the heart, several cautious conclusions can be drawn from the evidence currently available. Conditioning may allow the heart to maintain mechanical function under certain stress situations, although under normal conditions bradycardia may be the most significant functional change. Cardiomegaly and increased coronary vascularization represent important structural changes. On the molecular level, there is almost certainly no adaptive increase in mitochondrial ATP production as a result of conditioning, although there may be changes in the rate of ATP utilization via myosin ATPase. The role of nonoxidative metabolism, particularly as related to the function of the conditioned heart in ischemia, remains to be established. Without doubt, a complex interplay of hormones stimulated by conditioning affects the entire organism, including the heart. The metabolic and functional consequences of these interrelationships provide a fertile and exciting field for future research.

References

1. Åstrand PO, Rodahl K: *Textbook of Work Physiology*, New York: McGraw-Hill, 1970.
2. Tipton CM: Training and bradycardia in rats. *Amer J Physiol* 209:1089-1094, 1965.
3. Hughson RL, Sutton JR, Fitzgerald JD, et al: The effect of physical training on intrinsic heart rate and response of the isolated sinoatrial node to noradrenaline (abstract). *Med Sci Sports* 7:69, 1975.
4. Badeer HS: The genesis of cardiomegaly in strenuous athletic training: a new look. *J Sports Med* 15:57-67, 1975.
5. Morganroth J, Maron BJ, Henry WL, et al: Comparative left ventricular dimensions in trained athletes. *Ann Intern Med* 82:521-524, 1975.
6. Wyatt HL, Mitchell JH: Influences of physical training on the heart of dogs. *Circ Res* 35:883-889, 1974.
7. Mole PA, Rabb C: Force velocity relations in exercise-induced hypertrophied rat heart muscle (abstract). *Med Sci Sports* 5:69, 1973.
8. Bloor CM, Leon AS: Interaction of age and exercise on the heart and its blood supply. *Lab Invest* 22:160-165, 1970.
9. Amsterdam EA, Choquet Y, Segel L, et al: Response of the rat heart to exercise conditioning: physical, metabolic, and functional correlates (abstract). *Clin Res* 21:399, 1973.
10. Grimm AF, Kubota R, Whitehorn WV: Properties of myocardium in cardiomegaly. *Circ Res* 12:118-124, 1963.
11. Hearn GR, Wainio WW: Succinic dehydrogenase activity of the heart and skeletal muscle of exercised rats. *Amer J Physiol* 185:348-350, 1956.
12. Scheuer J, Stezoski SW: The effect of physical training on the mechanical and metabolic response of the rat heart to hypoxia. *Circ Res* 30:418-429, 1972.
13. Carew TE, Dennis CA, Covell JW: Left ventricular function in exercise induced hypertrophy (abstract). *Fed Proc* 33:380, 1974.
14. Nutter D, Fuller E, Watt E, et al: Myocardial mechanics in exercise trained and detrained rats (abstract). *Fed Proc* 34:462, 1975.
15. Oscai LB, Mole PA, Brei B, et al: Cardiac growth and respiratory enzyme levels in male rats subjected to a running program. *Amer J Physiol* 220:1238-1241, 1971.
16. Dowell RT, Cutilletta AF, Rudnik MA, et al: Heart functional responses to pressure overload in exercised and sedentary rats. *Amer J Physiol* 230:199-204, 1976.
17. DeSchryver C, DeHerdt P, Lammerant J: Effect of physical training on cardiac catecholamine concentrations. *Nature* 214:907-908, 1967.
18. DeSchryver C, Mertens-Strythagen J, Becsei I, et al: Effect of training on heart and skeletal muscle catecholamine concentration in rats. *Amer J Physiol* 217:1589-1592, 1969.
19. DeSchryver C, Mertens-Strythagen J: Intensity of exercise and heart tissue of catecholamine content. *Pflueger Arch* 336:345-354, 1972.
20. Crews J, Aldinger EE: Effect of chronic exercise on myocardial function. *Amer Heart J* 74:536-542, 1967.
21. Penpargkul S, Scheuer J: The effect of physical training upon the mechanical and metabolic performance of the rat heart. *J Clin Invest* 49:1859-1868, 1970.
22. Carey R, Tipton CM, Lund DR: Influence of training on myocardial responses of rats subjected to conditions of ischaemia and hypoxia. *Cardiovasc Res* 10:359-367, 1976.
23. Bhan AK, Scheuer J: Effects of physical training on cardiac actomyosin adenosine triphospha-

tase activity. *Amer J Physiol* 223:1486-1490, 1972.

24. Medugorac I, Kammereit A, Jacob R: Influence of long-term swimming training on the structure and enzyme activity of myosin in the rat myocardium. *Hoppe Seyler Z Physiol Chem* 356:1161-1171, 1975.

25. Medugorac I: Relationship between Ca-ATPase activity and subunits of myosin in the myocardium of rats conditioned by swimming. *Experientia* 31:941-942, 1975.

26. Bhan AK, Scheuer J: Effects of physical conditioning on cardiac myosin. *Circulation* 45 (suppl II):II-131, 1972.

27. Bhan AK, Scheuer J: Effects of physical training on cardiac myosin ATPase activity. *Amer J Physiol* 228:1178-1182, 1975.

28. Baldwin KM, Winder WW, Holloszy JO: Adaptation of actomyosin ATPase in different types of muscle to endurance exercise. *Amer J Physiol* 229:422-426, 1975.

29. Wilkerson JE, Evonuk E: Changes in cardiac and skeletal muscle myosin ATPase activities after exercise. *J Appl Physiol* 30:328-330, 1971.

30. Gollnick PD, Ianuzzo CD: Hormonal deficiencies and the metabolic adaptations of rats to training. *Amer J Physiol* 223:278-282, 1972.

31. Dohm GL, Huston RL, Askew EW, et al: Effects of exercise on activity of heart and muscle mitochondria. *Amer J Physiol* 223:783-787, 1972.

32. Sembrowich WL, Shepherd RE, Gollnick PD: The effects of exhaustive exercise on heart mitochondria from trained and sedentary rats (abstract). *Med Sci Sports* 7:69, 1975.

33. Kraus H, Kirsten R: Influence of exercise upon energy production of heart and liver mitochondria. *Pflueger Arch* 320:334-347, 1970.

34. Arcos JC, Sohai RS, Sun S-C, et al: Changes in ultrastructure and respiratory control in mitochondria of rat heart hypertrophied by exercise. *Exp Molec Path* 8:49-65, 1968.

35. Holloszy JO: Adaptation of skeletal muscle to endurance exercise. *Med Sci Sports* 7:155-165, 1975.

36. Sobel BE: Salient biochemical features in ischemic myocardium. *Circ Res* 34 (suppl III) 173-181, 1974.

37. Barnard RJ, Duncan HW: Heart rate and ECG responses of fire fighters. *J Occup Med* 17:247-250, 1975.

38. Poland JL, Blount DH: Glycogen depletion in rat ventricles during graded exercise. *Proc Soc Exp Biol Med* 121:560-562, 1966.

39. Terjung RL, Baldwin KM, Winder WW, et al: Glycogen repletion in different types of muscle and in liver after exhausting exercise. *Amer J Physiol* 226:1387-1391, 1974.

40. Segel LD, Chung A, Mason DT, et al: Cardiac glycogen in Long-Evans rats: diurnal pattern and response to exercise. *Amer J Physiol* 229:398-401, 1975.

41. Lamb DR, Peter JB, Jeffress RN, et al: Glycogen, hexokinase, and glycogen synthetase adaptations to exercise. *Amer J Physiol* 217:1628-1632, 1969.

42. Blount DH, Meyer DK: Effects of cardiac work on glycogen fractions of the heart. *Amer J Physiol* 197:1013-1016, 1959.

43. Poland LJ, Trauner DA: Adrenal influence on the supercompensation of cardiac glycogen following exercise. *Amer J Physiol* 224:540-542, 1973.

44. Simon LM, Scheuer J, Robin ED: Cytochrome oxidase and pyruvate kinase changes in the chronically exercised rat (abstract). *Clin Res* 19:340, 1971.

45. York JW, Penney DG, Oscai LB: Effects of physical training on several glycolytic enzymes in rat heart. *Biochim Biophys Acta* 381:22-27, 1975.

46. Scheuer J, Kapner L, Stringfellow CA, et al: Glycogen, lipid, and high energy phosphate stores in hearts from conditioned rats. *J Lab Clin Med* 75:924-929, 1970.

47. Conlee RK, Tipton CM: Influence of fasting and hormone deficiency on myocardial glycogen levels in rats. *Proc Soc Exp Biol Med* 149:473-475, 1975.

48. Shelley WB, Code CF, Visscher MB: The influence of thyroid, dinitrophenol, and swimming on the glycogen and phosphocreatine level of the rat heart in relation to cardiac hypertrophy. *Amer J Physiol* 138:652-658, 1943.

49. Poland JL, Blount DH: The effects of training on myocardial metabolism. *Proc Soc Exp Biol Med* 129:171-174, 1968.

50. Aldinger EE, Sohal RS: Effects of digitoxin on the ultrastructural myocardial changes in the rat subjected to chronic exercise. *Amer J Cardiol* 26:369-374, 1970.

51. Edington DW, Cosmas AC: Effect of maturation and training on mitochondrial size distributions in rat hearts. *J Appl Physiol* 33:715-718, 1972.

52. Peterson RA: Effect of training on myocardial mitochondria (abstract). *Med Sci Sports* 4:64, 1972.
53. King DW, Gollnick PD: Ultrastructure of rat heart and liver after exhaustive exercise. *Amer J Physiol* 218:1150-1155, 1970.
54. Maher JT, Goodman AL, Francesconi R, et al: Responses of rat myocardium to exhaustive exercise. *Amer J Physiol* 222:207-212, 1972.
55. Terjung RL, Klinkerfuss GH, Baldwin KM, et al: Effect of exhausting exercise on rat heart mitochondria. *Amer J Physiol* 225:300-305, 1973.
56. Tomanek RJ, Banister EW: Myocardial ultrastructure after acute exercise stress with special reference to transverse tubules and intercalated discs. *Cardiovasc Res* 6:671-679, 1972.
57. Laguens RP, Gomez-Dumm CLA: Fine structure of myocardial mitochondria in rats after exercise for one-half to two hours. *Circ Res* 21:271-279, 1967.
58. Laguens RP, Lozada BB, Gomez-Dumm CL, et al: Effect of acute and exhaustive exercise upon the fine structure of heart mitochondria. *Experientia* 22:244-246, 1966.
59. Gale JB: Mitochondrial swelling associated with exercise and method of fixation. *Med Sci Sports* 6:182-187, 1974.
60. Gale JB: Effects of fixatives and buffers upon the morphology of heart and skeletal muscle mitochondria from exhausted rats (abstract). *Med Sci Sports* 7:69, 1975.
61. Banister EW, Tomanek RJ, Cvorkov N: Ultrastructural modifications in rat heart: responses to exercise and training. *Amer J Physiol* 220:1935-1940, 1971.
62. Cvorkov N, Banister EW, Liskop KS: Effect of high-protein diet on rat heart mitochondria after exhaustive exercise. *Amer J Physiol* 226:996-1000, 1974.
63. Sim DN, Neill WA: Investigation of the physiological basis for increased exercise threshold for angina pectoris after physical conditioning. *J Clin Invest* 54:763-770, 1974.
64. Stevenson JA, Feleki V, Rechnitzer P, et al: Effect of exercise on coronary tree size in the rat. *Circ Res* 15:265-269, 1964.
65. Tipton CM, Taylor B: Influence of atropine on heart rates of rats. *Amer J Physiol* 208:480-484, 1965.
66. Raab W: Prevention of degenerative heart disease by neurovegetative reconditioning. *Public Health Rep* 78:317-327, 1963.
67. Barrett AM, Stockham MA: The response of the pituitary-adrenal system to a stressful stimulus: the effect of conditioning and pentobarbitone treatment. *J Endocr* 33:145-152, 1965.
68. Ostman I, Sjostrand NO, Swedin G: Cardiac noradrenaline turnover and urinary catecholamine excretion in trained and untrained rats during rest and exercise. *Acta Physiol Scand* 86:299-308, 1972.
69. Ostman I, Sjostrand NO: Effect of heavy physical training on the catecholamine content of the heart and adrenals of the guinea pig. *Experientia* 27:270-271, 1971.
70. Ostman I, Sjostrand NO: Effect of prolonged physical training on the catecholamine levels of the heart and adrenals of the rat. *Acta Physiol Scand* 82:202-208, 1971.
71. Leon AS, Horst WD, Spirt N, et al: Heart norepinephrine levels after exercise training in the rat. *Chest* 67:341-343, 1975.
72. Crout JR, Creveling CR, Udenfriend S: Norepinephrine metabolism in rat brain and heart. *J Pharmacol Exp Ther* 132:269-277, 1961.
73. Salzman SH, Hirsch EZ, Hellerstein HK, et al: Adaptation to muscular exercise: myocardial epinephrine-^{3}H uptake. *J Appl Physiol* 29:92-95, 1970.

7

Experimental Observations on the Effects of Physical Training Upon Intrinsic Cardiac Physiology and Biochemistry

James Scheuer, MD
Somsong Penpargkul, MD
Ashok K. Bhan, PhD

Epidemiologic studies suggest that sedentary persons tend to have increased morbidity from cardiovascular diseases. Many investigations have demonstrated the effects of physical training on the integrated function of the cardiovascular system. The trained subject can attain a higher level of exercise and a greater maximal oxygen consumption than the untrained subject. This improved performance is achieved by way of increased cardiac output and peripheral oxygen extraction. The increased maximal cardiac output is associated with a lower heart rate at any level of exercise, but with the same maximal heart rate after physical training as before. Stroke volume is greater at any level of cardiac output in the physically trained state than in the sedentary state. In patients with coronary artery disease, physical training causes heart rate and cardiac output responses similar to those of normal persons. Some early results of training programs in patients who have recovered from myocardial infarction indicate that training may reduce the likelihood of reinfarction or sudden cardiac death.

Although the studies in intact man and animals are informative on the general effects of physical training, studies that elucidate some of the effects on physical training on the heart itself have only recently been conducted. The investigations described here were performed to determine whether physical training in rats affects intrinsic cardiac function, metabolism or biochemistry.

The Training Program

Male rats weighing 200 to 240 gm were made to swim 75 minutes twice a day, 5 days a week, usually for 8 weeks. Matched sedentary control rats from the same shipment as the swimming animals were kept at normal cage activity for the same periods. Except for the swimming protocol the two groups were treated identically. The details of this protocol have been published previously.[1]

Perfused Heart Studies

To study the intrinsic mechanical function of these hearts as a pump and as a muscle, hearts were perfused in an isolated working rat heart apparatus with a bicarbonate buffer containing 5 mM glucose.[2] The apparatus permits evaluation of cardiac function in the presence of a fixed aortic pressure and a controlled left atrial pressure, with the heart rate regulated by pacing and measurements made of coronary flow, cardiac output, left ventricular pressure and maximal rate of pressure rise (dP/dt), myocardial oxygen consumption and lactate and pyruvate production.

Cardiac Function Under Steady-State Conditions—In the first series of experiments, hearts were perfused under steady-state conditions for periods of 1 hour. Although the trained intact rats had bradycardia, when the hearts were perfused in the isolated perfusion apparatus without control of heart rate, the rates of hearts from sedentary animals and from conditioned animals were virtually identical. Under these steady-state conditions, hearts from trained rats had greater cardiac output and external cardiac work than hearts of sedentary animals. Of more significance, the hearts of conditioned rats responded to a 15% increase in heart rate by an increase in cardiac work, whereas hearts of sedentary animals did not respond to tachycardia. With the increment in heart rate, myocardial oxygen consumption increased only in hearts of trained rats, whereas the production of lactate and pyruvate, products of glycolytic metabolism, increased with tachycardia only in hearts of sedentary animals.

Effect of Increasing Left Atrial Pressure—Figure 1 demonstrates the effects of increasing left atrial pressure on hearts of sedentary and conditioned animals in the working rat heart apparatus. The increase was associated with increased coronary flow only in hearts of conditioned animals. Cardiac output increased in both groups, but was significantly greater in hearts of conditioned rats than in hearts of sedentary control animals. Peak left ventricular systolic pressure and maximal dP/dt also increased to a greater extent in hearts of conditioned animals. When the heart was made to contract isovolumically by clamping the aortic tubing, the left ventricular pressure and dP/dt levels were higher in hearts of conditioned rats. In terms of cardiac output, pressure and dP/dt, hearts of conditioned animals had a greater cardiac reserve capacity to respond to the stress of increasing preload or afterload. Since hearts were contracting from the same end-diastolic pressure, the greater pressure and dP/dt achieved during isovolumic beats implies increased contractility in hearts of conditioned rats.

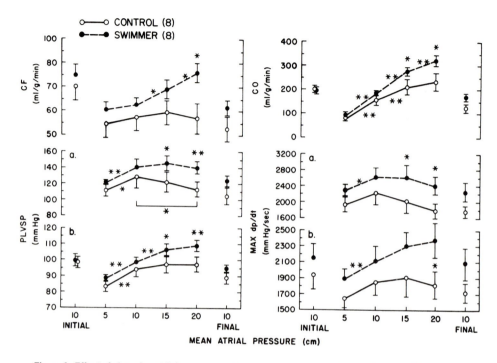

Figure 1. Effect of changing atrial pressure on dynamic performance of hearts from conditioned rats (swimmers) and control animals. a indicates values obtained when the aortic tubing was clamped. b indicates values with an aortic pressure of 85 cm of fluid. Asterisks along the lines indicate that mean points among swimmers or controls are significantly different. Asterisks above the points indicate that at that atrial pressure the difference between swimmers and controls is significant. * = $P < 0.05$; ** = $P < 00.1$. CF = coronary blood flow; CO = cardiac output; Max dp/dt = maximal rate of pressure rise; PLVSP = peak left ventricular systolic pressure. Reproduced with permission from Penpargkul S, Scheuer J: The effect of physical training upon the mechanical and metabolic performance of the rat heart. *J Clin Invest* 49:1859-1868, 1970.

Figure 2 shows the results of the same experiments in terms of calculated work, mean left ventricular systolic pressure and metabolic measurements. With increasing atrial pressure, external work and mean pressure were greater in hearts of conditioned rats, as was myocardial oxygen consumption. Lactate production, the product of nonoxidative metabolism, tended to be greater in hearts of sedentary animals. Although cardiac efficiency increased with increasing atrial pressure in both groups, there was no significant difference between hearts of sedentary and conditioned rats.

Mechanism of Oxygen Delivery—Figure 3 shows the mechanism of oxygen delivery in these experiments.[3] Although oxygen consumption increased significantly with increasing atrial pressure in both groups, the increase was greater in hearts of conditioned rats. This increase in the conditioned animals was achieved by the increase in coronary flow and no change in the extraction of oxygen across the myocardium. In hearts of control animals, the increased oxy-

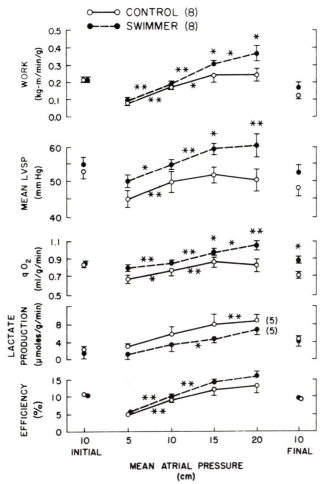

Figure 2. Effect of changing atrial pressure upon work, mean left ventricular systolic pressure (LVSP), oxygen consumption (qO_2), lactate production and efficiency. Designations as in Figure 1. Work and metabolic values are per gram dry weight. Reproduced with permission from Penpargkul S, Scheuer J: The effect of physical training upon the mechanical and metabolic performance of the rat heart. *J Clin Invest* 49:1859-1868, 1970.

gen delivery was achieved by a greater oxygen extraction and was not associated with an increase in coronary flow. This finding of increased oxygen extraction in hearts of sedentary rats without augmented coronary flow implies a limitation in coronary flow reserve in these animals and is consistent with previous observations of increased myocardial vascularity induced in rats by physical training.[4-6]

The ratio of oxidative to glycolytic adenosine triphosphate (ATP) formation was higher at all levels of cardiac work in the hearts of conditioned rats.[2]

Implications of Studies—These studies in isolated perfused working rat hearts demonstrated that hearts from conditioned rats have a greater intrinsic cardiac

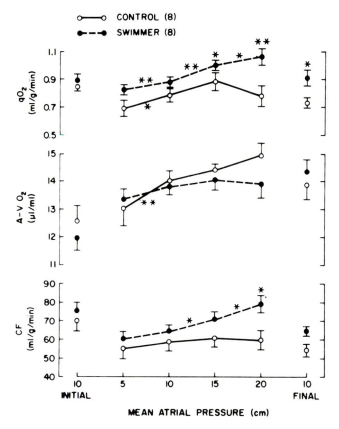

Figure 3. Mechanisms of oxygen delivery to the myocardium with increasing atrial pressure. A-V O_2 = extraction of oxygen across the myocardium; CF = coronary flow per gram dry weight; qO_2 = myocardial oxygen consumption per gram dry weight. Symbols as in Figure 1.

reserve capacity to respond to tachycardia, increasing preload and increasing afterload in terms of cardiac output, pressure development and maximal rate of pressure development. The results imply improved potential function of the heart both as a pump and as a muscle. The mechanism of increased reserve appears to be in part a greater capacity for increasing coronary flow and oxygen delivery in hearts of conditioned rats.

Studies on Energy-Related Metabolism

Energy Stores and Energy Release: To determine if some other cause for increased energy availability could be found, hearts from conditioned and sedentary animals were analyzed for glycogen, lipids and high energy phosphates.

Cardiac Glycogen—Figure 4 shows the effects of physical training on endogenous cardiac glycogen stores. Cardiac glycogen serves as an endogenous substrate store and reservoir for emergency energy formation. Hearts of conditioned

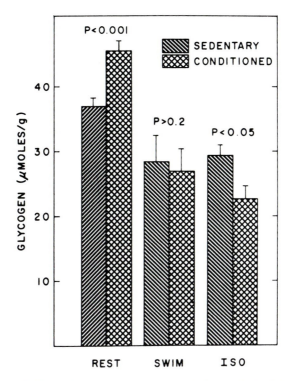

Figure 4. Effects of swimming upon myocardial glycogen levels. Values for rest were taken 36 hours after the last swim (conditioned rats). Values for swimming were taken immediately after a 75-minute swim (sedentary and conditioned rats). Values for isoproterenol (ISO) were taken 30 minutes after subcutaneous injection of 50 μg/kg in both groups.

rats had greater endogenous glycogen stores than hearts of sedentary animals. Figure 4 also demonstrates that this glycogen could be mobilized for exercise during a short swim or with the beta adrenergic stimulus of parenterally administered isoproterenol. This modest increase in cardiac glycogen availability would not deliver a great deal of energy but could be important in borderline hypoxic states.

Lipids and High Energy Phosphates—Endogenous triglycerides are also a potential reservoir for energy formation, and these lipids were slightly decreased in the hearts of conditioned animals.[1, 7] Studies of the metabolic conversion of glucose to lactate or carbon dioxide showed no difference between hearts of sedentary and conditioned animals during aerobic conditions, but during hypoxia there was a tendency for greater conversion to lactate in hearts of conditioned animals.[3] Studies of free fatty acid metabolism by conditioned hearts also showed a slight increase in turnover of fatty acid through the triglyceride pool.[3, 7] The levels of high energy phosphate stores, creatine phosphate and adenosine triphosphate, were similar in hearts of sedentary and conditioned animals.[1]

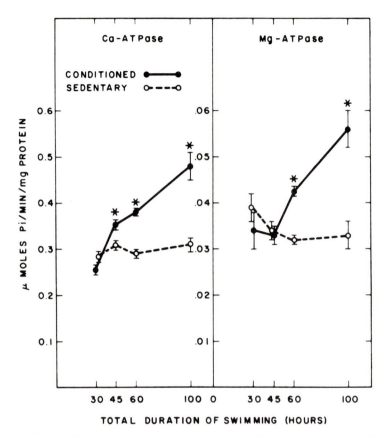

Figure 5. Effect of total duration of swimming on calcium (Ca^{++})- and magnesium (Mg^{++})-stimulated ATPase activities of cardiac actomyosin. Data are means ± standard error. Asterisk indicates $P < 0.01$ when comparing hearts from control and conditioned animals. 30, 45 and 60 hours represent swimming 90 min/day for 4, 6 and 8 weeks, respectively; 100 hours represents swimming 150 min/day for 8 weeks. Swimming was conducted 5 days/week. Reproduced with permission from Bhan AK, Scheuer J: Effects of physical training on cardiac actomyosin adenosine triphosphatase activity. *Amer J Physiol* 223:1486-1490, 1972.

Therefore, in terms of metabolism of fatty acids and glucose, the main sources of cardiac energy, and of high energy phosphate stores, there appeared to be no major difference in hearts of physically trained animals and of sedentary animals that could account for the difference in cardiac performance.

Pyruvate Kinase and Cytochrome Oxidase—The question remained whether there were alterations in the pathways of energy liberation. To investigate this possibility, the activity levels of pyruvate kinase, a marker for the glycolytic pathway, and cytochrome oxidase, a marker for the oxidative pathway, were measured in hearts of sedentary and conditioned rats.[8] Cytochrome oxidase levels were not different in the two groups of hearts, whereas pyruvate kinase values were 50% higher in hearts of conditioned than in sedentary animals. This finding confirmed the work of Oscai et al,[9] who demonstrated no increase in oxidative enzymes in hearts of trained animals. Therefore, we concluded that the beneficial effects of physical training probably cannot be attributed to an increase in the capacity of the myocardial cell for aerobic energy formation.

Energy Utilization: Since the studies of the energy production pathways provided evidence for only modest potential increases in energy delivery it became important to investigate some of the mechanisms of energy utilization. For these studies animals swam 90 minutes a day, 5 days a week for periods of 4, 6 and 8 weeks; an additional group swam 75 minutes twice daily for 8 weeks.

Calcium and Magnesium ATPase—Figure 5 demonstrates the effects of these swimming programs on the enzymatic capacity to split ATP by actomyosin (ATPase) extracted from hearts of conditioned and sedentary animals.[10] Calcium ATPase studied in the presence of high ionic strength solutions showed increased activity after 6 and 8 weeks of the swimming program. The magnitude of increase was linearly related to the total number of hours that the animals swam. Magnesium ATPase, studied at lower ionic strengths, also increased with the swimming program.

Superprecipitation of Actomyosin—Another measurement of actomyosin activity is the rate at which an actomyosin gel superprecipitates in the presence of ATP. Figure 6 shows that the rate of superprecipitation of actomyosin gels was significantly higher in preparations from hearts of conditioned animals than in those from hearts of sedentary animals. The increased actomyosin ATPase activity and the faster rate of superprecipitation correlate well with the suggested increased contractility of the hearts from conditioned rats as demonstrated in the isolated working perfused heart apparatus.

In these studies of actomyosin the heart weights were the same in control and trained animals except in the group that swam 8 weeks for 150 minutes daily. The conditioned rats in this group had cardiac hypertrophy.[10] Thus, these studies demonstrate an increase in ATPase activity that occurs before the onset of hypertrophy but continues into the hypertrophic phase. This finding is in contrast with the reduced ATPase activity that accompanies decreased contractility when hearts are made hypertrophic with hemodynamic overload.[11]

Pure Myosin ATPase Activity—To validate the enzymatic changes in the contractile proteins, pure myosin was isolated from hearts of conditioned rats, and the ATPase activity was studied.[12] Physical training was associated with a 30% increase in pure myosin ATPase activity. To elucidate the mechanism of this increased activity, the myosin was reacted with a number of agents that changed the conformation of the active site of the enzyme. It was demonstrated that ethylene glycol, which disrupts some of the bonds at the active site, had a more powerful effect on myosin from control than from conditioned hearts. Iodoacetamide and 5,5'-dithiobis-(2-nitrobenzoic acid), both agents that bind sulfhydryl groups at the active site, also had a greater effect on myosin from control hearts than from conditioned hearts. These results are consistent with the inter-

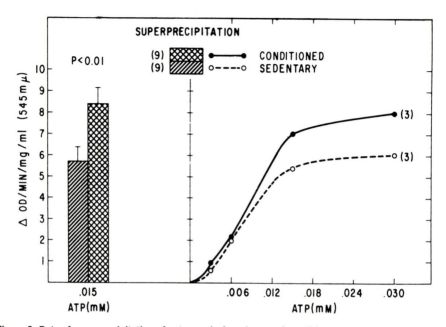

Figure 6. Rate of superprecipitation of actomyosin from hearts of conditioned rats. Curves on right show rate of superprecipitation (ΔOD/mg per ml per min) as a function of adenosine triphosphate (ATP) concentration. Bars on left show mean rates of superprecipitation for nine hearts at 0.0015 mM ATP. Reproduced with permission from Bhan AK, Scheuer J: Effects of physical training on cardiac actomyosin adenosine triphosphatase activity. *Amer J Physiol* **223:1486-1490, 1972.**

pretation that a conformational change at the active site of myosin is induced by physical training in hearts of conditioned rats and is responsible for an alteration in the enzymatic activity. This change appears to be closely related to the availability of sulfhydryl groups at the active site. Therefore, these studies on the energy utilization phase of cardiac metabolism demonstrate a change in the enzymatic activity of the proteins that might be partially responsible for increased cardiac reserve in the hearts of animals that have been conditioned.

Effects of Hypoxia on Function and Metabolism of Conditioned Hearts

Since epidemiologic evidence suggests that one effect of physical training may be to increase the resistance of the heart to myocardial ischemia, but not to prevent the development of atherosclerosis, we conducted further experiments in the isolated heart apparatus to investigate how hearts from conditioned rats respond to hypoxia.[13] The first studies were performed in an apparatus in which the heart beats isovolumically. These demonstrated that hearts of conditioned rats tended to have a smaller increase in end-diastolic pressure than hearts of sedentary rats during hypoxia but that developed left ventricular systolic pres-

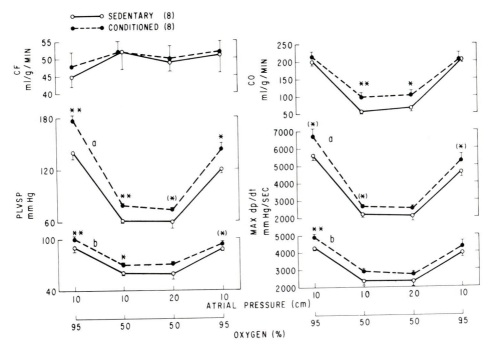

Figure 7. Effects of hypoxia on the performance of conditioned hearts in the working rat heart apparatus. Symbols as in Figure 1. Reproduced with permission of the American Heart Association, Inc. from Scheuer J, Stezoski SW: Effect of physical training on the mechanical and metabolic response of the rat heart to hypoxia. *Circ Res* 30:418-429, 1972.

sure and maximal dP/dt were not improved by physical training. There were no differences in values for oxygen delivery, lactate production, lactate/pyruvate ratio and accumulation of the reduced form of nicotinamide adenine dinucleotide (NADH), as measured by epicardial fluorimetry during hypoxia in hearts of sedentary and conditioned rats.

Hypoxia and Cardiac Performance—Figure 7 shows the effect of hypoxia on hearts in the isolated working rat heart apparatus. Here the hearts were perfused first under aerobic conditions at 10 cm atrial pressure and then underwent hypoxic conditions while the atrial pressure remained at 10 cm and was then raised to 20 cm. A recovery period followed during which perfusion conditions were the same as in the control period. During hypoxia, cardiac output was almost twice as high in hearts of conditioned rats as in those of sedentary control rats. There was a slightly greater left ventricular pressure development but no significant difference during hypoxia in maximal dP/dt. Also the pressure and dP/dt failed to respond to an increase in preload or afterload, indicating that the heart had lost its reserve capacity to respond to stress.

Cardiac Work and Metabolism During Hypoxia—Figure 8 shows the external work and pressure relations in these hearts together with the metabolic findings.

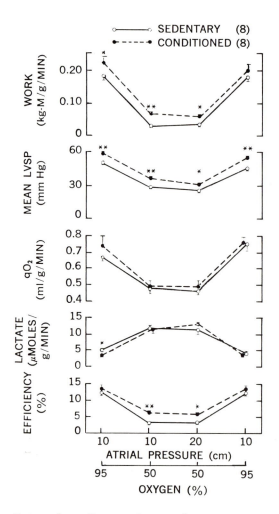

Figure 8. Cardiac work and metabolism in conditioned hearts during hypoxia in the working rat heart apparatus. Designations as in Figure 2. Work, qO_2 and lactate output are per gram dry weight. Reproduced with permission of the American Heart Association, Inc. from Scheuer J, Stezoski SW: Effect of physical training on the mechanical and metabolic response of the rat heart to hypoxia. *Circ Res* 30:418-429, 1972.

External cardiac work was almost twice as great during hypoxia in hearts of conditioned rats as in those of sedentary rats, and mean left ventricular systolic pressure, which relates to wall tension, was only slightly greater during hypoxia in the conditioned rats. There was no difference during hypoxia between the two groups in myocardial oxygen consumption or lactate production values, thus suggesting that energy delivery during hypoxia was the same in hearts of sedentary and conditioned animals. External efficiency was twice as great during hypoxia in hearts of conditioned animals as in hearts of sedentary animals. Thus, hearts of conditioned animals had greater cardiac output, cardiac work and mean pressure performance than hearts of sedentary animals during hypoxia without any evidence of an increase in energy production. High energy phosphate stores and glycogen levels were the same during hypoxia in hearts of conditioned and sedentary rats.[13]

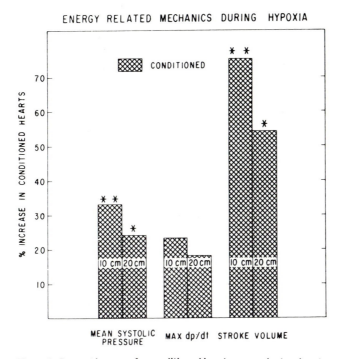

Figure 9. Percent increase for conditioned hearts over sedentary hearts in energy-related functions. Asterisks indicate statistical significance as in previous figures. Max dp/dt = maximal rate of pressure rise.

Figure 9 shows the percent increase of performance of hearts of conditioned animals over the control level during hypoxia. There was a 20 to 30% greater mean systolic pressure in hearts of conditioned rats during hypoxia but a 55 to 70% greater stroke volume. There was no significant difference in maximal dP/dt. When the end-diastolic pressure is the same, as it was in these experiments, mean systolic pressure relates most closely to wall tension, maximal dP/dt correlates with contractility and stroke volume correlates with extent of fiber shortening. These three factors are primary determinants of energy utilization in the myocardium per heartbeat. Tension and contractility are the major determinants of energy consumption, whereas fiber shortening against a load costs very little energy. Therefore, by increasing the stroke volume, and thus its fiber shortening, the conditioned heart would increase its cardiac work efficiently with little change in energy utilization.

Discussion

Aerobic performance of hearts of conditioned rats in the working rat heart apparatus was improved as measured by the responses to rapid pacing and to increased preload or afterload. This improvement was related in part to a greater capacity for increased coronary flow and oxygen delivery to the myocardium.

Hearts from conditioned rats had a slight increase in endogenous glycogen stores, which could be mobilized by stressful stimuli. Triglyceride levels were slightly depressed in hearts of conditioned animals, and levels of high energy phosphate compounds were normal. When studied in the arrested state, conditioned hearts appeared to have a faster turnover of the triglyceride fatty acid pool but no other differences in basal glucose or fatty acid metabolism.

Oxidative enzymes were not increased in hearts of conditioned rats, but actomyosin and myosin ATPase activity levels in these hearts were increased in proportion to the severity and duration of the conditioning process. This increase in ATPase activity was associated with a higher rate of actomyosin superprecipitation.

When studied in the working rat heart apparatus, the performance of hearts of conditioned rats appeared to be relatively resistant to hypoxia. This appeared to be due not to an improvement in energy formation but to more efficient mechanisms of energy utilization.

Many questions remain unanswered by these investigations. In most of the studies hypertrophy of the heart was absent. Therefore, the information may not be relevant to the subject who undergoes an extreme training program and manifests cardiac hypertrophy. It is possible that some training programs may be beneficial and others deleterious to the heart. We do not know the optimal program for promoting cardiac benefits or how the effects of training can be maintained once they have been developed. Finally, the experiments described were performed in young to middle-aged rats with a normal heart. Extrapolation of these in vitro results to intact human subjects who may have cardiac disease must be made with caution.

Summary

Hearts of rats conditioned by a moderate swimming program for 8 weeks were compared with hearts of sedentary animals. Hearts of conditioned rats had greater mechanical responses to tachycardia and to increases in preload and afterload, in part because of improved coronary blood flow and oxygen delivery. Energy stores and intermediary metabolism could not account for improved performance of conditioned hearts. Changes in the properties of myocardial contractile proteins with conditioning were characterized by increased adenosine triphosphatase (ATPase) activity and rates of superprecipitation of actomyosin and by alterations in the availability of sulfhydryl groups at the active site of myosin. Hearts of conditioned rats were partially resistant to hypoxia. During hypoxia they converted chemical energy to external work with greater efficiency than hearts of sedentary rats.

The studies indicate that a moderate conditioning program in rats improves potential aerobic cardiac performance. Factors in this improvement include increased capacity for coronary flow and oxygen delivery and higher levels of actomyosin and myosin ATPase activity. Conditioning also confers partial resistance to hypoxia, apparently as a result of improved mechanisms of energy utilization.

Acknowledgment—Mr. S. William Stezoski and Ms. Patricia Pisanelli provided technical assistance.

This study was supported by American Heart Association Grant 70-738, Western Pennsylvania Heart Association Grant 1971-1972 and U.S. Public Health Service Research Grant HL 15498 from the National Heart and Lung Institute, National Institutes of Health, Bethesda, Maryland.

References

1. Scheuer J, Kapner L, Stringfellow CA, et al: Glycogen, lipid and high energy phosphate stores in hearts from conditioned rats. *J Lab Clin Med* 75:924-929, 1970.
2. Penpargkul S, Scheuer J: The effect of physical training upon the mechanical and metabolic performance of the rat heart. *J Clin Invest* 49:1859-1868, 1970.
3. Scheuer J, Penpargkul S, Bhan AK: "The Effect of Physical Conditioning Upon Metabolism and Performance of the Rat Heart," in Dhalla NS (Ed): *Myocardial Metabolism*, vol 3, pp 145-159, Baltimore: University Park Press, 1973.
4. Tepperman J, Pearlman D: Effects of exercise and anemia on coronary arteries of small animals as revealed by the corrosion-cast technique. *Circ Res* 9:576-584, 1961.
5. Stevenson JAF, Feleki V, Rechnitzer P, et al: Effect of exercise on coronary tree size in the rat. *Circ Res* 15:265-269, 1964.
6. Bloor CM, Leon AS: Interaction of age and exercise on the heart and its blood supply. *Lab Invest* 22:160-165, 1970.
7. Fröberg SO: Effects of training and of acute exercise in trained rats. *Metabolism* 20:1044-1051, 1971.
8. Simon LM, Scheuer J, Robin ED: Cytochrome oxidase and pyruvate kinase changes in the chronically exercised rat (abstract). *Clin Res* 19:340, 1971.
9. Oscai LB, Mole PA, Brei B, et al: Cardiac growth and respiratory enzyme levels in male rats subjected to a running program. *Amer J Physiol* 220:1238-1241, 1971.
10. Bhan AK, Scheuer J: Effects of physical training on cardiac actomyosin adenosine triphosphatase activity. *Amer J Physiol* 223:1486-1490, 1972.
11. Scheuer J: Metabolism of the heart in cardiac failure. *Prog Cardiovasc Dis* 13:24-54, 1970.
12. Bhan AK, Scheuer J: Effects of physical conditioning on cardiac myosin (abstract). *Circulation* 46 (suppl II): 131, 1972.
13. Scheuer J, Stezoski SW: Effect of physical training on the mechanical and metabolic response of the rat heart to hypoxia. *Circ Res* 30:418-429, 1972.

8

Effect of Exercise on
Hemostatic Mechanisms

Garrett Lee, MD
Ezra A. Amsterdam, MD
Anthony N. DeMaria, MD
Gerald Davis, PhD
Teresa LaFave
Dean T. Mason, MD

During the past two decades data have been accumulated regarding the influence of physical activity on hemostatic mechanisms of the circulating blood. This subject has important implications, both for normal physiological function and in ischemic heart disease since blood coagulation, platelet function and fibrinolysis have been implicated as potential factors in vascular thrombosis and atherosclerosis. There is also considerable current interest in possible means of altering blood hemostasis as one approach to the treatment of ischemic heart disease.

Mechanisms of Blood Coagulation

When a vessel wall is injured or altered, a series of interactions among plasma proteins in the blood coagulation pathway takes place.[1] In the intrinsic pathway, factor XII is activated, initiating a continuous chain of reactions involving factors VIII, IX, XI, platelets and calcium ions. The common pathway is then initiated: factor X is activated which, with factor V, converts prothrombin to thrombin. Under the influence of thrombin, fibrinogen, a soluble protein, can be converted to fibrin, an insoluble protein. In the extrinsic pathway, which bypasses the foregoing intrinsic route, factor X is activated through a series of reactions involving factors III and VII (Figure 1).

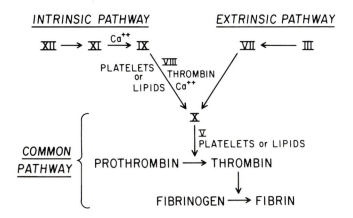

Figure 1. Mechanisms of blood coagulation.

Effects of Exercise on Blood Coagulation

Physical exertion is known to enhance blood coagulability.[2] We have exercised 28 patients to greater than 70% of their maximal heart rates in a multi-stage treadmill protocol. In clotting studies performed immediately before and after stress testing, we have found a slight but significant shortening of the partial thromboplastin time (PTT) following the exercise. The prothrombin time (PT) in the same patients was unaltered (Figure 2). The latter finding is consistent with several published studies of individuals undergoing strenuous exercise testing.[3] Enhanced clotting ability, as reflected in the shortened PTT, was also noted in normal subjects following strenuous treadmill exercise,[4] standardized bicycle exercise,[5] moderate exercise such as walking up and down steps,[6] and in men who were physically active during work hours as compared to a group of less active men.[7] The shortened PTT and normal PT may reflect an increase in one or more of the coagulation factors in the intrinsic pathway, while factors in the extrinsic and common pathways remain unaltered following exercise.

Assays of clotting factors by several investigators have consistently revealed increased factor VIII activity following exercise. One study demonstrated that the effect of strenuous treadmill exercise in male subjects yielded an average increase in factor VIII of 188%.[4] In another investigation factor VIII elevations of two to three times over baseline levels occurred following a strenuous, rapid run up and down a staircase for three minutes.[8] Increased factor VIII concentration was also found in subjects exercised by running a distance of half a mile at maximum speed.[9] The mechanism controlling the regulation of factor VIII activity following exercise is not well understood. The rise in factor VIII may be due to release from stores or activation of factor VIII already present in the circulation. It has been found that the spleen is not an important storage organ

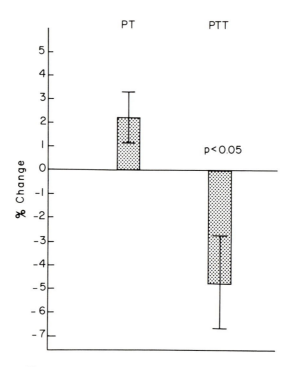

Figure 2. Change in prothrombin time (PT) and partial thromboplastin time (PTT) following treadmill exercise.

for factor VIII released during exercise, since an increase in its activity was seen in both normal individuals and asplenic patients.[9] Studies using factor VIII antibodies suggest that the elevation of its activity during exercise represents a true increase.[10] The administration of adrenalin can also increase VIII activity and a beta blocker such as propranolol can prevent the exercise-induced rise in factor VIII.[11-13] Of interest, exercising patients with von Willebrand's disease can also increase VIII activity and decrease bleeding time.[14]

There have been no consistent reports of significant increases in other coagulation factors of the intrinsic, extrinsic or common pathways following exercise. Ikkala et al [15] noted a rise in V as well as VIII but no change in fibrinogen, factor VII complex or IX. Iatridis et al [4] reported elevations in VIII and XII, but no increase in fibrinogen, prothrombin, factors V, VII or X. Egeberg [8] and Cohen et al [12] independently demonstrated increased VIII activity after exercise while fibrinogen, prothrombin, V, VII, IX, X, XI and XII were unaltered.

Physical Conditioning and Blood Coagulation

Although acute exercise results in a decrease in clotting time and an increase in one or more clotting factors, physical conditioning may lessen the magni-

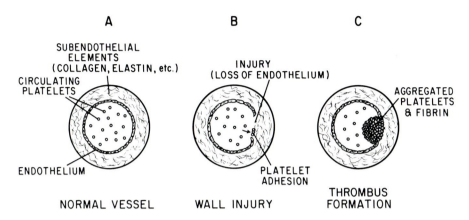

Figure 3. Schematic representation of the role of platelets in response to injury of vascular wall.

tude of the decreased clotting time following acute exercise. Ferguson and Guest [16] performed strenuous treadmill testing in male volunteers and discovered, in the same subjects, significantly less reduction of clotting time after exercise in the conditioned state compared to the unconditioned state.

Role of Platelets in Blood Coagulation

Platelets participate in blood coagulation by providing a lipid or lipoprotein surface that catalyzes one or more reactions in the clotting process. Phospholipids or lipoproteins present in platelet membranes are required in both the reaction by which factors VIII, IX and calcium activate factor X and in the reaction by which factors V, X and calcium activate prothrombin (Figure 1). In addition, platelets, normally 250,000/mm^3 of which are freely circulating and non-adherent to the vascular endothelium, can undergo a series of reactions among themselves when the vessel is disrupted and the blood comes into contact with the perivascular tissue (Figure 3). The circulating platelets adhere to the subendothelial elements such as collagen which can result in structural and metabolic changes in platelets, causing release of adenosine diphosphate (ADP) from platelet storage granules. The ADP that is released induces platelet aggregation. Further, as noted earlier, platelets provide phospholipid that catalyzes one or more reactions in the coagulation pathway producing thrombin, which is important not only in the conversion of fibrinogen to fibrin resulting in a firm platelet-fibrin mass, but can also induce further platelet aggregation.[17]

Platelet Function Tests

There are three basic tests available to study platelet function: platelet count, platelet adhesion and platelet aggregation. Platelets can be counted electroni-

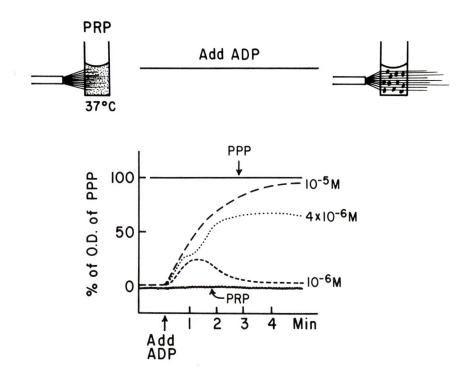

Figure 4. Adenosine diphosphate (ADP)-induced platelet aggregation (O.D. = optical density, PPP = platelet poor plasma, PRP = platelet rich plasma).

cally or by phase contrast microscopy.[18, 19] Platelet adhesion is measured by initially counting platelets and then allowing them to adhere to a material such as glass in a rotating bulb or glass bead column and then recounting them.[20, 21] Platelet adhesion is expressed as a percentage of the platelet count before and after contact with a material such as glass. Platelet aggregation is determined by centrifuging citrated whole blood to separate the platelet rich plasma from the platelet poor plasma. A cuvette of each of the separately spun solutions is placed in a platelet aggregometer and, by means of a light source and a photoelectric cell, the difference in optical density of the two plasma samples is tested. Platelet poor plasma is clear and interferes little with light transmission to the photoelectric cell, while platelet rich plasma is turbid and results in reduced light transmission. The addition of an aggregating agent such as ADP, epinephrine or collagen can induce platelet aggregation so that the platelet rich solution becomes clearer, resulting in increased light transmission through the plasma. Platelet aggregates induced by low concentrations of exogenously added ADP may be unstable and are reversible, and disaggregation can occur. Higher concentrations of exogenously added ADP can initiate the primary phase of platelet aggregation and cause further release of endogenous ADP, resulting in an irreversible secondary phase of aggregation (Figure 4).[22, 23] This method is

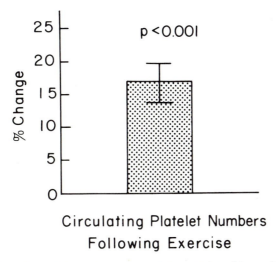

Figure 5. Quantitative change in circulating platelets with exercise.

used to measure the "aggregability" of platelets from a given patient's serum in the normal state and/or in response to interventions such as drugs, exercise or disease states.

Effects of Exercise on Platelet Function

Studies performed in our laboratory on 25 subjects after vigorous exercise on a treadmill, to greater than 85% of maximal heart rate, demonstrated a significantly elevated platelet count compared to the resting level (Figure 5). The finding that strenuous activity can significantly raise platelet numbers in the circulation was supported by Ferguson and Guest [16] in subjects vigorously exercised on a treadmill and by Warlow and Ogston [24] who studied the effects of rapid running on platelet count. Dawson and Ogston,[25] using a bicycle ergometer to regulate work performed, found that a critical amount of exercise is required to produce a detectable rise in platelet count. At a moderate workload, healthy women had significantly elevated platelet counts immediately after exercise and a return to pre-exercise values after a brief rest.[25] At the same level of work, platelet counts did not rise in healthy men. However, after a higher workload there was a significant rise in platelet numbers which did not return to baseline values following the same rest period as in the women after a moderate workload.[25] Independent investigations by Sarajas et al [26] of strenuous bicycle exercise in one group of subjects and mild exercise such as walking in another group, and by Bennett,[27] who studied strenuous exercise such as walking up and down steps in one group and mild or mild, prolonged exercise in another group, showed significantly elevated platelet counts following strenuous activity but no significant thrombocytosis after mild or mild, prolonged activity. Further, Pegrum et al [28] discovered that platelet counts were unchanged in many of their subjects after mild, prolonged activity such as walking.

The source of the increase in circulating platelets with exercise is obscure. It has been postulated that the pulmonary vascular bed harbors platelets and leukocytes and that any accelerated circulatory activity from exercise may cause their release.[26, 29] The hemoconcentration, reflected by a slight rise in the hematocrit, with physical exertion cannot account for the elevated platelet count.[26] The spleen is not the source of increased platelets since it has been demonstrated that exercise-induced thrombocytosis is also present in asplenic subjects.[25] Of interest, epinephrine has been shown to stimulate thrombocytosis but beta adrenergic blockade by propranolol does not prevent the exercise-induced rise in circulating platelets.[25]

Physical training may attenuate the degree of thrombocytosis from exercise at the same workload as prior to training. Ferguson and Guest [16] performed strenuous exercise on a treadmill in a group of pre-conditioned subjects and found that the mean increase in platelet count was 26%. Following a one-month conditioning program, the same level of exercise induced a rise in platelet count of only 14%.

Pegrum found that platelet adhesiveness decreased after mild, prolonged physical activity such as walking.[28] Bennett [27] also reported significantly less platelet adhesion after mild or mild, prolonged activity such as walking; he further performed strenuous activity such as walking up and down steps in another group of subjects and noted no change in platelet adhesiveness immediately following exercise as compared to pre-exercise control values. Warlow and Ogston [24] demonstrated no alteration in platelet adhesiveness after a strenuous, fast run. It appears that strenuous activities produce no change in platelet adhesion while mild or mild, prolonged activities such as walking may decrease platelet adhesiveness.

We examined ADP-induced platelet aggregation in 12 normal subjects using a multistage treadmill protocol. There was a gradual decrease in platelet aggregation at the completion of the first stage (1.7 mph, 10% grade), a significant fall at the end of the second stage (2.5 mph, 12% grade) and a further reduction at the end of the third stage (3.4 mph, 14% grade). Platelet aggregation remained significantly lower than baseline even after a 10-minute rest period following exercise (Figure 6). In eight patients with angiographically documented coronary artery disease there was also a significant drop in platelet aggregation at the completion of the first and second stage of treadmill exercise which remained lower than pre-exercise aggregation even after a 10-minute rest period (Figure 7). These findings are in accord with those of Simpson et al [30] who exercised subjects on a treadmill to greater than 90% of their maximal heart rate, corresponding to an oxygen consumption of approximately 33 to 40 ml/kg/min. The subjects had been previously classified by behavior pattern analysis into coronary prone (type A) or noncoronary prone (type B) individuals.[31] Type B subjects had a slight decrease in platelet aggregation after exercise, which was ab-

NORMAL SUBJECTS

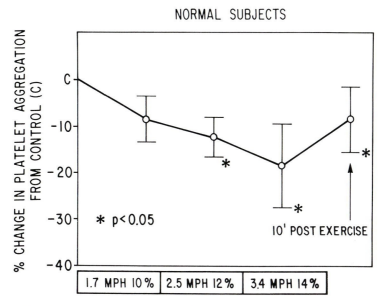

Figure 6. Platelet aggregation in normal subjects measured at end of each level of multistage treadmill exercise test and at 10 minutes postexercise (MPH = miles per hour). Statistical tests based on comparison with control data.

CAD PATIENTS

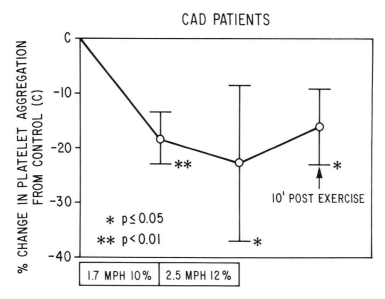

Figure 7. Platelet aggregation in coronary artery disease (CAD) patients measured at end of each level of multistage treadmill exercise test and at 10 minutes postexercise. (MPH = miles per hour). Statistical tests based on comparison with control data.

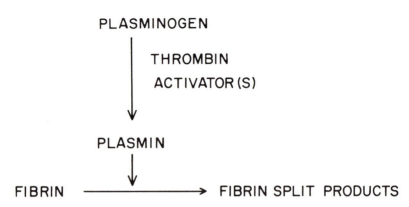

Figure 8. Mechanism of fibrinolysis.

sent in type A subjects. Yamazaki et al [32] performed the Master "2-step" exercise test in one group of normal subjects and found no change in platelet aggregation after exercise; however, in patients with coronary artery disease platelet aggregation increased following exercise. Strenuous exercise reported by Ikkala et al [15] using the bicycle ergometer and Prentice et al [9] and Warlow and Ogston [24] who subjected their volunteers to a fast run resulted in increased platelet aggregation following the physical stress. Hence, there is much conflicting data regarding platelet aggregation. It is possible that the reported discrepancies in platelet adhesion and aggregation may be partly related to the increase in platelet count during exercise. It has been shown that change in platelet count may itself alter aggregability.[29, 33] In this regard, it is important to emphasize that in our studies of the relation of platelet aggregability to exercise stress, aggregation studies were performed after dilution of exercise plasma samples to attain a platelet count equivalent to that of pre-exercise plasma, thereby obviating the effect of exercise-induced thrombocytosis on aggregability. In summary, current data suggest that platelet aggregation is probably decreased or is unaltered following mild exercise while variable results, which appear to be at least partially due to changes in platelet count, are found after strenuous activity.

Mechanisms of Fibrinolysis

Although the hemostatic response to vascular injury is activation of the coagulation mechanism and formation of fibrin, the blood also contains a potent proteolytic system which can digest fibrin and thus reestablish circulation. Plasminogen, present in serum globulin, can interact with activators found in tissue, vascular wall or plasma to form plasmin, a proteolytic enzyme which can digest fibrin to form fibrin split products (Figure 8).[1] The fibrinolytic and blood coagulation systems are intimately related; tissue damage and activation

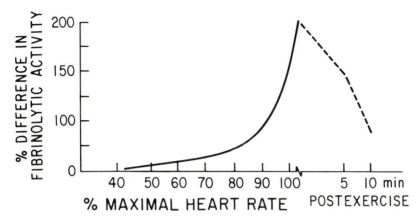

Figure 9. Fibrinolytic activity during increasing intensity of exercise and following exercise.

of XII can trigger both systems. Thrombin, important in the conversion of fibrinogen to fibrin, factor VIII to its activated state and in increasing platelet aggregation, also enhances conversion of plasminogen to plasmin.

Fibrinolytic activity can be measured on fibrin plates prepared with bovine fibrinogen clotted with thrombin. The human plasma is treated, diluted and added to the fibrin plate and the fibrinolytic activity is expressed as the diameter product in square millimeters of the lysed zone.[34, 35] Fibrinolytic activity can also be assessed by euglobulin lysis time—the shorter the lysis time, the greater the fibrinolytic activity.[36]

Exercise and Fibrinolysis

There is general agreement that exercise enhances the fibrinolytic activity of blood.[2, 37-41] In general, fibrinolytic activity increases as the intensity and duration of exercise rise. However, it has been shown that the magnitude of the increase in fibrinolysis with exercise is related to the intensity of the exercise relative to the individual's maximal exercise capacity.[42] Thus, short duration and low intensity of activity may produce a marked rise in fibrinolytic activity in one individual while a longer duration and higher exercise intensity may be required to induce a similar amount of fibrinolytic activity in another. We have observed that an exercise intensity resulting in achievement of 80 to 85% predicted maximal heart rate is required to initiate a marked response in fibrinolytic activity (Figure 9), which usually returned to normal within 30 minutes. Moreover, it has been shown that fibrinolysis is influenced by time of day, being greater in late afternoon and evening and lower in the morning.[7, 42, 43]

The mechanism of exercise-induced fibrinolysis is thought to be due to an increased plasminogen activator and not to increased levels of circulating plasmin.[4, 12, 44] Since the rise in plasminogen activator is speculative, a possible alternative explanation is a reduction in antiactivator or antiplasminogen.[38, 45] Of interest, epinephrine can stimulate both factor VIII and fibrinolytic activity.[46] However, it appears that the exercise-induced rise in VIII and fibrinolysis act through different mechanisms since beta adrenergic blockade with propranolol can prevent the elevation in factor VIII but not fibrinolysis.[12]

Fibrinolysis and Physical Conditioning

Physical conditioning not only diminishes the exercise-related acceleration of clotting factors, but also maintains the responsiveness of fibrinolytic activity to exercise. Following conditioning, Ferguson and Guest [16] demonstrated a reduced fibrinolytic activity at rest, but with exercise, fibrinolytic responsiveness was similar to that of the unconditioned state. There are no current data available to clearly indicate that resting fibrinolytic activity is augmented following physical conditioning. Moxley et al [47] demonstrated no statistically significant differences in resting fibrinolytic activity between inactive men and those who participated in a regular exercise program. Initial testing in an untrained individual following maximal exercise may demonstrate a large increase in fibrinolytic activity. However, following daily physical conditioning, a repeat test at the same level of exercise may result in a significantly decreased enhancement of fibrinolytic response to exercise, again emphasizing that the degree of fibrinolysis is determined by the intensity of activity relative to each individual's maximal effort.[42]

Effect of Age on Exercise-Induced Fibrinolysis

Age has been shown to influence fibrinolytic activity. Although a hypercoagulable state following exercise is found in healthy men, regardless of age, the rise in fibrinolytic activity is much greater in the young than in the aged,[6] suggesting one possible basis for the increased susceptibility of older individuals to vascular thrombosis.

Exercise, Physical Conditioning and Vascular Thrombosis

It has been hypothesized that atherosclerotic lesions may develop as a result of continuing deposition of microthrombi on the arterial intima in response to endothelial injury.[48] Vascular thrombosis associated with enhanced platelet aggregation has been documented in acute myocardial infarction,[49, 50] angina,[51] stroke,[49] familial hyperbetalipoproteinemia [52] and diabetes.[53] Impaired fibrinolysis has also been suggested in the pathogenesis of atheromata in the development of coronary artery disease and in the formation of occlusive intravascular thrombi.[54, 55] Indeed, impaired or decreased fibrinolytic response to exercise has been reported in atherosclerotic patients,[6] in patients with diabetes mellitus [56, 57] and in patients with type IV hyperlipidemia.[58] If there is some validity to this hypothesis, then physical conditioning may alter the development of atherosclerosis by affecting blood coagulation, platelet function and fibrinolysis.

Spontaneous blood coagulation due to a rise in factor VIII and an increase in circulating platelets as a result of moderate to strenuous exercise, would certainly be considered undesirable. However, it is not known whether the transient elevations in VIII and platelet number are detrimental in patients with vascular thrombosis. Fibrinolysis, which occurs almost simultaneously with enhanced coagulability in association with increased physical activity, would be regarded as a favorable process. As previously noted, however, the fibrinolytic system tends to become less responsive with aging. Mild or mild, prolonged activities such as walking have been shown to decrease platelet adhesiveness while platelet count remained the same. In our laboratory platelet aggregation tends to fall as intensity and duration of exercise increase, but there is not general agreement on this matter.[9, 15, 24] Indeed, epidemiologic studies have not implicated excessive physical activity, but lack of it, as a possible etiologic factor in ischemic heart disease.[59-62]

Physical conditioning, known to enhance exercise performance by diminishing the rise in heart rate and arterial pressure with exercise, hence reducing myocardial oxygen demand,[63] might also beneficially influence the course of ischemic heart disease by favorably altering blood coagulation. Thus, compared to the unconditioned state, a reduction in the magnitude of the decrease in clotting time has been demonstrated in conditioned subjects, while the responsiveness of their fibrinolytic systems remains intact.

Interestingly, the beta adrenergic blocking agent propranolol, which has gained wide use in the treatment of angina pectoris, also may have a potentially beneficial role in ischemic heart disease through its effects on the blood clotting mechanism. Propranolol can prevent the exercise-induced rise in factor VIII without inhibiting the fibrinolytic response to exercise.[12] Other drugs which may have a desirable role, and are currently undergoing investigation, include platelet-inhibiting agents such as aspirin, which can inhibit the secondary phase of platelet aggregation.[64]

Summary

Physical activity can enhance spontaneous blood coagulability, the mechanism of which appears to be related to an increase in measured factor VIII activity. The resultant hypercoagulable state is associated with a concomitant increase in fibrinolytic activity. The responsiveness of the fibrinolytic system to exercise varies with the intensity of exercise relative to the individual's maximal capacity, time of day (greater activity in the late afternoon than morning) and age (less responsive in the elderly). The number and function of circulating platelets can be altered by exercise. A critical degree of exertion is necessary to increase platelets; mild or mild, prolonged activity (eg, walking) does not appear to augment number of platelets while strenuous exercise (eg, rapid running) may induce a significant thrombocytosis. Platelet adhesiveness falls with mild activity and is unaltered with strenuous exercise. Platelet aggregability appears to remain unchanged or decreases with mild exertion but the effects of strenuous activity have been variable. Physical conditioning appears to attenuate the increased coagulability induced by exercise while the reactivity of the fibrinolytic system remains fully intact.

References

1. Wintrobe WM, Lee GR, Boggs DR, et al (Eds): "Blood Coagulation," in *Clinical Hematology*, pp 409-450, Philadelphia: Lea and Febiger, 1974.
2. Astrup T: "The Effects of Physical Activity on Blood Coagulation and Fibrinolysis," in Naughton JP, Hellerstein HK (Eds): *Exercise Testing and Exercise Training in Coronary Heart Disease*, p 169, New York: Academic Press, 1973.
3. Overman RS, Newman AA, Wright IS: Plasma prothrombin times in normal human subjects. The effect of certain factors on the prothrombin time. *Amer Heart J* 39:56-64, 1960.
4. Iatridis SG, Ferguson JH: Effect of physical exercise on blood clotting and fibrinolysis. *J Appl Physiol* 18:337-344, 1963.
5. Finkel A, Cumming GR: Effects of exercise in the cold on blood clotting and platelets. *J Appl Physiol* 20:423-424, 1965.
6. Berkarda B, Akokan G, Derman U: Fibrinolytic response to physical exercise in males. *Atherosclerosis* 13:85-91, 1971.
7. Korsan-Bengtsen K, Wihelmsen L, Tibblin G: Blood coagulation and fibrinolysis in relation to degree of physical activity during work and leisure time. *Acta Med Scand* 193:73-77, 1973.
8. Egeberg O: The effect of exercise on the blood clotting system. *Scand J Clin Lab Invest* 15:8-13, 1963.
9. Prentice CRM, Hassanein AA, McNicol GP, et al: Studies on blood coagulation, fibrinolysis and platelet function following exercise in normal and splenectomized people. *Brit J Haematol* 23:541-552, 1972.
10. Rizza CR, Eipe J: Exercise, factor VIII and the spleen. *Brit J Haematol* 20:629-635, 1971.
11. Egeberg O: Changes in the activity of antihemophilic A factor and in the bleeding time associated with muscular exercise and adrenalin infusion. *Scand J Clin Lab Invest* 15:539-549, 1963.
12. Cohen RJ, Epstein SE, Cohen LS, et al: Alterations of fibrinolysis and blood coagulation induced by exercise and the role of beta-adrenergic receptor stimulation. *Lancet* II:1264-1266, 1968.
13. Ingram GIC: Increase in antihaemophilic globulin activity following infusion of adrenaline. *J Physiol* 156:217-224, 1961.
14. Egeberg O: The effect of muscular exercise on hemostasis in Von Willebrand's disease. *Scand J Clin Lab Invest* 15:273-283, 1963.
15. Ikkala E, Myllyla G, Sarajas HSS: Hemostatic changes associated with exercise. *Nature* 199:459-461, 1963.
16. Ferguson E, Guest MM: Exercise, physical conditioning, blood coagulation and fibrinolysis. *Thromb Diath Haemorrh* 31:63-71, 1974.
17. Weiss HJ: Platelet physiology and abnormalities of platelet function (first of two parts). *New Eng J Med* 293:531-541, 1975.
18. Simmons A, Schwabbauer ML, Earhart CA: Automated platelet counting with autoanalyzers. *J Lab Clin Med* 77:656-660, 1971.
19. Brecher G, Cronkite EP: "Estimation of the Number of Platelets by Phase Microscopy," in Tocantins LM, Kazal LA (Eds): *Blood Coagulation, Hemorrhage and Thrombosis*, New York: Grune and Stratton, 1964.
20. Wright HP: The adhesiveness of blood platelets in normal subjects with varying concentrations of anti-coagulants. *J Path Bact* 53:255-262, 1941.
21. Hirsh J, McBride JA, Dacie JV: Thrombo-embolism and increased platelet adhesiveness in postsplenectomy thrombocytosis. *Aust Ann Med* 15:122-128, 1966.
22. Born GVR, Cross MJ: The aggregation of blood platelets. *J Physiol* 168:178-195, 1963.
23. O'Brien JR: Platelet aggregation. II: Some results from a new method of study. *J Clin Pathol* 15:452-455, 1962.
24. Warlow CP, Ogston D: Effects of exercise on platelet count, adhesion and aggregation. *Acta Haemat* 52:47-52, 1974.

25. Dawson AA, Ogston D: Exercise-induced thrombocytosis. *Acta Haemat* 42:241-246, 1969.
26. Sarajas HSS, Konttinen A, Frick MH: Thrombocytosis evoked by exercise. *Nature* 192:721-722, 1961.
27. Bennett PN: Effect of physical exercise on platelet adhesiveness. *Scand J Haemat* 9:138-141, 1972.
28. Pegrum GD, Harrison KM, Shaw S, et al: Effect of prolonged exercise on platelet adhesiveness. *Nature* 213:301-302, 1967.
29. Sarajas HSS: Reaction patterns of blood platelets in exercise, characteristics, origin and possible coronary implications. *Adv Cardiol* 18:176-195, 1976.
30. Simpson MT, Olewine DA, Jenkins CD, et al: Exercise-induced catecholamines and platelet aggregation in the coronary-prone behavior pattern. *Psychosom Med* 36:476-487, 1974.
31. Rosenman RH, Brand RJ, Jenkins CD, et al: Coronary heart disease in the western collaborative group study: Final follow-up experience of 8 ½ years. *JAMA* 233:872-877, 1975.
32. Yamazaki H, Kobayashi I, Shimamoto T: Enhancement of ADP-induced platelet aggregation by exercise test in coronary patients and its prevention by pyridinolcarbamate. *Thromb Diath Haemorrh* 24:438-449, 1970.
33. Haanen C, Holorinet A: Blood platelet aggregation under various conditions and in some diseases. *Exp Biol Med* 3:164-174, 1968.
34. Astrup T, Mullertz S: The fibrin plate method for estimating fibrinolytic activity. *Arch Biochem* 40:346-351, 1952.
35. Brakman P: *Fibrinolysis. A Standardized Fibrin Plate Method and A Fibrinolytic Assay of Plasminogen*, Amsterdam: Scheltema and Holkema, NV, 1967.
36. Chakrabarti R, Bielawiec M, Evans JF, et al: Methodological study and a recommended technique for determining the euglobulin lysis time. *J Clin Path* 21:698-701, 1968.
37. Biggs R, MacFarlane RG, Pilling J: Experimental production of increased fibrinolysis by exercise and adrenalin. *Lancet* I:402-405, 1947.
38. Sherry S, Lindemeyer RI, Fletcher AP, et al: Studies on enhanced fibrinolytic activity in man. *J Clin Invest* 38:810-822, 1959.
39. Cash JD: Effect of moderate exercise on the fibrinolytic system in normal young men and women. *Brit Med J* 2:502-506, 1966.
40. Menon IS, Burke F, Dewar HA: Effect of strenuous and graded exercise on fibrinolytic activity. *Lancet* I:700-703, 1967.
41. Cash JD, Woodfield DG: Fibrinolytic response to moderate exercise in 50 healthy middle-aged subjects. *Brit Med J* 2:658-661, 1968.
42. Rosing DR, Brakman P, Redwood DR, et al: Blood fibrinolytic activity in man diurnal variation and the response to varying intensities of exercise. *Circ Res* 27:171-184, 1970.
43. Fearnley GR, Balmforth G, Fearnley E: Evidence of a diurnal fibrinolytic rhythm; with a simple method of measuring natural fibrinolysis. *Clin Sci* 16:645-650, 1957.
44. Sawyer WD, Fletcher AP, Alkjaersig N, et al: Studies on the thrombolytic activity of human plasma. *J Clin Invest* 39:426-434, 1960.
45. Ogston D, Fullerton HW: Changes in fibrinolytic activity produced by physical activity. *Lancet* II:730-733, 1961.
46. Cash JD, Allan AGE: The fibrinolytic response to moderate exercise and intravenous adrenalin in the same subjects. *Brit J Haemat* 13:376-383, 1967.
47. Moxley RT, Brakman P, Astrup T: Resting levels of fibrinolysis in blood in inactive and exercising men. *J Appl Physiol* 28:549-552, 1970.
48. Duguid JB: Thrombosis as a factor in the pathogenesis of coronary atherosclerosis. *J Path Bact* 58:207-212, 1946.
49. Sano T, Boxer MGJ, Boxer LA, et al: Platelet sensitivity to aggregation in normal and diseased groups: A method for assessment of platelet aggregability. *Thromb Diath Haemorrh* 25:524-531, 1971.
50. Salky N, Dugdale M: Platelet abnormalities in ischemic heart disease. *Amer J Cardiol* 32:612-617, 1973.
51. Frishman WH, Weksler B, Christodoulou JP, et al: Reversal of abnormal platelet aggregability and change in exercise tolerance in patients with angina pectoris following oral propranolol. *Circulation* 50:887-896, 1974.
52. Carvalho ACA, Colman RW, Lees RS: Platelet function in hyperlipoproteinemia. *New Eng J Med* 290:434-438, 1974.

53. Sagel J, Colwell JA, Crook J, et al: Increased platelet aggregation in early diabetes mellitus. *Ann Intern Med* 82:733-738, 1975.
54. Chakrabarti R, Hocking ED, Fearnley GR, et al: Fibrinolytic activity and coronary artery disease. *Lancet* I:987-990, 1968.
55. Cash JD: A new approach to studies of the fibrinolytic enzyme system in man. *Amer Heart J* 75:424-428, 1968.
56. Seth HN: Fibrinolytic response to moderate exercise and platelet adhesiveness in diabetes mellitus. *Acta Diabet Lat* 10:306-314, 1973.
57. Cash JD, McGill RC: Fibrinolytic response to moderate exercise in young male diabetics and non-diabetics. *J Clin Path* 22:32-35, 1969.
58. Epstein SE, Rosing DR, Brakman P, et al: Impaired fibrinolytic response to exercise in patients with Type IV hyperlipoproteinemia. *Lancet* II:631-634, 1970.
59. Morris JN, Crawford MD: Coronary heart disease and physical activity of work: Evidence of a national necropsy survey. *Brit Med J* 2:1485-1496, 1958.
60. Kahn HA: The relationship of reported coronary heart disease to physical activity of work. *Amer J Public Health* 53:1058-1067, 1963.
61. Fox SM III, Haskell WL: Physical activity and the prevention of coronary artery disease. *Bull NY Acad Med* 44:950-967, 1968.
62. Hellerstein HK: Exercise therapy in coronary artery disease. *Bull NY Acad Med* 44:1028-1047, 1968.
63. Redwood DR, Rosing DR, Epstein SE: Circulatory and symptomatic effects of physical training in patients with coronary artery disease and angina pectoris. *New Eng J Med* 286:959-965, 1972.
64. Davies T, Lederer DA, Davies JA, et al: The effect of aspirin on the exercise-induced changes in platelet function and blood coagulation. *Thromb Res* 5:69-81, 1974.

9

Coronary and Systemic Circulatory Adaptations to Exercise Training and Their Effects on Angina Pectoris

William A. Neill, MD

The rate at which muscular work can be carried out steadily over an extended period is limited, and for a given individual quite reproducible from one time to the next. This applies to both healthy subjects and patients with symptomatic ischemic coronary heart disease. Healthy subjects and patients both may practice exercise in order to increase their exercise capacity or their endurance. The basis of their improvement, however, is not the same in the two instances. Changes in skeletal muscle metabolism and peripheral blood flow that are important in expanding the limits of performance in normal individuals do not apply equally to patients whose exercise is restricted specifically by coronary circulatory abnormalities resulting in angina pectoris. The principle aim of this chapter is to clarify this distinction, *ie*, to define the particular aspects of the overall normal cardiovascular adaptations to training that are pertinent for the patient limited by angina pectoris.

Normal Adaptation to Endurance Training

Skeletal Muscle Metabolism and Blood Flow—Training by endurance exercises, such as running or swimming, increases the functional capacity of the oxidative enzyme systems responsible for energy transfer in the skeletal muscles. These changes occur without significant skeletal muscle hypertrophy (in contrast to heavy isometric work); therefore, the maximum oxygen (O_2) consumption per gram of muscle is higher in endurance-trained muscles. The specific activity expressed per gram of muscle tissue is higher for a variety of mitochondrial enzymes responsible for substrate catabolism, oxidative phosphorylation and ATP hydrolysis.[1-4] The functional capacity of the glycolytic enzymes is not proportionately augmented.[2,5] As a result, the ability to dispose of pyruvate increases out of proportion to its formation by glycolysis. Repeated exposure of muscles to endurance-type exercise alters their metabolism from anaerobic towards aerobic energy turnover, which is more suited to sustained steady-state exercise. This relative shift in enzyme activities in skeletal muscle is probably a major reason for the smaller rise in blood lactate level during exercise in trained subjects.[6,7]

The increased metabolic capacity of trained muscles is accompanied by a modest increase in the maximum blood flow attained through their vascular bed. The augmented capacity for blood flow is not utilized, however, at submaximum work loads. At a given work level, muscle blood flow is less and arteriovenous O_2 difference wider following training.[8-10] The explanation of the lower blood flow in proportion to metabolism and work is unknown, but it suggests that the increased capacity of the mitochondrial respiratory enzyme system enables the muscles to utilize O_2 more easily at a lower O_2 concentration.

Cardiac Output—Exercise causes a profound redistribution of systemic blood flow so that the working muscles receive most of the cardiac output. If the exertion is strenuous enough, blood flow to the viscera and nonworking muscles may actually decrease. The diminished need for blood flow to the working skeletal muscles following training provides a potential opportunity to reduce cardiac work during exercise: a given level of submaximum work might be achieved at a lower cardiac output. This does not take place, however. Instead, the redistribution of cardiac output which shifts blood flow preferentially from nonworking to working regions is less intense in trained subjects,[11,12] and total cardiac output for a given work load is unchanged. Training does not alter the relationship between the work done and O_2 consumed by the body [9,13] nor the relationship between the O_2 consumed and the cardiac output.[9,13,14] Therefore, in performing a given task, the trained individual has the same overall demands for blood flow as the untrained individual. A trained person is capable of carrying out a heavier maximum work load, but in doing so, he requires a higher systemic blood flow or cardiac output.

The altered metabolic and circulatory responses to exercise induced by endurance training appear to arise from changes in the trained muscles themselves, and they are not transferrable to untrained muscles in the same individual. Suppose that a person trains his leg muscles, for example, by repetitive bicycle exercise. With subsequent testing, blood flow to the exercising muscles is less at a given work load and greater at the maximum load for leg exercise but not for arm exercise.[14] Moreover, the rise in blood lactate concentration then is less during exercise of the trained leg muscles but is the same as before conditioning if the individual engages in exercise of his untrained arm muscles.[15]

Exercise conditioning may also increase blood hemoglobin concentration and decrease blood O_2 affinity. These changes in the composition of blood could lower cardiac work by facilitating O_2 transport to the working muscles. This effect does not appear to be sufficient, however, to significantly alter the observed relationship between cardiac output and systemic O_2 consumption.

Heart Rate and Blood Pressure—Physical training decreases the heart rate that occurs in the resting state and at each level of work. The highest heart rate that can be attained during exertion is approximately the same after training; therefore, the same pretraining maximal rate then occurs at a higher work load.[13, 14] The lower heart rate is accompanied by a larger stroke volume (cardiac output remaining nearly constant).

The basis of the relative bradycardia is not thoroughly established, but it is apparently related to a shift in the balance between sympathetic and vagal influences on the sinus node. The Wenckebach phenomenon occasionally provoked by training is thought to represent enhanced vagal tone,[16] and the bradycardia is especially sensitive to vagal inhibition by atropine.[17] Myocardial catecholamine concentration has been found to be reduced in trained rats, which may reflect decreased sympathetic nerve activity.[18] As with the adaptation in skeletal muscle blood flow provoked by training, the relative bradycardia seems to depend upon some alteration in the trained skeletal muscles themselves. When the training exercises are limited to specific muscle groups, the heart rate is subsequently lower when those muscles work but not during exercise involving other muscles which were not included in the training process.[19] Training causes no consistent change in arterial blood pressure at rest or during exercise.[6, 20, 21]

Cardiac Muscle—Endurance training leads to cardiac hypertrophy [22-24] and increase in maximum work and metabolic rate of the heart.[25] In contrast to skeletal muscle, energy turnover capacity per gram of myocardium as judged by specific activities of enzyme systems, remains nearly constant.[22] This difference in adaptive response between cardiac and skeletal muscle may be related to the proportionately higher metabolic rate per gram that is maintained by the myocardium throughout the day in the initial untrained state.

Coronary Arteries—The myocardium must rely on the coronary circulation for transport of substances needed in its metabolism, as well as for disposal of metabolic end products. The coronary circulation responds faithfully to transient fluctuations in myocardial blood flow needs by moment-to-moment adjustment of coronary arteriole resistance. The coronary blood vessels are also capable of growth as a means of adapting to sustained increase in needs for blood flow. The large conducting coronary arteries enlarge in patients with left ventricular hypertrophy due to aortic valve disease. In rats, physical training increases the total bulk of the coronary arteries [26] and increases the maximum blood flow which can be carried through the coronary vascular system.[25]

Essential Features in Normal Subjects—The most important factors responsible for increased performance after exercise training in normal subjects are increased skeletal muscle aerobic energy turnover capacity; increased skeletal muscle blood flow capacity; and increased myocardial mass and work capacity.

Nature of the Limiting Factor in Exertion

Physical training augments endurance exercise capacity in normal subjects by expanding those factors that normally determine maximum steady state exercise, namely the capacity of the exercising skeletal muscles for oxidative energy turnover and, probably of lesser importance, the transport of O_2 to the muscles by the circulatory system. The higher myocardial O_2 consumption needed during exercise is met satisfactorily by coronary vasodilation and increased coronary blood flow and is not normally a limiting variable.

The parameters which determine the maximum exercise attainable by patients with exertional angina pectoris are quite different. In this case, physical activity is interrupted prematurely because of chest pain. Obstructive coronary artery disease limits coronary blood flow; and when the rising myocardial O_2 consumption rate during exercise exceeds the maximum ability of the coronary circulation to deliver O_2 (and remove metabolites), myocardial hypoxia (and acidosis) occurs. The chest pain presumably is an external manifestation of myocardial hypoxia or some related chemical change. The onset of the pain, then, is a sign that O_2 supply to the myocardium is no longer adequate in relation to O_2 needs by the myocardium. In these patients the limiting factor in exertion can be expressed as: myocardial O_2 supply/myocardial O_2 consumption requirements for a given task to be performed. Under these conditions, any change which either increases O_2 supply or decreases O_2 consumption requirements of the myocardium *for a given task* should enable the patient to improve his capacity for exertion. If the O_2 supply increases or the O_2 requirements decrease, the same task that formerly caused angina can be carried out without angina, and the magnitude of physical task required to provoke angina will be higher (increased exercise angina threshold).

Patients who are limited specifically by angina pectoris and cannot make use of their skeletal muscle capabilities to begin with would not benefit from an increase in the capacity for energy turnover in the skeletal muscles. In fact, any increased peripheral metabolism that did occur would demand more cardiac work for transporting substances to and from the skeletal muscles, and the heart could not respond to the greater demands unless O_2 supply to the heart were increased concurrently. Also, one could not expect any benefit from cardiac hypertrophy or from a metabolic adaptation within the heart muscle which simply increased its capacity for O_2 transport by the respiratory enzyme system since it is the supply of O_2, not its turnover rate, which is abnormally limited.

Task Performance and Angina Threshold

The level of physical activity that usually precipitates angina pectoris represents the exercise angina threshold for that patient. The patient expresses his angina threshold in terms of a task within his routine, eg, carrying packages upstairs at his home. The investigator may express it as a work level on a treadmill. In any case, the exercise angina threshold is a quantification of body activity, not of heart work or coronary blood flow.

Physical training by endurance exercise does increase the exercise angina threshold of most patients who adhere to the program.[9, 20, 27-29] The patient is apt to state that he has pain less often or can perform asymptomatically some task which formerly caused chest pain. The higher angina threshold has been documented by demonstrating that after conditioning angina develops at a higher work level during treadmill or bicycle ergometer testing. We will now consider the aspects of normal adaptation to endurance training that might explain the increased exercise angina threshold in patients with coronary heart disease.

Basis of the Increased Exercise Angina Threshold

Decreased Myocardial O_2 Consumption—Myocardial O_2 consumption increases during exercise in proportion to the increases which occur in heart rate and systolic blood pressure.[30, 31] This is a very useful observation from a practical standpoint, because it enables one to estimate indirectly quantitative changes in myocardial O_2 consumption from a readily measured parameter: the product of heart rate and systolic blood pressure (HR × BP) under conditions in which it would be very difficult to determine myocardial O_2 consumption by more direct invasive catheterization procedures. It has been further noted that an individual patient with angina tends to experience his chest pain from one time to another at a consistent HR × BP.[32-34] This pair of observations, the correlation between myocardial O_2 consumption and HR × BP and the occurrence of angina at a consistently reproducible HR × BP, taken together support the contention that angina occurs when the maximum myocardial O_2 consumption has been reached. Maximum myocardial O_2 consumption for an individual patient is fixed because maximum coronary blood flow is pathologically limited, O_2 extraction from the coronary blood remaining nearly constant.

It was pointed out previously that endurance training normally causes a relative bradycardia. This physiologic effect also occurs in patients with coronary heart disease, and several studies have shown that the HR × BP value at a given work level or task is lower in patients following training.[9, 20, 28] One can safely assume that the lower HR × BP indicates lower myocardial O_2 consumption needs. This change undoubtedly at least partly explains the increase in exercise angina threshold experienced by the patient.

Although important, the lower HR × BP during exercise probably is not the entire explanation for the increased angina threshold. Trained patients not only lower their HR × BP at a given work level, but they also apparently are able to attain a higher maximum HR × BP before angina occurs [28, 29] (different results have also been reported [21]). There are two possible interpretations of the higher maximum HR × BP (which are not necessarily mutually exclusive): (1) The maximal myocardial O_2 consumption is higher or (2) The normal relationship between myocardial O_2 consumption and HR × BP has been altered in a manner which conserves O_2. See Part III for supporting evidence for possible higher maximum myocardial O_2 consumption. Changes which should be considered as likely means of disrupting the expected relationship between O_2 consumption and HR × BP are diminished left ventricular volume, decreased contractile state (inotropy) and supplemental anaerobic metabolism.

Systemic arterial blood pressure influences myocardial metabolic rate through its effect on left ventricular wall tension. Therefore, diminished left ventricular volume during exertion would be expected to decrease myocardial O_2 consumption relative to HR × BP (which explains the influence of acute alterations in blood volume on angina threshold [35, 36]). Chest X rays [6, 13, 20] and left ventricular angiograms [29] performed in patients at rest before and after conditioning show no evidence of decrease in cardiac or left ventricular volume, at least in the resting state.

Contractile state of the myocardium exerts an independent effect on myocardial O_2 consumption. Diminished contractility decreases myocardial O_2 consumption even when HR × BP is kept constant and could, therefore, explain a disproportionately low myocardial O_2 consumption in relation to concurrent HR × BP. Although unproven, a decrease in sympathetic outflow to the heart during exercise is a strong possibility following conditioning. The relative bradycardia and diminished myocardial catecholamine concentration have already been mentioned as evidence of attenuated sympathetic activity. On the other hand, sympathetic inhibition in patients by propranolol administration differs from the effect of training. Although propranolol treatment increases exercise angina threshold, the patients experience angina at a lower, not higher maximum HR × BP.[37, 38] The outcome may be a question of magnitude. In the studies with propranolol, opposing wasteful effects of cardiac dilatation on myocardial O_2 consumption may have outweighed the economizing effects of diminished contractility.

The need for ATP regeneration by substrate catabolism presumably underlies the observed relationship between HR × BP and myocardial O_2 consumption. Since the source of ATP seems to be immaterial, any supplemental ATP contributed anaerobically by glycolysis can be expected to reduce by an equivalent amount the requirements of oxidative phosphorylation and, therefore, to decrease O_2 consumption relative to HR × BP. Anaerobic glycolysis does not normally occur in the myocardium but can be temporarily induced by acute hypoxia. Exercise training has been shown not to increase the capacity for anaerobic glycolysis: hearts from trained rats produce no more lactate when subjected to acute hypoxic or work stress than do hearts of sedentary rats.[25, 39] These results, however, may not be very relevant to patients with coronary ischemia. The coronary circulation is perfectly capable of meeting myocardial O_2 needs during exercise in normal rats, and it is questionable whether a significant hypoxic stimulus for enzyme change occurred during training in these experiments. The results of experiments with chronic systemic hypoxic exposure are perhaps more pertinent. In rats adapted to simulated high altitude, maximum myocardial lactate production during an acute anoxic stress was twice as great as the lactate production in control rats.[40]

In patients with ischemic coronary heart disease, exercise training did not increase maximum myocardial lactate production induced by atrial pacing, as judged by mixed coronary venous blood sampled from the coronary sinus during angina.[29] Thus, the training did not bring about myocardial enzyme changes which allowed anaerobic glycolysis to make a new significant contribution to the overall energy balance of the heart. On the other hand, this approach is incapable of eliminating a different important possibility. If a small hypoxic region of the myocardium is responsible for the angina, a substantial increase in anaerobic metabolism in that region (as seen in the altitude adapted rats) might supplement local ATP formation enough to delay exertional angina without creating a detectable change in lactate concentration in a sample of mixed coronary venous blood.

Increased Myocardial O_2 Supply—The bradycardia resulting from training clearly contributes to the increase that occurs in exercise angina threshold. Other potential changes which might also spare myocardial O_2 consumption needs were discussed. The question to be considered now is whether decreased O_2 consumption needs are solely responsible for the increased angina threshold or whether training also augments O_2 supply to the heart muscle for its metabolism.

Under normal circumstances, the myocardium extracts most of the O_2 from the blood in transit through the coronary circulation. Training does not seem to increase O_2 extraction [29]; therefore, increased myocardial O_2 supply must depend upon increased coronary blood flow. The presence of coronary collateral blood vessels in patients is correlated quantitatively with the severity of underlying ischemic coronary disease, and as pointed out earlier, endurance training stimulates enlargement of coronary arteries. These phenomena suggest that coronary vessel growth is regulated to maintain adequate myocardial O_2 supply. Collateral development seems to be capable of responding rapidly to an ischemic stimulus,[41, 42] and it seems reasonable that even brief repeated episodes of myocardial hypoxia experienced during a training program might enhance coronary collateral development. The effect of exercise training on coronary collateral growth in response to gradual left circumflex coronary artery occlusion was studied in dogs.[43] Coronary collateral perfusion to the occluded circumflex artery was quantified in these experiments by measuring the coronary arterial pressure distal to the occlusion. The pressure was higher in dogs which regularly exercised than in sedentary dogs. These experiments, which have not been confirmed by other investigators, provide essentially the only direct evidence that training does augment coronary collaterals.

There is no obvious difference in the angiographic visualization of coronary collaterals between physically active or sedentary patients,[44] and coronary arteriograms obtained in patients or dogs before and after completion of an exercise training program disclosed no systematic change in the appearance of coronary collaterals.[6, 29, 45, 46] New collaterals were evident only in response to new coronary arterial obstructive lesions. The information gained by this approach, however, must be regarded as unsatisfyingly crude. Collaterals are difficult to quantify by angiography, and no additional assessment can be made of the functional capabilities of the collaterals during exercise.

A potentially important lead was uncovered by comparing the results of exercise training on exercise-induced angina and pacing-induced angina. The same patients were able to achieve a higher maximum HR × BP before angina occurred during exercise testing, but not during pacing.[29] This observation, which needs to be confirmed, suggests that exercise training brings about a functional adaptation which is specific for exercise. It recurs when the patient exercises but cannot be counted on to emerge in the face of a different type of stress to myocardial O_2 supply, eg, pacing-induced tachycardia. If this is the case, then the physiologic explanation for the increased exercise angina threshold is likely to be discovered only by studying the patient while he is exercising.

Investigations made during exercise, employing newer techniques to assess coronary function, seem to offer the most promising approach to the question of how training effects coronary collaterals. For example, focal myocardial ischemia provoked by exercise can be identified from precordial scintiscans representing heterogeneous uptake of radioactive cations by the unevenly perfused myocardium.[47] Also, scintiscans could locate radioactive metabolites signifying regions of abnormal myocardial metabolism which result from underlying focal ischemia.[48] These methods could be used to determine whether endurance training reduces focal myocardial ischemia occurring in coronary patients during exercise. Coronary blood flow distribution within the heart, including focal myocardial ischemia brought about during acute hemodynamic stress,[49] can be studied very effectively in animals by the radioactive labeled microsphere technique. This technique could be applied to the study of the training effect on collateral function during exercise in animals with experimental coronary occlusion.

Essential Features in Coronary Disease Patients—The most important factors which are responsible for the increase in exercise angina threshold following endurance training in coronary patients, based on information currently available are as follows: (1) Decreased myocardial O_2 consumption needed for task which includes lower heart rate and possibly lower cardiac contractility; and (2) Possibly increased coronary collateral blood flow.

Summary

Repetitive bouts of endurance exercise induce adaptations which enhance the ability of the body to carry out the exercise. In normal subjects, the most important adaptations are: increased metabolic turnover and work capacity of the trained skeletal muscles, increased maximum circulatory support available to these trained muscles and increased capacity of the heart to meet the trained body's higher circulatory needs.

In patients limited by exertional angina pectoris, the limiting factor determining their angina threshold can be expressed as myocardial O_2 consumption requirements relative to myocardial O_2 supply for a given task to be performed. Endurance training raises their exercise angina threshold. One important mechanism is decrease in myocardial O_2 consumption due to the relative bradycardia induced by training. Decrease in myocardial O_2 consumption from decreased myocardial contractility and increased myocardial O_2 supply from augmented coronary collateral function may also contribute to the increased angina threshold.

References

1. Holloszy JO: Biochemical adaptations in muscle. Effects of exercise on mitochondrial oxygen uptake and respiratory enzyme activity in skeletal muscle. *J Biol Chem* 242:2278-2282, 1967.
2. Morgan TE, Cobb LA, Short FA, et al: "Effect of Long-term Exercise on Human Muscle Mitochondria," in Pernow B, Saltin B (Eds): *Muscle Metabolism During Exercise*, pp 87-95, New York: Plenum, 1971.
3. Oscai LB, Holloszy JO: Biochemical adaptations in muscle. II: Response of mitochondrial adenosine triphosphatase, creatine phosphokinase, and adenylate kinase activities in skeletal muscle to exercise. *J Biol Chem* 246:6968-6972, 1971.
4. Gollnick PD, Armstrong RB, Saltin B, et al: Effect of training on enzyme activity and fiber composition of human skeletal muscle. *J Appl Physiol* 34:107-111, 1973.
5. Baldwin KM, Winder WW, Terjung RL, et al: Glycolytic enzymes in different types of skeletal muscle: adaptation to exercise. *Amer J Physiol* 225:962-966, 1973.
6. Varnauskas E, Bergman H, Houk P, et al: Hemodynamic effects of physical training in coronary patients. *Lancet* II:8-12, 1966.
7. Saltin B, Hartley LH, Kilbom A, et al: Physical training in sedentary middle-aged and older men. II: Oxygen uptake, heart rate, and blood lactate concentration at submaximal and maximal exercise. *Scand J Clin Lab Invest* 24:323-334, 1969.
8. Grimby G, Häggendal E, Saltin B: Local xenon-133 clearance from the quadriceps muscle during exercise. *J Appl Physiol* 22:305-310, 1967.
9. Clausen JP, Larsen OA, Trap-Jensen J: Physical training in the management of coronary artery disease. *Circulation* 40:143-154, 1969.
10. Varnauskas E, Björntorp P, Fahlen M, et al: Effects of physical training on exercise blood flow and enzymatic activity in skeletal muscle. *Cardiovasc Res* 4:418-422, 1970.
11. Grimby G: Renal clearances during prolonged supine exercise at different loads. *J Appl Physiol* 20:1294-1298, 1965.
12. Clausen JP, Trap-Jensen J: Effects of training on the distribution of cardiac output in patients with coronary artery disease. *Circulation* 42:611-624, 1970.
13. Hartley LH, Grimby G, Kilbom A, et al: Physical training in sedentary middle-aged and older men. III: Cardiac output and gas exchange at submaximal and maximal exercise. *Scand J Clin Lab Invest* 24:335-344, 1969.
14. Saltin B, Blomqvist G, Mitchell JH, et al: Response to exercise after bed rest and after training. *Circulation* 38 (suppl 7):1-78, 1968.
15. Klausen K, Rasmussen B, Clausen JP, et al: Blood lactate from exercising extremities before and after arm or leg training. *Amer J Physiol* 227:67-72, 1974.
16. Meytes I, Kaplinsky E, Yahini JH, et al: Wenckebach a-v block: a frequent feature following heavy physical training. *Amer Heart J* 90:426-430, 1975.
17. Frick MH: The effect of physical training in manifest ischemic heart disease. *Circulation* 40:433-434, 1969.
18. DeSchryver C, De Herdt P, Lammerant J: Effect of physical training on cardiac catecholamine concentrations. *Nature* 214:907-908, 1967.
19. Clausen JP, Klausen K, Rasmussen B, et al: Central and peripheral circulatory changes after training of the arms or legs. *Amer J Physiol* 225:675-682, 1973.
20. Frick MH, Katila M: Hemodynamic consequences of physical training after myocardial infarction. *Circulation* 37:192-202, 1968.

146   *Neill*

21. Clausen JP, Trap-Jensen J: Heart rate and arterial blood pressure during exercise in patients with angina pectoris: effects of training and of nitroglycerin. *Circulation* 53:436-442, 1976.
22. Oscai LB, Molé PA, Brei B, et al: Cardiac growth and respiratory enzyme levels in male rats subjected to a running program. *Amer J Physiol* 220:1238-1241, 1971.
23. Wyatt HL, Mitchell JH: Influences of physical training on the heart of dogs. *Circ Res* 35:883-889, 1974.
24. Roeske WR, O'Rourke RA, Klein A, et al: Noninvasive evaluation of ventricular hypertrophy in professional athletes. *Circulation* 53:286-292, 1976.
25. Penpargkul S, Scheuer J: The effect of physical training upon the mechanical and metabolic performance of the rat heart. *J Clin Invest* 49:1859-1868, 1970.
26. Stevenson JA, Felcki V, Rechnitzer P, et al: Effect of exercise on coronary tree size in the rat. *Circ Res* 25:265-269, 1964.
27. Hellerstein HK: Exercise therapy in coronary disease. *Bull N Y Acad Med* 44:1028-1074, 1968.
28. Redwood DR, Rosing DR, Epstein SE: Circulatory and symptomatic effects of physical training in patients with coronary artery disease and angina pectoris. *New Eng J Med* 286:959-965, 1972.
29. Sim DN, Neill WA: Investigation of the physiological basis for increased exercise threshold for angina pectoris after physical conditioning. *J Clin Invest* 54:763-770, 1974.
30. Holmberg S, Serzysko W, Varnauskas E: Coronary circulation during heavy exercise in control subjects and patients with coronary heart disease. *Acta Med Scand* 190:465-480, 1971.
31. Nelson RR, Gobel FL, Jörgensen CR, et al: Hemodynamic predictors of myocardial oxygen consumption during static and dynamic exercise. *Circulation* 50:1179-1189, 1974.
32. Robinson BF: Relation of heart rate and systolic blood pressure to the onset of pain in angina pectoris. *Circulation* 35:1073-1083, 1967.
33. Wahren J, Bydgeman S: Onset of angina pectoris in relation to circulatory adaptation during arm and leg exercise. *Circulation* 44:432-441, 1971.
34. Cokkinos DV, Voridis EM: Constancy of pressure-rate product in pacing-induced angina pectoris. *Brit Heart J* 38:39-42, 1976.
35. Parker JO, Case RB, Khaja F, et al: The influence of changes in blood volume on angina pectoris. *Circulation* 41:593-604, 1970.
36. Khaja F, Sanghvi V, Mark A, et al: Effect of volume expansion on the anginal threshold. *Circulation* 43:824-835, 1971.
37. Goldbarg AN, Moran JF, Butterfield TK, et al: Therapy of angina pectoris with propranolol and long-acting nitrates. *Circulation* 40:847-853, 1969.
38. Dagenais GR, Pitt B, Ross RS: Exercise tolerance in patients with angina pectoris. *Amer J Cardiol* 28:10-16, 1971.
39. Scheuer J, Stezoski SW: Effect of physical training on the mechanical and metabolic response of the rat heart to hypoxia. *Circ Res* 30:418-429, 1972.
40. Bowers WD Jr, Burlington RF, Whitten BK, et al: Ultrastructural and metabolic alterations in myocardium from altitude-acclimated rats. *Amer J Physiol* 220:1885-1889, 1971.
41. Khouri EM, Gregg DM, McGranahan GM Jr: Regression and reappearance of coronary collaterals. *Amer J Physiol* 220:655-661, 1971.
42. Schaper W, Pasyk S: Influence of collateral flow on the ischemic tolerance of the heart following acute and subacute coronary occlusion. *Circulation* 53 (suppl 1):57-62, 1976.
43. Eckstein RW: Effect of exercise and coronary artery narrowing on coronary collateral circulation. *Circ Res* 5:230-235, 1957.
44. Helfant RH, Vokonas PS, Gorlen R: Functional importance of the human coronary collateral circulation. *New Eng J Med* 284:1277-1281, 1971.
45. Kaplinsky E, Hood WB Jr, McCarthy B, et al: Effects of physical training in dogs with coronary artery ligation. *Circulation* 37:556-565, 1968.
46. Ferguson RJ, Petitclerc R, Choquette G, et al: Effect of physical training on treadmill exercise capacity, collateral circulation and progression of coronary disease. *Amer J Cardiol* 34:764-769, 1974.
47. Zaret BL, Strauss HW, Martin ND, et al: Noninvasive regional myocardial perfusion with radioactive potassium. *New Eng J Med* 288:809-812, 1973.
48. Weiss ES, Hoffman EJ, Phelps ME, et al: External detection and visualization of myocardial ischemia with ^{11}C-substrates *in vitro* and *in vivo*. *Circ Res* 39:24-32, 1976.
49. Neill WA, Oxendine J, Phelps N, et al: Subendocardial ischemia provoked by tachycardia in conscious dogs with coronary stenosis. *Amer J Cardiol* 35:30-36, 1975.

PART III

Coronary Heart Disease Diagnosis: Methodological & Interpretive Aspects

10

Methods of Exercise Testing:
Step Test, Bicycle, Treadmill, Isometrics

Robert A. Bruce, MD

Appraisal of exercise testing methods properly requires consideration of physiologic types of exercise, clinical applications and objectives, physiologic differences between major classes of dynamic tests, comparison of oxygen requirements and circulatory responses, recommended objectives and rationale, experience with general application and clinical evaluation of therapeutic intervention.

Physiologic Types of Muscular Exercise and Circulatory Implications

Basically, there are three types of skeletal muscle contractions. The first type is dynamic with rhythmical contractions of extensor and flexor muscle groups. Examples of dynamic exercise include walking, stepping, pedaling, jogging and running. The alternating contractions of these muscle groups facilitate arterial inflow to the working muscles and venous return to the right heart chambers. The second type is isometric, or sustained muscle contraction. Examples of isometric exercise include handgrip, isometric weight lifting and waterskiing. These sustained contractions limit arterial inflow by compressing small arteries and do not facilitate venous return. The third type represents the combination of the first two. Examples of this type of exercise include carrying a heavy load while walking or executing vigorous handgrips while pedaling a bicycle.

Dynamic vs. Isometric Exercise—Of the two major physiologic types of exercise stress, dynamic exercise is clearly preferred because the circulatory responses are directly proportional to relative aerobic requirements. In a comparative study of the two types of exercise in the same four normal subjects,

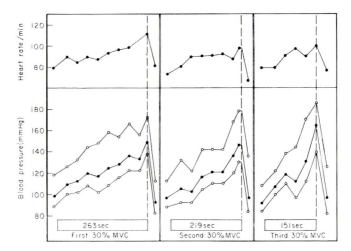

Figure 1. Heart rate and blood pressure responses to isometric handgrip exercise at 30% of maximal voluntary contraction (MVC) in four normal subjects. Note reproducibility of responses when repeated after 10 minutes (center panel) and after only 3 minutes (right panel) of recovery. Reproduced with permission from Bruce RA et al: The effects of digoxin on fatiguing static and dynamic exercise in man. *Clin Sci* 34:29-42, 1968.

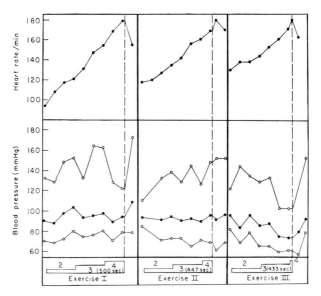

Figure 2. Heart rate and blood pressure responses to multistage treadmill test of dynamic exercise to maximal limits in the same four normal subjects. Again note reproducibility on repetition after only 10 minutes (center panel) and only 3 minutes (right panel) of recovery. Reproduced with permission from Bruce RA et al: The effects of digoxin on fatiguing static and dynamic exercise in man. *Clin Sci* 34:29-42, 1968.

TABLE I

Circulatory Reponses to Voluntary Handgrip, 30% of Maximal, Held to Limit of Fatigue

	At Rest	Peak Response		% Change
Cutaneous circulation	Normal	Intensely hyperemic		—
Blood pressure (mm Hg)	112/82	206/142	(+94/+60)	83/73
Heart rate (beats/min)	77	92	(+15)	19

blood pressure responses were exaggerated with isometric exertion (Figure 1) and heart rate responses were greater with dynamic exercise (Figure 2).[1] Even when each type of exertion was repeated after inadequate time for recovery, there was no significant change in these patterns. Accordingly, isometric exertion, especially if performed at a level more than 25% of maximal voluntary contraction, can be hazardous because the acute increases in blood pressure are greatly in excess of aerobic requirements [2] (Table I). Anecdotal data indicate hazards of acute pulmonary edema, arrhythmias, myocardial infarction and even sudden death (two instances during waterskiing) in patients with heart disease. Whatever type of stress test is used, it is important not to limit observations to electrocardiographic changes of possible myocardial ischemia of diagnostic significance, but also to note changes in rhythm, heart rate and blood pressure as indicators of circulatory impairment.

Physiologic Differences Between Major Types of Conventional Tests of Dynamic Exercise

Conventional tests of dynamic exercise can be subdivided into two major categories with important pathophysiologic differences.

Submaximal Tests—These may be single stage or multistage, with continuous or discontinuous work loads and *predetermined, arbitrary* end points. These end points may be the number of trips on standardized steps (even when adjusted for sex, age and weight), work load, oxygen requirement or, more commonly, a target heart rate based upon a percentage of estimated maximal heart rate. The latter is obtained from age and activity status then compared with average values of "normal" persons. All these criteria fail to consider that maximal heart rate is distinctly lower in patients with heart disease, especially those with myocardial ischemia, and that the range of normal responses clearly documented by the 95% confidence intervals is fairly broad. Furthermore, when one of these arbitrary end points is attained, it is necessary to rely upon the subjective assessment of the patient to determine whether that arbitrary level of activity represents a low, intermediate or high fraction of his capacity. Accordingly, exercise capacity is poorly defined and, consequently, reserve function is uncer-

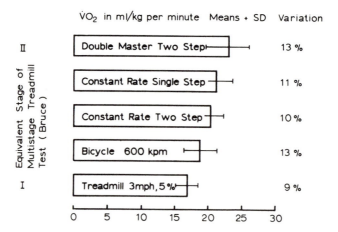

Figure 3. Aerobic costs of five commonly used submaximal tests. $\dot{V}O_2$max = maximal oxygen uptake. Adapted with permission from Blackburn H et al: "Exercise Tests: Comparison of the Energy Cost and Heart Rate Response to Five Commonly Used Single-stage, Non-steady-state, Submaximal Work Procedures," in Brunner D, Jokl E (Eds): *Medicine and Sport, Vol 4: Physical Activity and Aging*, pp 28-36, Basel: Karger, 1970.

tain. The majority of submaximal test procedures take into consideration that their arbitrary limits exceed the capabilities of the more impaired patient and include a variety of other indications for stopping stress, some of which may be ambiguous.

Maximal Tests—Individualized, self-determined symptomatic end points of *maximal possible performances* permit each subject to attain his physiologic limit while the various symptoms, signs and circulatory, electrocardiographic and metabolic responses are observed and recorded. With a multistage treadmill protocol, this procedure has been feasible in more than 97% of more than 20,000 tests in our experience. These end points are more reproducible than the responses at any submaximal work load. Furthermore, with this protocol, maximal oxygen uptake and its relation to expected normal values (adjusted for sex, age and activity status) can be readily defined from elapsed time in minutes and a nomogram.

Comparison of Oxygen Requirements and Circulatory Responses

Oxygen requirements of five different submaximal exercise tests, defined by measurements in the same normal subjects, are shown in Figure 3. The greatest energy expenditure in these five tests occurred with the double Master two-step test, which required 23 ml/kg body weight per minute.[3] Results of this test also exhibited the greatest variability in the relation of standard deviation to the means. The least variable, and therefore most reproducible, results were found at a low level of energy expenditure on the treadmill.

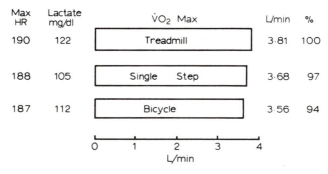

Max HR	Lactate mg/dl	$\dot{V}O_2$ Max	L/min	%
190	122	Treadmill	3·81	100
188	105	Single Step	3·68	97
187	112	Bicycle	3·56	94

Figure 4. Comparison of maximal exercise performances obtained by three different discontinuous test methods in the same normal men aged 20 to 40 (mean 26.4) years. HR = heart rate; Max = maximal. Adapted with permission from Shephard RV et al: The maximum oxygen intake. An international reference standard of cardiorespiratory fitness. *Bull WHO* **38**:757-764, 1968.

Peak Oxygen Uptake—Maximal tests should define the peak oxygen uptake, but when the same men are tested by different methods to a level of maximal exertion, values for oxygen uptake differ [4] (Figure 4). The lowest value was obtained with the bicycle ergometer, and the highest with a multistage treadmill.[5] Other studies of patients with coronary artery disease indicate that ventilation as well as heart rate, arterial pressure, pressure-rate product and systemic resistance are greater in the same patients during bicycle exercise than during treadmill testing.[6] These differences are attributed to more vigorous muscle contractions with the ergometer, particularly in persons not conditioned to bicycling.

Maximal Oxygen Uptake ($\dot{V}O_2$ max)—When a multistage treadmill test of maximal exercise is used, and the subject continues exertion until a self-determined

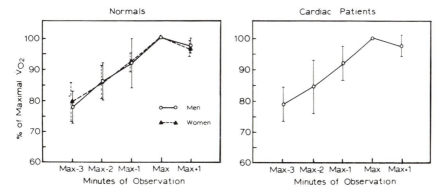

Figure 5. Approach to maximal oxygen uptake in normal subjects and patients with heart disease during multistage treadmill test. Reproduced with permission from Bruce RA et al: Maximal oxygen intake and nomographic assessment of functional aerobic impairment in cardiovascular disease. *Amer Heart J* **85**:546-562, 1973.

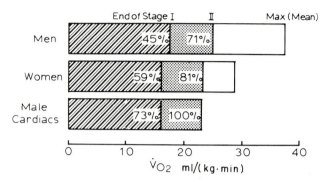

Figure 6. Relative aerobic requirements of submaximal exercise using multistage tread-mill protocol, scaled to absolute values of maximal oxygen uptake. Reproduced with permission from Bruce RA: Exercise testing of patients with coronary heart disease: principles and normal standards for evaluation. *Ann Clin Res* 3:323-332, 1971.

end point of fatigue or other limiting symptoms, it is remarkable that the approach to maximum appears similar in all ambulatory persons (provided that subjects do not use the handrails for partial support of body weight [7,8] (Figure 5). This applies even though there are striking differences in weight-adjusted $\dot{V}O_2$ max. Thus, at 1 or 2 minutes before $\dot{V}O_2$ max the average percent $\dot{V}O_2$ max is similar for normal subjects and patients with heart disease. For the one in five subjects who continue for 1/2 to 1 minute beyond the point of $\dot{V}O_2$ max by greater utilization of anaerobic glycolysis for the source of additional energy, $\dot{V}O_2$ max is reduced about 3 to 5%. Hemodynamic studies clearly indicate that this fall is due to a further decrease in stroke volume rather than to a reduction in either heart rate or arterial-mixed venous O_2 difference.[9-12]

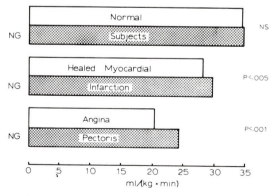

Figure 7. Comparison of effects of nitroglycerin on maximal oxygen uptake of patients with coronary artery disease and normal subjects. Reproduced with permission from Detry J-MR, Bruce RA: Effects of nitroglycerin on "maximum" oxygen intake and exercise electrocardiogram in coronary heart disease. *Circulation* 43:155-163, 1971.

$\dot{V}O_2$ max in milliliters per minute per kilogram is greater in men than in women (Figure 6); accordingly, the relative aerobic costs for a given submaximal exertion are greater in women than in men. They are still greater in men with cardiac disease than in either normal men or normal women, because the weight-adjusted value of $\dot{V}O_2$ max is even lower in patients with cardiac disease.

$\dot{V}O_2$ max can be increased acutely with nitroglycerin in patients with coronary heart disease, but not in normal subjects [13] (Figure 7). Thus, in the presence of myocardial ischemia, work capacity is enhanced transiently when the preload and afterload imposed on the ischemic myocardium are reduced by peripheral vasodilatation; then the available coronary flow of oxygenated blood is more nearly adequate for the reduced hemodynamic stress applied.

Oxygen costs of isometric work, even when forced to maximal limits, do not approach the values obtained with dynamic exercise. Thus, isometric exercise is useless for testing functional aerobic capacity, just as it is useless for acquiring the benefits of endurance training obtained by dynamic exercise conditioning.

Recommended Objectives and Rationale of Testing

The goals of exercise testing should not be restricted to electrocardiographic observations of myocardial ischemia as possible evidence of coronary vascular disease. Instead, the objectives should be to define functional aerobic capacity, the magnitude of its deviation from appropriate normal standards, and the car-

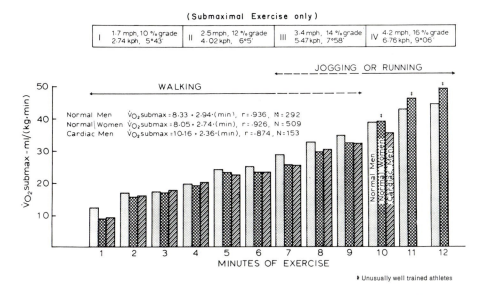

Figure 8. Aerobic requirements of healthy middle-aged men and women with cardiac disease during submaximal exercise in multistage treadmill test, in absolute values, weight-adjusted. Reproduced with permission from Bruce RA et al: Maximal oxygen intake and nomographic assessment of functional aerobic impairment in cardiovascular disease. *Amer Heart J* 85:546-562, 1973.

diovascular mechanisms of any impairment.

These objectives can be met rapidly, reliably and safely with a multistage treadmill test that encompasses submaximal and maximal exercise.[14] The oxygen requirements for the first four stages or 12 minutes are shown in Figure 8, and average values for maximal oxygen uptake are shown in Figure 6. In meeting these requirements, it is important that none of the body weight be supported by leaning on the handrails; this reduces oxygen requirement and increases variability of measurements of both intensity and duration. In our setting, each subject undergoes a medical examination and a resting electrocardiogram to detect contraindications before testing, and the patient and the electrocardiogram are monitored during and immediately after testing. As a result of these precautions we have observed a morbidity rate of less than 0.1% and no mortality in more than 20,000 tests. This experience compares favorably with that of the national experience surveyed by Rochmis and Blackburn,[15] who reported respective morbidity and mortality rates of 2.4 and 1 per 10,000 tests, in a survey of 170,000 exercise tests. Despite these precautions, we have witnessed three nonfatal myocardial infarctions; the first was in a normal subject who after exercise testing became acutely ill while taking a hot shower [16]; the others were in patients with coronary heart disease. There have also been five cases of immediately postexertional cardiac arrest (2%) in men with prior myocardial infarction or angina pectoris who also developed exertional hypotension.[17]

With this protocol, the $\dot{V}O_2$ max and functional aerobic impairment can be derived by regression equations or nomogram from the total duration of exercise.

Clinical Application of Maximal (Treadmill) Exercise Testing

In July 1971, a prospective study of exercise testing was initiated in 15 testing sites in the Seattle area. These included four hospital laboratories, the medical department in a major industry, and ten private clinics and offices of physicians and cardiologists. The objectives were to test the hypothesis that specific individuals at risk could be detected earlier and more frequently by maximal exercise testing, and that the mechanisms of clinical events might be predicted in terms of angina or infarction from ischemia or sudden death from arrhythmia. In the first 4½ years, nearly 9,000 persons have been tested with only three morbid complications and no mortality. Analysis of the men reveals interesting findings in relation to chest pain (Figure 9) and other responses to exercise in those who were classified as normal ("inapparent") vs. patients with "possible," "probable" or "definite" coronary heart disease (Figure 9 and 10). Among the normal men, $\dot{V}O_2$ max estimated from duration of multistage exercise treadmill protocol [14] averaged 35 ml/min. Accordingly, functional aerobic impairment of only 1.9% represents remarkable validation of the principle and nomographic technique for assessment of functional aerobic capacity. Functional aerobic impairment increased with clinical severity of disease from 12.5 to 13%. Furthermore, determinations of the changes in heart rate from electrocardiogram and changes

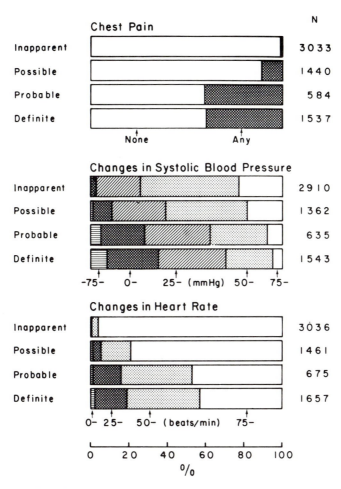

Figure 9. Percentage prevalences, with maximal exertion, of chest pain and changes in two hemodynamic variables in 6,594 men, stratified in relation to clinical detection of heart disease.

in systolic blood pressure by sphygmomanometry provided significant insights into the circulatory mechanisms of impairment (Figure 9). The rate changes averaged 106 in normal men and fell progressively to 91, 72 and 67 as severity of disease increased. The pressure changes averaged 63 mm Hg in normal men and fell with increasing severity of disease to 57, 43 and 36 mm Hg. The former represents the chronotropic reserve and the latter an index of inotropic reserve of the left ventricle. Actually, since peripheral vascular resistance diminishes markedly with maximal exercise, the change in pressure underestimates the inotropic reserve of the ventricle. Representative differences in electro-cardiographic responses, including arrhythmia, conduction defects and ST dis-

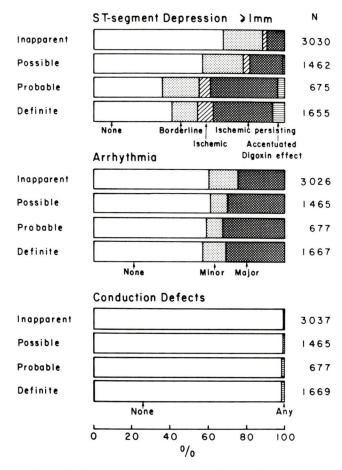

Figure 10. Percentage prevalences of ≥ 1 mm ST-segment depression, arrhythmia and conduction defects with maximal exertion among 6,450 men, in relation to clinical detection of heart disease.

placement in relation to the clinical certainty of coronary heart disease are illustrated in Figure 10.

With regression analysis of the variation in heart rate, systolic pressure and the product of rate and pressure $\times 10^{-2}$ at maximal exercise with age in healthy men, it has been possible to derive estimates of predicted normal values and the percentage deviation of observed values from age-predicted standards.[18] This latter can then be expressed as heart-rate impairment and functional left ventricular impairment at maximal exercise (Figure 11), which provide insights into the relative importance of these hemodynamic mechanisms in relation to the functional aerobic impairment for the whole body.

In conclusion, some of the salient principles of exercise testing of ambulatory

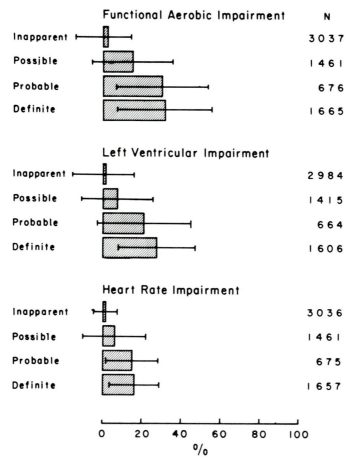

Figure 11. Manifestations of decreased ventricular capacity among 6,839 men, expressed in percentage impairment in functional aerobic capacity, inotropic capacity and chronotropic capacity, respectively.

normal subjects and patients with heart disease have been reviewed briefly. Isometric exercise may be hazardous; dynamic exercise offers greater benefits and fewer risks. Experience with the multistage treadmill test indicates that it is a practical, reliable and safe method of testing, with the distinct advantage that its use permits definition of the functional capacity of the cardiovascular system.

Summary

Methods of exercise testing are considered in relation to physiologic types, clinical applications and objectives, physiologic differences in end points and inferences, and comparison of oxygen requirements and circulatory responses.

Hazards and safety precautions are cited.

The multistage treadmill test of submaximal and maximal exercise is described in terms of oxygen requirements, measurement of maximal oxygen uptake, approach to maximal uptake, determination of functional aerobic impairment and assessment of circulatory and electrocardiographic responses. Initial findings are presented of a new, prospective community study ("Seattle Heart Watch") designed to test the hypothesis that specific persons at risk for future angina pectoris, myocardial infarction or sudden death can be identified by this method.

Acknowledgment—Alison Ross provided substantial assistance in revising this paper.

References

1. Bruce RA, Lind AR, Franklin D, et al: The effects of digoxin on fatiguing static and dynamic exercise in man. *Clin Sci* 34:29-42, 1968.
2. Lind AR: Cardiovascular responses to static exercise. (Isometrics, anyone?) *Circulation* 41:173-176, 1970.
3. Blackburn H, Winkler C, Vilandré J, et al: "Exercise tests: Comparison of the Energy Cost and Heart Rate Response to Five Commonly Used Single-stage, Non-steady-state, Submaximal Work Procedures," in Brunner D, Jokl E (Eds): *Medicine and Sport, vol 4: Physical Activity and Aging*, pp 28-36, Basel: Karger, 1970.
4. Shephard RV, Aleen C, Benade AJS, et al: The maximum oxygen intake. An international reference standard of cardiorespiratory fitness. *Bull WHO* 38:757-764, 1968.
5. Bruce RA, Jones JW, Strait GB: Anaerobic metabolism and related factors in cardiac surgery. *Amer Heart J* 67:643-650, 1964.
6. Niederberger M, Bruce RA, Kusumi F, et al: Disparities in ventilatory and circulatory responses to bicycle and treadmill exercise. *Brit Heart J* 36:377-383, 1974.
7. Bruce RA: Exercise testing of patients with coronary heart disease: principles and normal standards for evaluation. *Ann Clin Res* 3:323-332, 1971.
8. Bruce RA, Kusumi F, Hosmer D: Maximal oxygen intake and nomographic assessment of functional aerobic impairment in cardiovascular disease. *Amer Heart J* 85:546-562, 1973.
9. Bruce RA, Petersen JL, Kusumi F: "Hemodynamic Responses to Exercise in the Upright Posture in Patients with Ischemic Heart Disease," in Dhalla NS (Ed): *Myocardial Metabolism*, pp 849-865, Baltimore: University Park Press, 1973.
10. Bruce RA, Kusumi F, Niederberger M, et al: Cardiovascular mechanisms of functional aerobic impairment in patients with coronary heart disease. *Circulation* 49:696-702, 1974.
11. Bruce RA, Kusumi F, Culver BH, Butler J: Cardiac limitations to maximal oxygen transport and changes in components after jogging across the US. *J Appl Physiol* 39:958-964, 1975.
12. Kusumi F, Bruce RA, Ross MA, et al: Elevated arterial pressure and postexertional ST-segment depression in middle-aged women. *Amer Heart J* 92:576-583, 1976.
13. Detry J-MR, Bruce RA: Effects of nitroglycerin on "maximum" oxygen intake and exercise electrocardiogram in coronary heart disease. *Circulation* 43:155-163, 1971.
14. Bruce RA, Gey GO, Cooper MN, et al: The Seattle Heart Watch: initial clinical, circulatory and electrocardiographic responses to maximal exercise. *Amer J Cardiol* 33:459-469, 1974.
15. Rochmis P, Blackburn H: Exercise tests: a survey of procedures, safety, and litigation experience in approximately 170,000 tests. *JAMA* 217:1061-1066, 1971.
16. Bruce RA, Hornsten TR, Blackmon JR: Myocardial infarction after normal responses to maximal exercise. *Circulation* 38:552-558, 1968.
17. Irving JB, Bruce RA: Exertional hypotension and postexertional ventricular fibrillation in stress testing. *Amer J Cardiol* 39:849-851, 1977.
18. Bruce RA, Fisher LD, Cooper MN, et al: Separation of effects of cardiovascular disease and age on ventricular function with maximal exercise. *Amer J Cardiol* 34:757-763, 1974.

11

Exercise Electrocardiography: Recognition of the Ischemic Response, False-Positive and False-Negative Patterns

Albert A. Kattus, MD

Depression of the ST segment has been recognized as the electrocardiographic hallmark of myocardial ischemia since Feil and Siegel [1] recognized its association with angina pectoris in their classic observations published in 1928. They observed a man with a normal resting electrocardiogram who had a spontaneous attack of angina while an electrocardiogram was being taken. The tracing they recorded resembled that of Figure 1, which represents the sequential electrocardiographic changes seen in one of our patients who experienced an anginal attack, probably attributable to anxiety, as the tracing was being recorded. Depression of the ST segment with a horizontal configuration coincided with the development of anginal pain similar to the pain he customarily had during physical exertion. Relief of pain after sublingual administration of nitroglycerin was associated with return of the ST segment to the base line. This sequence of events with the association of angina and depressed ST segment, both reversed by the administration of nitroglycerin, constitutes very strong evidence, perhaps even proof, that the ST-segment depression was due to myocardial ischemia.

The impracticality of obtaining electrocardiographic monitoring of naturally occurring anginal attacks has led to the development of provocative tests among which the Master "2-step" exercise test [2] is the only one to have survived into the present era. This test, considered a single stage test since the work load remains constant throughout the duration of the exercise period, has been supplanted in our institution in recent years by a multistage treadmill exercise test. [3] The idea underlying multistage testing is that one can begin by subjecting a patient to a low level of work load not in excess of what he is customarily able to do without

SPONTANEOUS ANGINA ATTACK

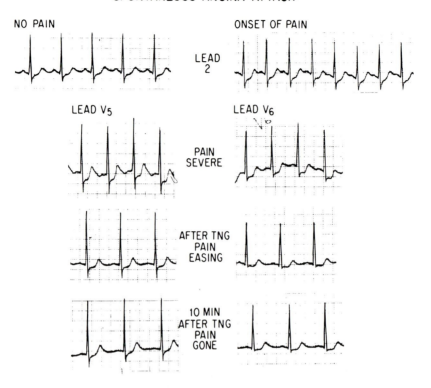

Figure 1. Electrocardiograms recorded during development of a spontaneous anginal attack and during its relief by administration of sublingual nitroglycerin (TNG). The fully developed ischemic response of horizontal depression of ST segments is seen during the height of the attack in lead V_6.

distress. The work load can then be increased in small increments during continuous electrocardiographic monitoring until ischemic manifestations in the form of anginal discomfort or ST-segment deviations, or both, make their appearance. In this way the work load imposed is tailored to the capacity of the patient and diagnostic accuracy is enhanced. Our test is designed to go beyond diagnostic capability to the determination of the patient's exercise tolerance as limited by the symptomatic manifestations of the disease—anginal pain, dyspnea, fatigue or leg pain. For this purpose, exercise is continued until the patient reaches a symptomatic end point score of 3+, indicating symptoms of moderately severe intensity (in our scoring system 1+ indicates mild, 2+ moderate, 3+ moderately severe and 4+ maximally severe intensity). This stopping point provides a tolerance test of good reproducibility that is useful for following up the course of the disease and the effects of therapeutic intervention drugs, surgery or exercise training.[4]

Intelligent use of exercise testing of any type requires an understanding of the

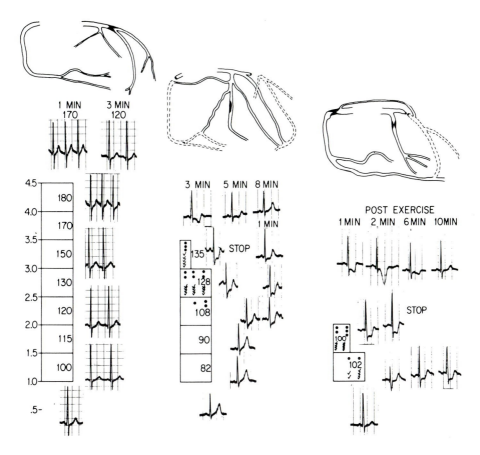

Figure 2. Three examples of standard treadmill tests showing diagrammatic representation of the test with each block representing 3 minutes of walking at 10% grade at the speed in miles/hour indicated by the top of the block. Maximal heart rate for each stage is inside each block. Dots at top of blocks indicate the severity of angina. The checks at bottom of blocks indicate millimeters of ST-segment depression. Electrocardiographic strips for appropriate stages are mounted to the right of the block diagrams. Sketches of coronary arterial anatomy as determined from coronary angiograms are above. Dotted lines indicate vessels filled by collateral vessels beyond the area of obstruction. Nonischemic response is shown on the left, ischemic responses in the center and on the right.

behavior of the electrocardiogram as it is influenced by exercise, recognition of the ischemic response, appreciation of the false-positive and false-negative response as well as the effects of certain electrocardiographic patterns that might distort the results.

The Ischemic Response

Figure 2 illustrates three treadmill tests performed in our laboratory. The graphic scheme representing the sequential stages is accompanied by electrocardiographic strips obtained with use of a bipolar transthoracic lead showing

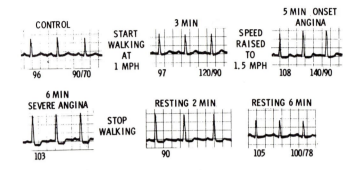

Figure 3. Sequential electrocardiographic strips from treadmill test of a patient with severe angina, poor exercise tolerance and extensive three vessel coronary obstructive disease. MPH= miles/hour.

the patterns at various stages, and drawings of the coronary arterial anatomy as disclosed by coronary cineangiograms. In the case illustrated on the left, exercise performance was normal, and there were no anginal symptoms or ischemic manifestations in the electrocardiogram. This patient had previously demonstrated Prinzmetal's variant angina [5] with nocturnal episodes of pain and ST-segment changes as well as mild angina at the 4 miles/hour stage of the treadmill test. The normal response illustrated occurred after 1 year of daily walking exercise. The local stenotic lesions in the left anterior descending coronary artery remained the same upon repeat study. Completion of the 4 or 4.5 miles/ hour stage of the test at 10% upgrade represents a performance equal to a maximal effort for the average sedentary adult American man. No deviation of the T waves or ST segments occurred either during or after exercise in this high work load test.

The *center panel of Figure 2* illustrates an ischemic response in a man who has achieved an improvement of capacity during a program of daily walking exercise. He was stopped by 3+ angina at the 3.5 miles/hour stage. Ischemic depression of the ST segment appears coincident with the onset of anginal distress, and the degree of depression increases as the intensity of the pain builds up to the 3+ end point. The postexercise recovery period is associated with deep T-wave inversion and then gradual return to the normal pattern. The arteriogram demonstrated total occlusions in both the left anterior descending and the right coronary arteries with collateral filling beyond the occlusions. Severely ischemic ST depression is usually seen over areas of myocardium supplied primarily by collateral circulation.

The *third panel* of Figure 2 illustrates a poor performance by a severely disabled man who was halted by 3+ angina in the second stage of the test at a low work level. Very severe ischemic depression is seen during exercise and very marked T inversion is seen during the recovery period. Total occlusion of the left anterior descending artery and severe stenoses in the left circumflex and right coronary arteries reduced coronary perfusion to all parts of the heart.

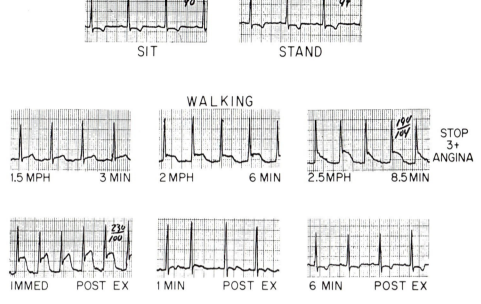

Figure 4. Electrocardiographic strips from treadmill test of a patient with angina whose ST segments became elevated during pain. Ischemia was caused by a single high grade stenosis of the left anterior descending coronary artery. IMMED = immediately; POST EX = postexercise.

The ischemic electrocardiographic responses shown in Figure 2 represent advanced and unmistakable changes. One cannot expect to find such typical changes in all cases, nor can one expect to find consistent relations between the degree of ST-segment depression and the intensity of anginal symptoms or the extent of impaired coronary perfusion. For example, the patient whose electrocardiograms are shown in Figure 3 had such severe anginal pain at a low working level that he could not progress beyond the 1.5 miles/hour stage of the standard treadmill test. With severe pain there was only 1 mm of horizontal ST-segment depression and no T-wave inversion in the postexercise recovery period. His coronary angiogram showed total occlusion of the right coronary artery with collateral filling distally, total occlusion of the left circumflex artery with preservation of a large marginal branch and severe stenosis in the proximal left anterior descending system—advanced three vessel disease yet minimal electrocardiographic changes provoked by exercise.

The ischemic response is not always manifested by ST-segment depression. Figure 4 displays electrocardiographic strips from an exercise test in which the angina was accompanied by marked ST-segment elevation. This response occurred in a man whose only coronary artery lesion was a single high grade stenosis in the proximal left anterior descending coronary artery. The pattern

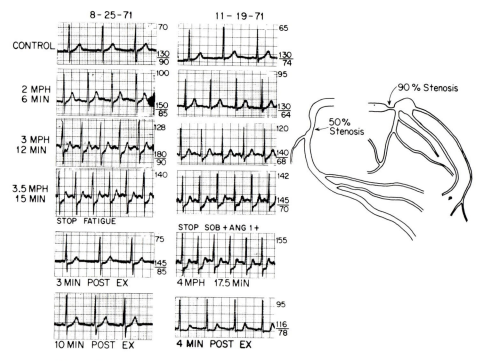

Figure 5. Two treadmill tests 3 months apart performed by a patient with mild angina. The first test resulted only in J-point depression, but the second test yielded a classic ischemic response. Coronary angiograms disclosed high grade stenosis of the left main coronary artery. ANG = angina; SOB = shortness of breath.

must be very rare; we have seen it only a few times, mostly in persons who have had a prior myocardial infarction. This patient had never had an infarct.

The Problem of J-Point Depression

The development of junctional or J-point depression with the ST segment remaining in an upward slanting orientation frequently causes uncertainty in interpretation of exercise electrocardiograms. This finding in the large series of subjects with long-term follow-up reported by Robb and Marks [6] was not associated with an increased prevalence of coronary events and thus has been regarded by many as a nonischemic or perhaps innocent electrocardiographic manifestation. In our experience, J-point depression is often a stage in the development of the ischemic response. Figure 5 illustrates two treadmill tests performed 3 months apart. In the first test the patient was stopped at the 3.5 miles/hour stage by fatigue, but he was experiencing mild substernal heaviness. In the second test, performed after a 10 lb weight loss and a program of a daily walking exercise, the pattern of J-point depression finally evolved into a clearly ischemic pattern as the ST segment became horizontal in the 4 miles/hour stage and he was stopped by

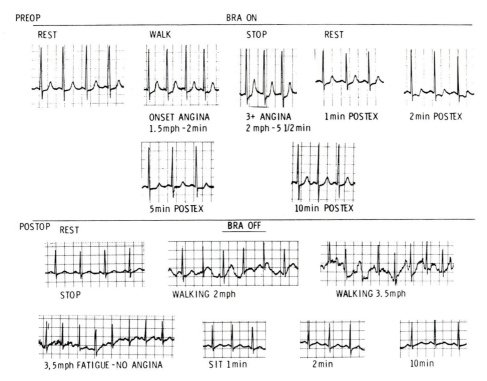

Figure 6. Electrocardiographic strips from two treadmill tests performed by a patient who had a good result from a saphenous vein bypass graft operation. In the preoperative test (top) the ischemic response emerges in the postexercise period. The postoperative test (bottom) demonstrates improved capacity and absence of ischemia, but the tracing is marred by motion artefact caused by uncontrolled motion of the bosom.

dyspnea and angina. The ischemic pattern persisted into the postexercise recovery period. Cause of the ischemia was a high grade stenosis of the left main coronary artery proximal to an aneurysmal poststenotic dilatation.

In some instances we have been able to confirm the ischemic origin of J-point depression by sublingual administration of nitroglycerin to the patient during treadmill walking and by observing the regression of this electrocardiographic pattern and disappearance of angina as walking continued at a steady pace. Thus, J-point depression may indeed be a manifestation of myocardial ischemia, but it cannot be interpreted with reliability unless confirmatory evidence can be generated: the presence of typical anginal distress, the eventual emergence of the typical ischemic pattern either during or after exercise, or the demonstrated presence of significant coronary artery obstruction.

Postexercise Ischemic Pattern

Ischemic ST depression sometimes emerges only in the recovery period after exercise. The top panel of Figure 6 shows the sequential electrocardiographic

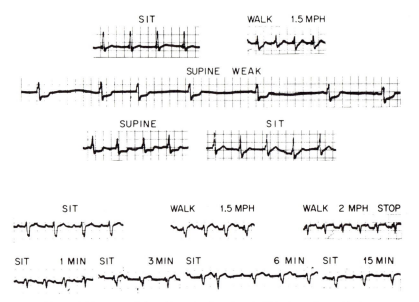

Figure 7. Electrocardiographic strips from treadmill tests performed by two subjects, one (top) demonstrating marked bradycardia in the postexercise period and the other (bottom) with first and second degree heart block.

changes during and after a standard treadmill test of a 54-year-old woman who was stopped at the 2 miles/hour stage with 3 + angina. J-point depression present at the end of exercise evolved into a clearly ischemic downslanting depression in the postexercise period, leaving no doubt about the ischemic nature of the response. Figure 6 also illustrates two other points. One is that treadmill testing is useful for assessing the results of coronary artery bypass graft surgery. The test at the bottom was conducted 3 months after a single saphenous vein graft bypassing a high grade stenosis in the left circumflex coronary artery. Great improvement in exercise tolerance is shown by completion of the 3.5 miles/hour stage of the test without ischemic manifestations. The second is that an important technology enters into the recording of adequate electrocardiographic tracings during exercise. The extensive low frequency motion artefact seen in the lower record occurred because the patient was not wearing a brassiere on the day of that test. Motion of the bosom during brisk walking causes pulling and tugging of the skin to which the electrode at the V_5 position is attached. Use of a brassiere usually avoids this form of motion artefact, as in the top record. Detailed instructions for placement and fixation of electrodes to obtain optimal recording fidelity have recently been published by the American Heart Association.[7]

In some patients with a severe ischemic response to exercise, the postexercise period is characterized by marked bradycardia. In Figure 7 a strong vagal influence is suggested by a series of junctional escape beats before the return of slow

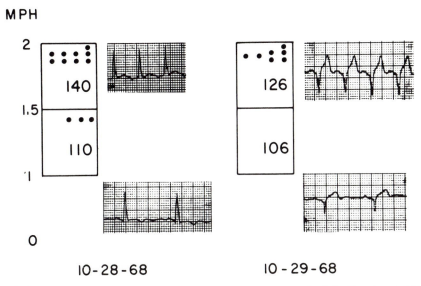

Figure 8. Treadmill test results of a man with angina and prior myocardial infarction. Inverted T wave became upright in lead V$_5$ during angina (left); ST segment became markedly elevated over the area of the infarction in lead V$_2$ (right). Reproduced with permission from Kattus AA, MacAlpin RN: Role of exercise in discovery, evaluation and management of ischemic heart disease. *Cardiovasc Clin* 1:255-279, 1969.

sinus rhythm and then a gradual reversion to a normal rate. The vast majority of bradycardiac responses do not progress to this extreme degree of slowing.

A rare cause of postexercise bradycardia is the development of atrioventricular block. The patient whose electrocardiogram is shown at the bottom of Figure 7 had first degree heart block during exercise with progressive PR prolongation in the postexercise period eventually leading to a brief episode of Wenckebach mechanism followed by recovery.

The Abnormal Resting Electrocardiogram

When a T wave inverted in the resting electrocardiogram becomes upright during exercise-induced angina the question arises whether this reversal of T-wave polarity represents an ischemic response. The problem is illustrated in Figure 8 in which the electrocardiogram of a patient with severe angina and an old anteroseptal myocardial infarct demonstrated a negative T wave in lead V$_5$ which became upright when the patient was stopped by 3+ angina. On the next day when the monitoring electrode was placed at the V$_3$ position, the site of the QS complex from the old infarct, striking ST-segment elevation was found at the time of 3+ angina. It was thus concluded that the strong influence of the repolarization potentials seen over the area of infarction were also influencing the surrounding areas. The significance of the ST-segment elevation is not entirely

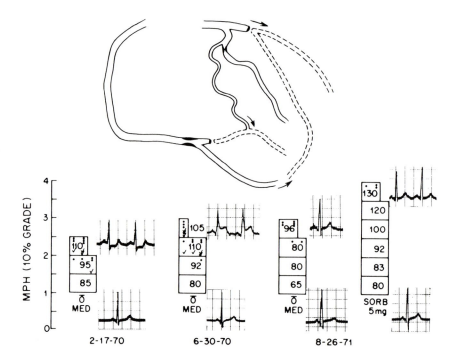

Figure 9. Sketch of coronary arterial anatomy (top) and sequential treadmill tests performed by a 50-year-old man with residual angina after an anteroseptal myocardial infarction in November 1969. In the first test, the ST segment is depressed; in the second test it is elevated; in subsequent tests, it is unchanged. O MED = no medication; SORB = premedication with isosorbide dinitrate.

clear. We have seen it in patients after infarction even though they have no symptoms with vigorous exercise. We believe that this response does not in itself indicate myocardial ischemia but is an electrical consequence of the physical forces that occur at the boundary between scar tissue and contracting myocardium as though there were a temporary ventricular aneurysm during exercise at the site of the healed infarct. Thus, reversal of T-wave polarity near the site of an old infarct cannot be regarded as reliable evidence of myocardial ischemia.

The series of tests recorded in a man with angina and a healed anteroseptal myocardial infarct (Figure 9) illustrate another perplexing problem. With all tests conducted using the same electrocardiographic lead system (negative electrode at RV_6 position and positive electrode at V_5) there was initially ST-segment depression with the occurrence of 3+ angina. Four months later, after an exercise training program there was slight improvement of exercise tolerance, but the ST segment was elevated when 3+ angina occurred. On the third test, the ST segment was unchanged with the same intensity of angina, and was also unchanged on a fourth test, when the patient had a greatly improved performance under the influence of isosorbide dinitrate absorbed from the buccal membrane. These findings suggest that the influence of ST-segment elevation from the region

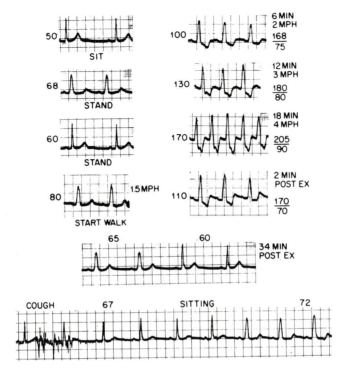

Figure 10. Electrocardiographic strips from a treadmill test performed by an asymptomatic man with rate-related left bundle branch block. He has good exercise tolerance and no coronary arterial obstruction.

of the healed infarct may have dominated the second test, whereas the subendo-cardial ischemia of the noninfarcted muscle may have dominated the first. In the third and fourth tests the two influences may have canceled out each other. It must be concluded that interruption of the normal pathways of depolarization as in myocardial infarction lead to abnormal pathways of repolarization; these alterations may distort the display of ST-segment changes during ischemia, thus rendering them uninterpretable.

Bundle Branch Block

Distortion of the repolarization pathway in bundle branch block may obscure the ischemic response or produce a deflection that resembles ischemia but is not. Figure 10 shows the development and regression of a rate-related left bundle branch block in an asymptomatic man who has excellent exercise tolerance, normal ventricular contractility and widely open coronary arteries. During exercise the ST segments are deeply depressed, but this alteration is due not to ischemia but to the abnormal pathway of repolarization secondary to the aberrant activation pathway.

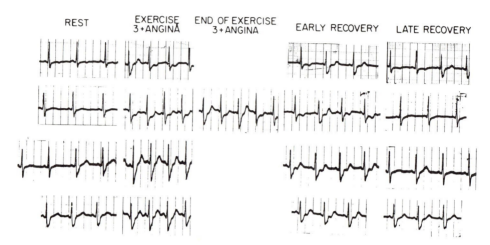

Figure 11. Electrocardiographic strips from four treadmill tests performed over a 2-year period by a man with severe angina and intermittent right bundle branch block which is at first exercise-induced but later becomes established. The ischemic response is readily seen in normally conducted beats but is obscured in the beats with bundle branch block.

Right bundle branch block also alters repolarization and thereby may obscure the ischemic effect on the ST segment. In Figure 11 a sequence of treadmill runs shows intermittent right bundle branch block finally evolving into fixed right bundle branch block. During the period of intermittency the ischemic pattern provoked by exercise can be seen in the normally conducted beats but not in the bundle branch blocked beats. Later downslanting of the ST segments is seen in the postexercise segments, but the classic ischemic pattern formerly present has been obscured by the conduction defect.

False-Positive Ischemic Responses

Drug Effects—ST-segment depressions closely resembling the ischemic pattern but not caused by ischemia have been recognized. Among the most common are those due to drug therapy. Digitalis glycosides may produce a pattern [9] such as that seen in Figure 12. On the left of the illustration are a resting electrocardiogram and strips from a double Master test in which an ischemic pattern was found. The tracings are from a healthy 21-year-old woman who had been taking weight-reducing pills, among which one turned out to be digitalis presumably given for its anorectic effect. A repeat two-step test performed 2 months after discontinuation of the drug yielded a normal response.

The studies shown in Figure 13 were performed in a young physician who had experienced an episode of sharp stabbing chest pain. The dramatic postexercise ST-T–wave inversions were not associated with discomfort. The rounded configuration of the trough of the inverted T wave resembled the pattern of digitalis

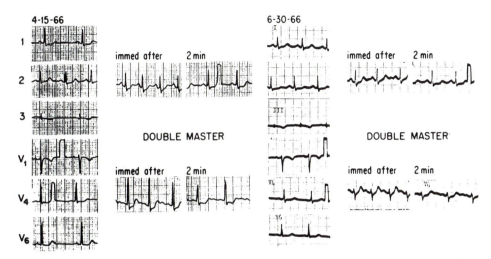

Figure 12. Electrocardiographic strips from double Master tests performed by a young woman at first when she was taking digitalis-containing reducing pills and again when she had discontinued these pills for 2 months. Reproduced with permission from Kattus AA et al: Spurious heart disease induced by digitalis-containing reducing pills. *Arch Intern Med* 122:298-304, 1968.

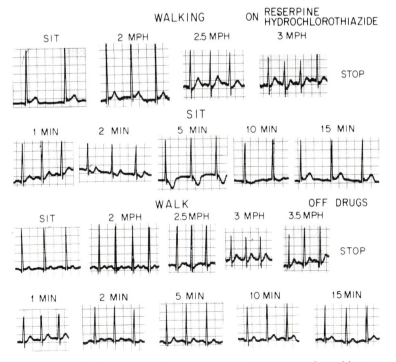

Figure 13. Electrocardiographic strips from treadmill tests performed by a young man who was taking reserpine and chlorothiazide during the first run and had discontinued these drugs for 2 months at the time of the second run.

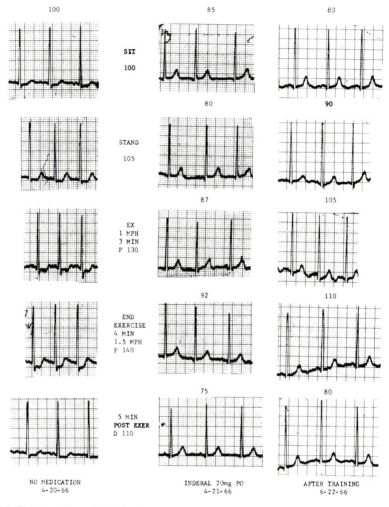

Figure 14. Electrocardiographic strips from three treadmill tests performed by a 63-year-old man who was stopped by leg claudication pain at a low work level but who had no anginal pain. During the first run, the patient was taking no medication. The second test was performed after oral administration of 20 mg of propranolol (Inderal ®) and the third after 2 months of a daily walking program of 1.5 miles/day performed in stages as permitted by leg pain. The changes in the first test are attributed to vasoregulatory asthenia. P and D = pulse rate. Reproduced with permission from Kattus AA et al: "Reversibility of Nonischemic Postural and Exercise-induced ECG Abnormalities of the T Waves and ST Segments by Beta Adrenergic Blockade," in Kattus AA, Ross G, Hall V (Eds): *UCLA Forum in Medical Sciences 13. Cardiovascular Beta Adrenergic Responses,* Copyright 1970 by The Reagents of the University of California.

effect. The patient denied taking digitalis but admitted that he had been treating himself for mild hypertension with reserpine and chlorothiazide. Several weeks after he stopped taking these agents, a normal exercise performance was elicited. It is believed that some degree of potassium depletion was responsible for the

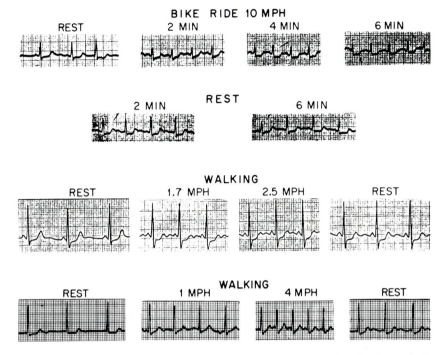

Figure 15. Top: electrocardiographic strips recorded before, during and after bicycle exercise in a patient who did not have pain during the test but stopped because of fatigue. She had marked pectus excavatum. Bottom: two treadmill tests performed by a patient with a short PR interval. The first test was conducted with the negative electrode on the manubrium and the positive electrode at the V_5 position. During the second test, the negative electrode was in the right axilla.

unusual T-wave pattern that emerged in the postexercise electrocardiogram.

Vasoregulatory Asthenia—A pattern that we have encountered at least three or four times a year is one that has often led to erroneous diagnoses of coronary artery disease. Holmgren et al [11] in Sweden have called it the syndrome of vasoregulatory asthenia. Its features are illustrated in Figure 14. The patient usually complains of ill-defined chest pains not well correlated with exertion and not usually convincing evidence of angina. The electrocardiogram often manifests ST sagging or T-wave inversion when the patient stands up. With exercise there is usually an inappropriate acceleration of the heart rate at low work levels, and the ST segments become depressed as in Figure 14. These changes are abolished or drastically modified by beta adrenergic blockade induced by propranolol. They may be entirely abolished by a period of mild exercise training such as walking 2 miles every day. Coronary arteriograms in patients with these findings disclose no obstructive disease in the blood vessels. The syndrome is believed to be due to excess adrenergic drive or perhaps excess responsiveness to adrenergic influence. In our experience it has a good prognosis, and we have never known a coronary event to occur in such a patient.[12]

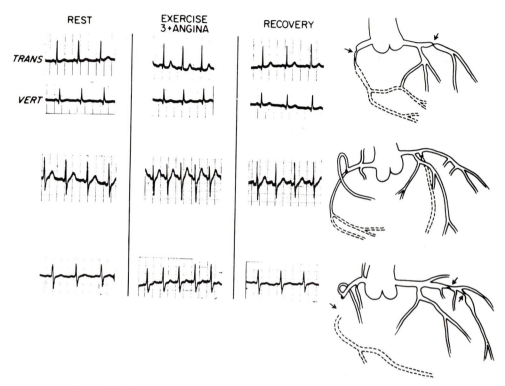

Figure 16. Electrocardiographic strips from treadmill tests performed by three patients who had no ST-segment shifts during 3 + angina. Transthoracic leads were recorded in all, and the first also had a vertical lead. All three subjects had prior inferior myocardial infarction. Sketches of the coronary arterial anatomy are at right.

Chest Deformity—Two uncommon causes for false-positive electrocardiographic responses to exercise are shown in Figure 15. At the top are strips from a bicycle exercise test in a woman who had vague chest pain. No pain was elicited during the test, and the ST-segment depression found was essentially similar before and after the exercise. Angiograms revealed normal coronary arteries. We believe her electrocardiographic pattern was due to a marked pectus excavatum. We have seen three other patients with this chest deformity who had similar electrocardiographic findings with exercise testing.

Effects of Atrial Potentials—The lower panel of Figure 15 represents a false-positive test due to the effect of the atrial repolarization wave on the ST segment. The patient, an asymptomatic woman, has a short PR interval of 0.11 second. In the first test the monitored electrocardiographic lead has the negative electrode on the manubrium and the positive electrode at the V_5 position. This lead is aligned along the axis of the P wave and tends to amplify the effects of the atrial potentials. Thus, the ST depressions associated with the amplified TA wave led to the appearance of an ischemic response. When the negative electrode was placed in the right axillary line, the lead axis became more perpendicular to the P-wave axis and the influence of the TA wave was greatly lessened in this patient with the Lown-Ganong-Levine syndrome.[13]

False-Negative Responses

False-negative electrocardiographic responses occur in about 10% of subjects who undergo testing. These patients have typical anginal distress during exercise without an accompanying pattern of ischemia on the electrocardiogram. The vast majority of these responses are found in subjects who have survived prior myocardial infarction. The tracings in Figure 16 are from three such subjects, all of whom had old healed inferior myocardial infarcts and Q waves in leads II, III and a VF but normal findings in the precordial leads. None of these patients had ST-segment deviation during exercise-induced 3+ angina. In each case multiple lead positioning did not reveal the expected changes. The coronary angiograms of these patients suggested that the angina was due to ischemia of the anterior myocardial wall since each had obstructive disease in the left anterior descending coronary system in addition to the total occlusion of the right coronary artery that had produced the previous infarcts. The reason for the failure of the ischemic electrocardiographic pattern to emerge is not apparent, but the typical character of the anginal pain, its relation to exercise and its response to nitroglycerin left no doubt about its ischemic origin. Thus in such cases when the presence of myocardial ischemia is clearly defined by other means including the resting electrocardiogram and arteriogram the classic ischemic electrocardiographic pattern is not a necessary component of a valid exercise test for exercise tolerance. In this situation the anginal symptom can be taken at face value even though the electrocardiographic proof is lacking.

Conclusions

This discussion has been concerned with the recognition of ischemic electrocardiographic responses as they are elicited by exercise testing under controlled conditions. Such changes have to do with the form of the depolarization and repolarization phases of the cardiac action potentials. The extensive problem of cardiac dysrhythmias as they are provoked by exercise have been purposely avoided since Chapter 14 is concerned with this subject.

The conclusions that may be drawn are: (1) The exercise electrocardiogram must be continuously monitored during testing since changes may be expected from moment to moment, and (2) Good fidelity of recording must be assured by careful attention to electrode placement and fixation to avoid motion and positional artefacts. When properly obtained, the exercise electrocardiogram is a powerful diagnostic tool for identifying myocardial ischemia and assessing its severity. Accurate interpretation demands an awareness of expected pattern variations, the possibilities of false-positive and false-negative responses and the misleading effects of pharmacologic and metabolic influences.

Summary

The ischemic electrocardiographic response is characterized by ST-segment depression in the left ventricular leads. When this response is elicited by exercise and is accompanied by anginal discomfort, it constitutes powerful diagnostic evidence of the presence of coronary artery obstructive disease. The amount of exercise required to elicit the response is closely related to the extent of the obstruction. ST-segment elevation provoked by exercise rarely occurs with proximal severe stenosis in the left anterior descending coronary artery or in leads exploring the region of healed myocardial infarcts. Depression of the J point may be an ischemic manifestation reversible by administration of nitroglycerin.

The ischemic electrocardiographic response may be obscured by conduction defects as in bundle branch block and healed myocardial infarcts. False-positive ischemic responses may be encountered in patients taking digitalis glycosides or potassium-depleting drugs, or in patients with hyperadrenergic states, pectus excavatum or short PR intervals.

This study was supported by U.S. Public Health Service Grants HE08470 and HE11634 from the National Heart and Lung Institute, National Institutes of Health, Bethesda, Maryland, and the Reschke-Binnay Memorial Research Fund and the Beaumont Foundation, Los Angeles, California.

References

1. Feil H, Siegel ML: Electrocardiographic changes during attacks of angina pectoris. *Amer J Med Sci* 175:255-261, 1928.
2. Master AM, Friedman R, Dack S: The electrocardiogram after standard exercise as a functional test of the heart. *Amer Heart J* 24:777-793, 1942.
3. Kattus AA, Alvaro AB, MacAlpin RN: Treadmill exercise tests for capacity and adaptation in angina pectoris. *J Occup Med* 10:627-635, 1968.
4. Smokler PE, MacAlpin RN, Alvaro AB, et al: Reproducibility of a multi-stage near maximal treadmill test for exercise tolerance in angina pectoris. *Circulation* 48:346-351, 1973.
5. Prinzmetal M, Kennamer R, Merliss R, et al: Angina pectoris. I: A variant form of angina pectoris. *Amer J Med* 27:375-388, 1959.
6. Robb GP, Marks HH: Postexercise electrocardiogram in arteriosclerotic heart disease. *JAMA* 200:918-926, 1967.
7. *Exercise Testing and Training of Apparently Healthy Individuals: A Handbook for Physicians*, pp 19-20, New York: American Heart Association, 1972.
8. Kattus AA, MacAlpin RN: Role of exercise in discovery, evaluation and management of ischemic heart disease. *Cardiovasc Clin* 1:255-279, 1969.
9. Kawal C, Hultgren HN: The effect of digitalis upon the exercise electrocardiogram. *Amer Heart J* 68:409-420, 1964.
10. Kattus AA, Biscoe BW, Dashe AW, et al: Spurious heart disease induced by digitalis-containing reducing pills. *Arch Intern Med* 122:298-304, 1968.
11. Holmgren A, Jonsson B, Levander M, et al: ECG changes in vasoregulatory asthenia and the effect of physical training. *Acta Med Scand* 165:259-271, 1959.
12. Kattus AA, MacAlpin RN, Alvaro AB: "Reversibility of Non-ischemic Postural and Exercise-induced ECG Abnormalities of the T Waves and ST Segments by Beta Adrenergic Blockade," in Kattus AA, Ross G, Hall V (Eds): *UCLA Forum in Medical Sciences 13. Cardiovascular Beta Adrenergic Responses*, pp 245-264, Los Angeles: University of California Press, 1970.
13. Lown B, Ganong WF, Levine SA: Syndrome of short P-R interval, normal QRS complex and paroxysmal rapid heart action. *Circulation* 5:693-706, 1952.

12

Computer Analysis of the Exercise Electrocardiogram

C. Gunnar Blomqvist, MD

Diagnostic analysis of the exercise electrocardiogram (ECG) is often a difficult task and there is usually a large variation between inter-observer and intra-observer interpretation.[1] Computer analysis methods offer attractive solutions to several technical problems and may produce significant gains in terms of diagnostic power. The following review considers measurement techniques, including methods for noise reduction, computer-based quantitative studies of the normal and abnormal exercise response, and diagnostic performance.

Measurement Methods

A significant portion of the observer variation in diagnostic interpretation can be attributed to the relatively poor technical quality of many ECG's recorded during exercise. It is difficult to obtain a noise-free recording even if great care is taken in the selection of electrodes and in the preparation of electrode sites. The average (root mean square) noise level in ECG's recorded during moderately heavy exercise approaches 30 μV with much larger peaks.[2] Computer processing as such does not eliminate measurement problems related to noise. On the contrary, analysis programs are generally more sensitive to noise than is the human reader. Preprocessing to significantly reduce the magnitude of unwanted extracardiac potentials, ie, transients associated with skeletal muscle activity and motion in the skin-electrode interphase, is therefore essential; effective methods have been developed.

Experienced human readers rely on a complex set of rules for wave recognition and amplitude measurements in noisy ECG's. The process is rarely defined in detail but often includes computation of rough averages and/or selection of typical or representative waveforms for measurement after a comparison of actual waveforms with expected waveforms. Although no direct attempts have been made to mimic this approach, the basic elements have all been utilized in computer programs.

Averaging of the ECG signal has proved an excellent method for noise reduction.[3-6] Summing the ECG over several cycles after careful alignment will eventually attenuate the extracardiac potentials, since they have no consistent time-amplitude relation to the ECG. The ECG signal/noise amplitude ratio improves by a factor equal to the square root of the number of beats included in the average. With the addition of each new beat, random noise is reduced and the ECG signal is reinforced. Averaging of 100 beats is likely to reduce the noise level to one-tenth of the amount present in the raw recording.

Use of averaging theoretically implies a steady state over the period of data collection. This condition is rarely completely satisfied, but the ECG response to exercise during a standard multilevel test develops gradually in both normal subjects and in patients with heart disease. Short-term variations are likely to be obscured by averaging, but their clinical significance is unknown.

Significant errors may be caused by improper alignment in time before averaging, inclusion of atypical beats (eg, premature beats with aberrant QRS and ST-T), beats with unusually large artifacts, or transient noise mistakenly identified as an ECG complex. Sophisticated procedures are available for precise alignment of beats and selective averaging.[7-10] Each new beat is stored temporarily in computer memory, characterized by multiple measurements and then classified as conforming to the typical or dominant pattern before being included in the average. Cross-correlation has proved to be a useful method for both classification and precise superimposition of beats.

Other methods for noise reduction have been used, but to a lesser extent. Computation of a *median* rather than an average waveform [11] has theoretical advantages. It may more closely approximate the approach of the human reader, but is often more cumbersome in terms of computation. Simple *filtering, ie,* elimination of components with a higher or lower frequency content than the signal to be analyzed, is a common processing technique, but is not applicable to the exercise ECG. The ECG and the noise have similar frequency spectra.[12] The introduction of filters to remove noise would inevitably cause significant loss of ECG information. The only exception is a narrow band-pass filter specifically designed to remove 60 cycles per second interference.

Effective noise reduction by a combination of selective averaging and optimal logical procedures for wave recognition makes it possible to define onset and offset of P, QRS and T with an error of less than 20, 15 and 30 msec, respectively, in more than 95% of ECG's recorded with a rate of amplitude measurement (analogue-to-digital conversion rate) of 200 per second in each lead. The precision of amplitude measurement is greater than 0.25 μV, corresponding to 0.25 mm at standard ECG sensitivity.[13]

TABLE I

Relation Between Heart Rate and ST-T Amplitudes at Rest and During Exercise

Measurement		Intercept (a) μV	Slope (b)	r	SEE (μV)
ST 1	X	108	-1.12	0.74	34
	Y	90	-0.84	0.67	32
	Z	-47	0.29	0.28	33
ST 2	X	94	-0.89	0.65	35
	Y	77	-0.69	0.61	31
	Z	-90	0.39	0.31	40
ST 3	X	94	-0.75	0.54	40
	Y	73	-0.57	0.50	33
	Z	-109	0.41	0.27	49
ST 4	X	106	-0.65	0.42	47
	Y	81	-0.51	0.43	37
	Z	-130	0.40	0.21	61
ST 8	X	384	-0.88	0.25	114
	Y	221	-0.69	0.28	73
	Z	-277	0.30	0.06	159

Linear regression with heart rate as independent variable, ST amplitude (μV) = a + b · heart rate. Based on 404 ECG's recorded in 56 normal men, age 23 to 62. ST 1, 2, etc, denote Frank lead amplitudes at points at 1/8, 2/8, etc, of the total interval between end of QRS and peak T. Positive polarity for lead X left, Y inferior, and Z posterior. Adapted with permission from Simoons.[10, 15]

Characterization of the Normal and Abnormal ECG Response to Exercise

Normal Response—Sjöstrand [14] demonstrated in an early quantitative study that normal ST and T amplitudes as measured by conventional techniques are closely related to heart rate during exercise. His findings have been confirmed and extended by a series of computer-based investigations of the normal exercise response.[4-6, 15-17] Vector lead systems have been used extensively during these studies. Their combined results provide a detailed description of the effects of exercise on all major components of the normal ECG. Quantitative information on the ECG response to maximal exercise in several groups of normal subjects has also been obtained by Bruce et al [18-21] utilizing analog computation of polar vector coordinates.

PR and QT intervals decrease linearly with increasing heart rates.[4, 15] Changes in *QRS duration* have been reported, but their significance is questionable. The magnitude is small [4, 15, 16] and the precise definition of the offset of QRS, *ie*, the QRS-ST junction, is difficult.

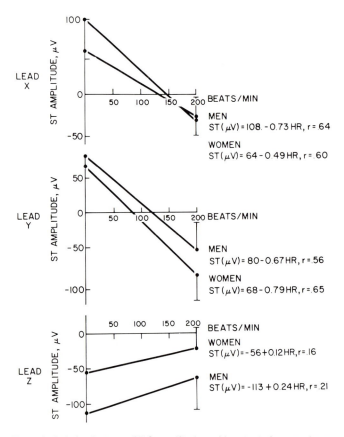

Figure 1. Relation between ST 2 amplitude and heart rate in normal men and women. ST 2 amplitudes are measured at 2/8 the interval between end of QRS and peak T. Linear regression analysis of 528 Frank lead ECG's recorded at rest and during exercise in 65 normal men and 45 normal women, age 18 to 29 years. Data from Blomqvist CG, Dunn RA, Pipberger HV, et al: Heart rate, sex, and QRS amplitude as determinants of normal ST amplitudes during exercise (abstract). *Circulation* 54 (suppl II):11, 1976.

Mean *P-wave* magnitude increases progressively with exercise without major changes in spatial orientation.[15, 16, 18] Rautaharju et al [16] found an increase in amplitude predominantly of the initial portion of the P wave, suggesting right atrial overload. A recent study from our laboratory [22] using a different reference level for amplitude measurements demonstrated changes in the terminal P wave toward a pattern of left atrial overload which is more consistent with the normal hemodynamic response to exercise.

The *mean QRS vector* shows a progressive shift to the right, superiorly, and, to a smaller extent, posteriorly.[4, 15, 23] The rightward-superior displacement is particularly prominent during the terminal portion of QRS. Spatial magnitude of the mean QRS vector decreases slightly.

With increasing heart rates, *ST-T changes*, with reference to the level of the PR segment, parallel the QRS changes. The correlation between heart rate and ST amplitudes is strongest during the early part of the ST segment in leads X (left-to-right) and Y (vertical).[10, 15, 25] Representative data are presented in Table I and Figure 1. The magnitude of the mean normal ST-segment vector at rest is small and is directed to the left, inferiorly and anteriorly. Increasing heart rates during exercise are associated with a progressive displacement to the right, superiorly, and to a lesser degree, posteriorly.

The effect of heart rate on *T-wave* amplitudes is relatively small with a slight rightward and superior T-vector displacement.

The results of cross-sectional studies of the effect of age on the normal ECG response [4, 18-21] are difficult to evaluate since it is practically impossible to exclude subclinical coronary heart disease in the older age groups. A recent study from our laboratory [25] has clearly demonstrated that *sex* is an important determinant of normal ST amplitudes at rest and at all levels of exercise. There are also differential spatial effects. ST amplitudes are lower in women at rest in leads X, Y and Z. Differences between mean values are abolished with increasing heart rates in lead X, but increase in lead Y. This may have important diagnostic implications, since common monitor leads include a significant vertical or Y component (Figure 1). Studies of the normal ST segment during exercise have demonstrated that the conventional criteria for abnormality, which assume a mean normal ST amplitude of zero irrespective of lead and heart rate and a maximal deviation of 1 mm or 0.1 mV in any direction, are inadequate. They represent an oversimplification and disregard the spatial distribution of the normal ST vector and the important effects of heart rate and sex.

Abnormal Response—Several studies based on computer-assisted evaluation of multiple leads have provided quantitative information on the ECG response to exercise in patients with verified coronary artery disease.[4, 8, 9, 20, 23-28] Orthogonal lead systems have been used extensively. The characteristic ischemic response in patients with normal ECG at rest consists of a progressive displacement of the ST segment to the right, superiorly and posteriorly. These changes are directionally similar to the normal response, but the magnitude tends to be greater at all heart rate levels. The larger magnitude of the changes in patients also applies to the middle and late portions of the ST segment. This results in abnormal ST vectors oriented to the right, superiorly and posteriorly. The correlate of this distribution is a variable degree of horizontal ST depression in the standard 12 leads (excluding a VR). Mean normal vectors during the late portion of the ST segment tend to remain leftward and anterior. The direction of the typical ischemic response closely parallels the electrical axis of lead V_5 and its variants with the negative electrode placed over the manubrium or in a right infrascapular or infraclavicular position. Quantitative spatial data are in agreement with the empirical selection of V_5-type leads for most single-lead exercise systems.

The exercise response in unselected groups of patients with angiographic

ST 2 DURING EXERCISE, HEART RATE <140
PATIENTS WITH ASHD vs. NORMAL SUBJECTS

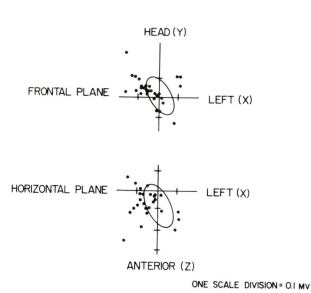

ONE SCALE DIVISION = 0.1 MV

Figure 2. Spatial distribution of normal and abnormal ST amplitudes. Spatial distribution of ST 2 amplitudes (measured at 2/8 of the interval between the end of QRS and peak T) during exercise in patients with arteriosclerotic heart disease (ASHD), *ie*, angiographic evidence of coronary disease. The ellipses describe the 95% confidence limits of the ST distribution in a series of 50 normal subjects, age range 18 to 29. Note that the points representing individual ST vectors in patients are scattered around the normal area. The anterior displacement of the mean normal ST vector is also readily apparent.

evidence of coronary artery disease, including patients with abnormal ECG at rest, is much more variable (Figure 2). The abnormal ST vectors form a scatter around the normal region. This corresponds to a wide variety of combinations of ST depression and ST elevation in standard leads. Several attempts have been made to relate the spatial distribution of the abnormal ST to specific anatomical data on the distribution of arterial lesions.[9, 10, 15, 25] The combined results suggest that the most common ischemic pattern with a rightward-superior-posterior displacement has no specific anatomical correlate. ST displacement anteriorly, inferiorly or to the left is usually associated with anterior, inferior or lateral transmural scars and wall motion abnormalities. Abnormal Q waves are usually present, but similar ST displacement conforming to the anatomical localization of the ischemic lesion is sometimes seen in patients without evidence of transmural infarction and a severe proximal stenosis of a major artery is usually present. It therefore seems likely that the common rightward-superior-posterior displacement reflects diffuse subendocardial ischemia and that leftward, inferior or anterior displacement is a sign of transmural ischemia in the corresponding area of the myocardium.

Computer-Assisted Diagnostic Evaluation

Conventional analysis methods require simple diagnostic rules as exemplified by the standard criteria for myocardial ischemia. Computer programs can easily accommodate multiple measurements and complex sets of criteria. A wide range of measurements and combinations of measurements derived from single and multiple leads have also been utilized. Univariate computer analysis methods based on single leads include measurement of a single ST-segment amplitude at a fixed interval from a QRS reference point [5] and evaluation of the integral of the negative portion of the ST segment.[11] The standard combination of amplitude and slope has also been translated into computer programs with quantitation of both variables [6] and derivation of a combined slope-amplitude index.[29] Multivariate analysis methods were introduced at an early stage,[4] but have been explored only to a limited extent.[10, 28] Proper assessment of their diagnostic potential requires very large well-defined groups of patients and normal subjects but superior performance has been demonstrated in the analysis of the ECG at rest.[28, 30, 31]

Comparative evaluation of diagnostic methods and criteria is a complex task. Two recent monographs from Holland by Ascoop [9] and Simoons [10] included extensive comparisons of criteria proposed by others as well as exploration of new techniques. Both authors carefully defined their patient groups and included angiographic studies. Ascoop [9] concluded that criteria based on the direction of instantaneous ST vectors (derived from Frank lead measurements), measurements of ST integrals and ST slope yielded a combined diagnostic gain (sensitivity and specificity) of 35, 13 and 36%, respectively, as compared to conventional visual analysis. Simoons [10] also reported that computer analysis improved diagnostic performance. The best results were obtained with a combination of two ST amplitudes from lead X, selected on the basis of linear discriminant analysis and normalized with respect to heart rate. This method increased sensitivity from 50% with visual analysis to 84% without loss in specificity. Use of other computer-based measurements, including ST-time integrals, various ST amplitudes at fixed and time-normalized intervals after the QRS, ST slopes and Chebyshev ST waveform vectors,[28] was also associated with improved performance relative to visual methods, but the gains were smaller.

Criteria for analysis of the exercise response in patients with abnormal ECG at rest remain tentative.[10]

Summary

Progress in the area of computer-assisted interpretation of the exercise ECG has been slow but significant. Highly effective methods for noise reduction and precise measurement of amplitudes and durations of waves have been developed. Detailed quantitative information on the normal and abnormal ECG response to exercise has been obtained. Recent objective evaluations of computer-based methods have demonstrated increased diagnostic power compared to visual analysis. It is likely that further gains can be realized with systems based on multivariate analysis and consideration of known determinants of the normal ST segment during exercise.

References

1. Blackburn HW, Blomqvist CG, Freiman A, et al: The exercise electrocardiogram—differences in interpretation. Report of a technical group on exercise electrocardiography. *Amer J Cardiol* 21:871-880, 1968.
2. Rautaharju PM, Friedrich H, Wolf H: "Measurement and Interpretation of Exercise Electrocardiograms," in Shepherd RJ (Ed): *Frontiers of Fitness*, pp 295-315, Springfield, Illinois: Charles C Thomas, 1971.
3. Rautaharju PM, Blackburn H: The exercise electrocardiogram. Experience in analysis of "noisy" cardiograms with a small computer. *Amer Heart J* 69:515-520, 1965.
4. Blomqvist CG: The frank lead exercise electrocardiogram. A quantitative study based on averaging technique and digital computer analysis. *Acta Med Scand* 178(suppl 440):1-98, 1965.
5. Bruce RA, Mazzarella JA, Jordan JW Jr, et al: Quantitation of QRS and ST segment responses to exercise. *Amer Heart J* 71:455-466, 1966.
6. McHenry PL, Stowe DE, Lancaster MC: Computer quantitation of the S-T segment response during maximal treadmill exercise. *Circulation* 38:691-701, 1968.
7. Brody DA: "The Laboratory Computer in Electrocardiography," in Caceres CA, Dreifus LS (Eds): *Clinical Electrocardiography and Computers*, p 401, New York: Academic Press, 1970.
8. Wolf H, MacInnes PJ, Stock J, et al: Computer analysis of rest and exercise electrocardiograms. *Comput Biomed Res* 5:329-346, 1972.
9. Ascoop CA: ST forces during exercise. Thesis, Groningen, The Netherlands.
10. Simoons ML: Computer-assisted interpretation of exercise electrocardiograms. Thesis, Utrecht, The Netherlands.
11. Sheffield LT, Holt JH, Lester FM, et al: On-line analysis of the exercise electrocardiogram. *Circulation* 40:935-944, 1969.
12. Winter DA, Rautaharju PM, Wolf HK: Measurement and characteristics of over-all noise content in exercise electrocardiograms. *Amer Heart J* 74:324-331, 1967.
13. Rautaharju PM, Warren J, Wolf HK: "Computer Analysis of Orthogonal and Multiple Scalar Lead Exercise Electrocardiograms," in Zywietz C, Schneider B (Eds): *Computer Application in ECG and VCG Analyses*, p 517, Amsterdam: North Holland Publishing Company, 1973.
14. Sjöstrand T: The relationship between heart frequency and the S-T level of the electrocardiogram. *Acta Med Scand* 138:201-210, 1950.
15. Simoons ML, Hugenholz PG: Gradual changes of ECG wave forms during and after exercise in normal subjects. *Circulation* 52:570-577, 1975.
16. Rautaharju PM, Punsar S, Blackburn H, et al: Waveform patterns in Frank-lead rest and exercise electrocardiograms of healthy elderly men. *Circulation* 48:541-548, 1973.
17. Davies CT, Kitchin AH, Knibbs AV, et al: Computer quantitation of ST segment response to graded exercise in untrained and trained normal subjects. *Cardiovasc Res* 5:201-209, 1971.
18. Bruce RA, Detry J, Early K, et al: Polarcardiographic responses to maximal exercise in healthy young adults. *Amer Heart J* 83:206-218, 1972.
19. Bruce RA, Yeou-Bing L, Dower G, et al: Polarcardiographic responses to maximal exercise and to changes in posture in healthy middle-aged men. *J Electrocardiology* 6:91-96, 1973.
20. Neiderberger M, Bruce RA, Dower GE, et al: Influence of age and ischemic heart disease on spatial ST-T magnitudes at rest and after maximal exercise. *J Electrocardiology* 6:279-284, 1973.
21. Bruce RA, Dower GE, Whitkanack S, et al: Polarcardiographic responses to maximal exercise in middle-aged women. *J Electrocardiology* 7:315-322, 1974.
22. Ahmad M, Blomqvist CG: P wave changes during exercise in normal subjects and in patients with hemodynamic evidence of left atrial overload. *J Electrocardiology*, to be published.

23. Smith RF, Wherry RJ: Quantitative interpretation of the exercise electrocardiogram. Use of computer techniques in the cardiac evaluation of aviation personnel. *Circulation* 34:1044-1055, 1966.
24. Blomqvist CG, Bergman SA, Hemming C, et al: "ST and T Wave Abnormalities at Rest and During Exercise in Patients with Arteriosclerotic Heart Disease," in Roskamm H, Reindell H (Eds): *Das chronisch kranke Herz*, p 205, Stuttgart and New York: FK Schattauer, 1973.
25. Blomqvist CG, Dunn RA, Pipberger HV, et al: Heart rate, sex, and QRS amplitude as determinants of normal ST amplitudes during exercise (abstract). *Circulation* 54(suppl II):11, 1976.
26. Dower GE, Bruce RA, Pool J, et al: Ischemic polarcardiographic changes induced by exercise: A new criterion. *Circulation* 48:725-734, 1973.
27. Ascoop CA, Distelbrink CA, DeLang P, et al: Quantitative comparison of exercise vectorcardiograms and findings at selective coronary arteriography. *J Electrocardiology* 7:9-16, 1974.
28. Dagenais GR, Villadiego RE, Rautaharju PM: "Characteristics of Normal and Abnormal Response to Exercise Quantified by Means of Waveform Vector Analysis," in Hoffman I, Hamby RI (Eds): *Vectorcardiography 3*, p 209, Amsterdam: North-Holland Publishing Company, 1976.
29. McHenry PL, Phillips JF, Knoebel SB: Correlation of computer-quantitated treadmill exercise electrocardiogram with arteriographic location of coronary artery disease. *Amer J Cardiol* 30:747-752, 1972.
30. Cornfield J, Dunn RA, Batchlor CD: Multigroup diagnosis of electrocardiograms. *Comput Biomed Res* 6:97-120, 1973.
31. Kornreich F, Block P, Brismee D: The missing waveform information in the orthogonal electrocardiogram (Frank leads). III: Computer diagnosis of angina pectoris from "maximal" QRS surface waveform information at rest. *Circulation* 49:1212-1222, 1974.

13

Use of the Exercise Electrocardiogram to Identify Latent Coronary Atherosclerotic Heart Disease

Victor F. Froelicher, MD

One of the greatest scientific accomplishments of the past two decades has been the identification of the risk factors related to the current epidemic of coronary atherosclerotic heart disease (CAD).[1-5] Analysis of the available data strongly suggests that modification of these factors might reduce the burden of this disease on our society. Because it will be some time before the primary prevention of CAD is a reality, it is advisable to evaluate screening methods for detecting asymptomatic CAD.[6,7] The relative value of techniques for identifying individuals who have asymptomatic CAD should be assessed in order to optimally direct preventive efforts to them. Also there is a necessity to evaluate individuals in whom sudden incapacitation could compromise public safety.[8] Two other concerns include the screening of individuals who plan to embark on an exercise program and the determination of the cost effectiveness of the available screening techniques. There is some hazard in beginning an exercise program,[9,10] and cost effectiveness is a practical concern in health care delivery.[11] The purpose of this chapter is to review data regarding the use of exercise testing in screening asymptomatic men for latent CAD. Three data sources will be used: (1) The United States Air Force School of Aerospace Medicine (USAFSAM) follow-up study; (2) Other follow-up studies; and (3) Coronary angiographic data from USAFSAM.

United States Air Force School of Aerospace Medicine Follow-up Study

At USAFSAM, maximal treadmill testing has been routinely performed in a consistent fashion on all consultation patients since 1965. A population of

1,390 asymptomatic USAFSAM aircrewmen who were evaluated from 1965 to 1968 and did not have any of the known causes for false-positive treadmill test were selected.[12, 13] Individuals with bundle branch block, Wolf-Parkinson-White syndrome, and valvular heart disease were among those excluded. At the time of evaluation their age range was 20 to 54 with a mean of 38 years. Ten percent had an abnormal exercise ST-segment response to maximal treadmill testing. They were identified in 1973 for a mean follow-up period of 6.3 years. Over the follow-up period, 3.3% of them developed an end point for CAD. Accepted end points for CAD included angina, acute myocardial infarction and sudden death. Abnormal coronary angiographic findings in asymptomatic men or autopsy findings of CAD in subjects who died of other causes were not used as end points. During evaluation in addition to other studies, a Master "2-step" exercise test was performed.

Methods

The following is a description of the methods used at USAFSAM as performed in the past and as currently modified. During the time of the follow-up study, the Balke-Ware protocol was used.[14, 15] Recently a shorter maximal treadmill test protocol has been adopted.[16, 17] Both protocols are shown in Figure 1. The 3.3 mile per hour constant speed has been used because of favorable experience with it for many years and because the constant speed helped to optimize the gathering of electrocardiographic data. The protocol was modified to 3-minute stages with 5% increases in grade mainly to shorten testing time after it was demonstrated that the physiological responses were comparable.

In the 1960's at USAFSAM, a standard 12-lead electrocardiogram (ECG) was obtained in the postexercise period in addition to bipolar lead CC_5. Obtaining

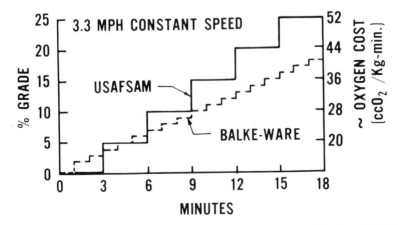

Figure 1. The Balke-Ware treadmill protocol and the subsequent modification (USAFSAM) to shorten testing time. The constant 3.3 mph speed is excellent for ECG signal gathering and the consistent increments in grade facilitate estimation of aerobic capacity.

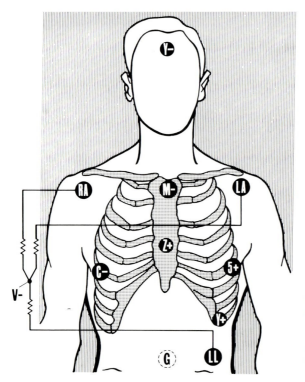

Figure 2. Placement of the silver foil or silver chloride pellet fluid-column adhesive electrodes for comparison of V$_5$ using Wilson's central terminal to left ventricular bipolar leads and for 3-dimensional computer ST-vector analysis.

the 12-lead ECG postexercise has been discontinued recently and bipolar inferior-superior and anterior-posterior leads have been included. The placement of the electrodes is shown in Figure 2. This electrode array makes possible comparison of multiple bipolar leads to V$_5$ using Wilson's central terminal as well as using three-dimensional techniques for computer ECG analysis. Using these techniques, bipolar lead CC$_5$ has been verified as comparable to V$_5$.[13, 18] Three-dimensional analysis would appear to solve the problem of how many electrodes to use since the entire repolarization process can be viewed spatially. Over 95% of the heart's electrical activity exists on a plane in space, called the eigenplane.[19] Using computer techniques, this plane can be reconstructed from three-dimensional leads and repolarization can be analyzed directly on this plane (Figure 3).

Subjects were encouraged to perform a maximal effort and the test was not stopped unless serious abnormalities occurred (Figure 4). In the recovery period ECG tracings were recorded with the subject supine for at least 8 minutes. The exercise ECG records were carefully reinterpreted and coded for the pattern and degree of ST-segment change and the leads involved.[20] Horizontal or downward sloping ST-segment depression of 0.1 mv or more in relation to the PR segment during or after exercise was considered an abnormal response. ST-

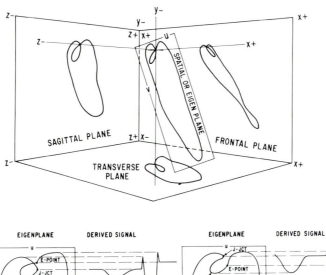

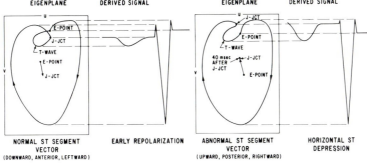

Figure 3. The top illustration is the spatial plane or eigenplane that contains 95% of the electrical energy of the heart. The eigenplane can be isolated by computer techniques, spatial ST-segment vectors constructed, and an optimal ECG signal derived. The bottom two illustrations show how normal and abnormal ST-segment changes are represented in this manner.

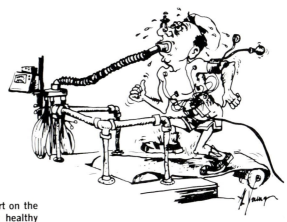

Figure 4. Example of the maximal effort on the treadmill of asymptomatic, apparently healthy aircrewmen during evaluation at USAFSAM.

TABLE I

Number, Mean Age and Incidence of Coronary Events in the
Groups of Asymptomatic Men in the USAFSAM Follow-up Study

Group	#	Mean Age (S.D.)	Incidence of CAD over the Follow-up Period
Astro	214	31 (2)	0%
Normal	710	37 (8)	1.0%
HBP	123	40 (7)	4.9%
NSTWC	186	41 (7)	4.3%
NSSTC	94	43 (7)	8.5%
CAD	63	46 (4)	27.0%
All	1390	38 (8)	3.3%

segment depression of 0.05 mv or more in the conventional leads after the Master "2-step" exercise test was interpreted as an abnormal response.

Subgroups

The medical records from the evaluations of the men were carefully reviewed and the men were placed into one of six groups according to the following order. The first group were those with probable CAD. Although they were totally asymptomatic at the time of evaluation, these were men who had either a history of symptoms consistent with CAD or who developed Q waves on serial ECG's. The second group were men with nonspecific ST-segment changes (NSSTC). They developed a serial change from a normal resting ECG to one showing minimal ST-segment depression. The third group were aircrewmen with nonspecific T-wave changes (NSTWC). They developed a serial change from a normal resting ECG to an ECG showing low amplitude T waves or rarely flat or inverted T waves. The fourth group were hypertensives (HBP). These were untreated labile hypertensives or mild essential hypertensives who did not fit into any of the prior groups. The fifth group were normal subjects. These were men referred for evaluation of possible minor medical, ophthalmological, psychiatric, otolaryngologic or flying problems. On routine evaluation, including history, physical examination, X rays, and resting electrocardiogram, they were considered free of any cardiovascular abnormality. The sixth group (Astro) included astronauts, test pilots and others referred for medical evaluation before entry into special projects who after routine evaluation were considered free of any cardiovascular abnormality.

Table I shows the number, age and incidence of CAD which occurred over the follow-up period in each of the six groups. Over one-half of the men were in

TABLE II

Calculation of Sensitivity, Specificity, Relative Risk and Predictive Value

$$\text{Sensitivity} = \frac{TP}{TP + FN} \times 100 \qquad \text{Relative Risk} = \frac{\dfrac{TP}{TP + FP}}{\dfrac{FN}{TN + FN}}$$

$$\text{Specificity} = \frac{TN}{FP + TN} \times 100 \qquad \text{Predictive value} \atop \text{of an abnormal} \atop \text{test} = \frac{TP}{TP + FP} \times 100$$

TP = true positives or those with abnormal test and disease
FN = false-negatives or those with normal test and with disease
TN = true negatives or those with normal test and no disease
FP = false-positives or those with abnormal test and no disease

the normal and Astro groups. The incidence of CAD in each group varied suggesting that the grouping had diagnostic significance. However, this conclusion was weakened by the fact that the mean age of the groups paralleled the CAD incidence.

Test Performance Definitions

Table II lists the terms that are used in describing the performance of any

TABLE III

The Results of Using Maximal Treadmill Testing (MTMT) to Screen for Latent CAD in the Groups of Asymptomatic Men in the USAFSAM Follow-up Study

Group	% with Abnormal MTMT	Sensitivity	Specificity	Relative Risk	Predictive Value
Astro	1.9	—	98%	—	—
Normal	2.7	28.6%	98%	14.5	10.5%
HBP	4.1	50.0%	98%	24.0	60.0%
NSTWC	18.3	75.0%	84%	13.5	17.6%
NSSTC	50.0	50.0%	50%	1.0	8.5%
CAD	49.2	76.5%	61%	3.4	41.9%
All	10.1	60.9%	92%	14.3	20.0%

diagnostic or screening test and shows how they are calculated.[21] Sensitivity is the percentage of times a test gives a positive result when those with the disease are tested. Specificity is the percentage of times the test gives a negative result when those without disease are tested. This is quite different from the conventional use of the word "specific." The predictive value of an abnormal test is the percentage of individuals with an abnormal test who have disease. The relative risk or risk ratio of an abnormal test response is the relative chance of having disease if the test is abnormal as compared to having disease if the test is normal.

Performance of Maximal Treadmill Test

Table III demonstrates how the maximal treadmill test is performed in each of the groups. There were no CAD events in the Astro group over the six-year follow-up. The 1.9% with an abnormal treadmill test were false-positives. The test had a high relative risk in the second, third and fourth groups. In the CAD group the relative risk was not as high but the predictive value was high, *ie*, there were less false-positives. This will be discussed further in this chapter. At the bottom of the table are the results of the test in the total population.

Table IV shows how maximal treadmill testing performed in the population subdivided by age. As in many other studies, the percentage of abnormal responders increased with age.[7, 20] Over the six-year follow-up there were no CAD events in the 20 to 29-year age group, and the 3.2% with an abnormal response were false-positives. It appears that exercise testing is not a very good screening tool for CAD in men less than 30 years of age. The prevalence of significant CAD is so low that tests screening for electrical or mechanical signs of dysfunction secondary to CAD are inappropriate. The ineffectiveness of electrocardiographic exercise testing was such that it would be much better to screen

TABLE IV

The Results of Using Maximal Treadmill Testing (MTMT) to Screen for Latent CAD in the USAFSAM Follow-up Study with the Men Grouped by Age

Age Group	Incidence of CAD	% with Abnormal MTMT	Sensitivity	Specificity	Relative Risk	Predictive Value
20 to 29 (n = 253)	0%	3.2	—	96.8%	—	—
30 to 39 (n = 563)	1.4%	5.5	50%	95.1%	17.2	12.9%
40 to 54 (n = 574)	6.6%	17.6	63%	85.6%	8.0	23.8%

TABLE V

USAFSAM Follow-up Study of 1,390 Asymptomatic Men Comparing the
Results of the Double Master's Test (DM) to the Maximal Treadmill Test (TM)

Exercise Test	% with Abnormal Response	Sensitivity	Specificity	Relative Risk	Predictive Value
DM	3.7	30.4%	97%	11.2	26.9%
TM	10.1	60.9%	92%	14.3	20.0%

for factors that appear to cause or accelerate the atherosclerotic process.[22] Such risk factor screening could be performed in children and young people with the goal of preventing CAD or forestalling it in its earliest stages.[23]

Comparison to Master "2-step" Exercise Test

Table V compares the results of Master testing to maximal treadmill testing. In all of the screening studies of asymptomatic men, the sensitivity of the Master test has been roughly one-half that of near maximal or maximal exercise testing.[7, 20] Because of the relatively low yield of the Master test without signifi-

TABLE VI

Results of Four Follow-up Studies Using Maximal or Near Maximal
Exercise Testing to Screen Asymptomatic Men for Latent CAD

Study and Years of Follow-up	Sensitivity	Specificity	Relative Risk for Developing CAD with Abnormal Exercise Test	Predictive Value of an Abnormal Exercise Test
Bruce [24] University of Washington, 1969 5 years	60%	91% $\left(\dfrac{197}{216}\right)$	13.6	13.6%
Aronow [25] Long Beach VA Hospital, 1975 5 years	67%	92% $\left(\dfrac{84}{91}\right)$	13.6	46%
Froelicher [12] USAFSAM, 1974 6.3 years	61%	92% $\left(\dfrac{1232}{1344}\right)$	14.3	20%
Cumming [26] University of Manitoba, 1975 3 years	58%	90% $\left(\dfrac{438}{484}\right)$	10	25%

cant improvement in specificity or predictive value, it has a limited role as a screening test. However in certain situations, its technical simplicity and safety make it a preferable alternative to not performing any type of exercise test. The Master test is still used to screen USAF aircrewmen with serial repolarization changes on their resting ECG. When they have abnormal responses to Master testing at their local USAF bases they are scheduled for referral to USAFSAM. Several months later during evaluation at USAFSAM, approximately half of these men have normal repeat Master tests and normal maximal treadmill tests. However, a small number of such men have had coronary angiography because of a previous markedly abnormal Master response (ST depression > 0.1 mv), in spite of currently normal exercise tests, and most of them have had significant CAD on coronary angiography.

Comparison of Follow-up Studies

There has been some skepticism concerning the results of maximal treadmill testing in asymptomatic USAF aircrewmen because of the high percentage of false-positives. This is counter to clinical experience in symptomatic populations. Table VI presents the results from the only follow-up screening studies of asymptomatic men using maximal or near maximal exercise.[12, 24-26] Unfortunately, the data cannot be presented as it should be, using age-adjusted survival curves. But the values for sensitivity, specificity, risk ratio and predictive value are strikingly similar.

Limitations of Screening with Exercise Testing

Some limitations of maximal or near maximal exercise testing for screening asymptomatic men are obvious. The sensitivity of exercise testing for detecting latent CAD in the four follow-up studies ranged from 58 to 67%. Only about 60% of those who were to develop CAD had an abnormal response when they were tested. Doyle and Kinch[27] and Bruce[28] have shown that the sensitivity of exercise testing can be increased by serially testing a population. Some of those who are going to develop CAD will change from a normal to an abnormal response when retested later. However, the exact predictive value of this change has not been determined. Thompson et al[29] reported an asymptomatic pilot who had a normal coronary angiogram but whose exercise test response changed from normal to abnormal.

Sensitivity

Table VII summarizes seven studies in which exercise testing was used to evaluate patients known to have clinical CAD.[30-36] This data has been selected from studies and presents the results of those with both clinical CAD and abnormal coronary angiography. These patients have been diagnosed as having CAD by two independent techniques—clinical judgment and coronary angiog-

TABLE VII

Sensitivity of Exercise Testing (Maximal or Near Maximal) in
Patients with Clinical CAD and Abnormal Coronary Angiograms

Study	% with Abnormal Test (Sensitivity)	
Mason [30] John Hopkins (1967)	78%	$\left(\dfrac{38}{49}\right)$
Kasselbaum [31] University of Oregon (1968)	50%	$\left(\dfrac{18}{36}\right)$
Roitman [32] University of Alabama (1970)	80%	$\left(\dfrac{24}{30}\right)$
Ascoop [33] Netherlands (1971)	59%	$\left(\dfrac{26}{44}\right)$
McHenry [34] University of Indiana (1972)	82%	$\left(\dfrac{70}{85}\right)$
Bartel [35] Duke University (1974)	65%	$\left(\dfrac{216}{332}\right)$
Borer [36] NIH (1975)	33%	$\left(\dfrac{13}{39}\right)$
Total	66%	$\left(\dfrac{405}{615}\right)$

Mean of percentages = 64%

raphy. It must be assumed that reasonable methods and criteria have been used by the different investigators. The studies are listed by the year and first author and place of origin. The denominators are the number of patients with both clinical CAD and abnormal coronary angiography. The numerators are the number of patients who had clinical CAD, abnormal coronary angiography and abnormal exercise tests. The sensitivity of exercise testing ranged from 33 to 82%. Bartel et al [35] studied the largest number of patients and their sensitivity of 65% was not much different from the mean sensitivity determined from the other six groups combined (64%). Case reports of individuals who had CAD events immediately following a normal maximal or near maximal exercise test emphasize the sensitivity limitations of exercise testing.[37, 38] Interestingly, the sensitivity results from incidence or follow-up studies (Table VI) have been very similar to the results of prevalence or coronary angiographic studies (Table VII).

Specificity

As previously defined, the specificity of a test is the percentage of those without the disease who have a negative test. It is difficult to find sufficient numbers of individuals without clinical CAD and with normal coronary angiography because there are few patients catheterized who do not have clinical CAD and do not have an abnormal exercise test. Therefore it is necessary to utilize data from follow-up studies. This involves using end points from an incidence study as opposed to using coronary angiography in a prevalence study. As shown in Table VI, in the four follow-up studies in which asymptomatic men were exercise tested and then followed for the manifestations of CAD, exercise testing demonstrated a specificity from 90 to 92%. To determine specificity, the number of subjects who did not develop CAD and had a normal test were divided by all of the subjects who did not develop CAD over the follow-up period.

Predictive Value

A major limitation of using exercise testing as a screening technique has been the low predictive value of about 30%, (ranging from 13.6 to 46%) in the four follow-up studies. Only that percentage of the abnormal responders developed CAD over the follow-up period and about 70% did not. That is, 70% of the abnormal responders were false-positives; they did not develop CAD over the follow-up period. Some of the individuals with false-positive responses have CAD that has not yet manifested itself and a longer follow-up may increase the predictive value. However this does not explain the majority of false-positives. As previously mentioned, individuals with any of the known causes of false-positive responses were excluded.[12, 13] Routine screening for hyperventilation and orthostatic repolarization changes in the USAFSAM exercise laboratory has not explained these false-positives.

Angiographic Findings

Because follow-up studies have demonstrated that an abnormal exercise test in asymptomatic men has a limited predictive value but a high relative risk for CAD, coronary angiography has been offered as an elective procedure to USAF aircrewmen with an abnormal test.[39, 40] This has been done for them to possibly be returned to flying status. One hundred and eleven asymptomatic aircrewmen with only an abnormal treadmill test have been studied (Table VIII). Using lesions $\geq$ 50% as an endpoint, a predictive value of approximately 31% was found for maximal treadmill testing (ie, 30.6% of the group had lesions $\geq$ 50% in one or more coronary arteries). Approximately 70% of the abnormal responders were probable false-positive for CAD. This confirms the percentage of false-positives found in the follow-up studies. There have not been any abnormalities of their left ventriculograms or left ventricular hemodynamics to explain their abnormal exercise tests.

Table IX lists some of the possible causes of an abnormal electrocardiographic response to exercise testing. CAD is listed first since it is today's major health problem and obviously the main diagnostic objective of exercise

TABLE VIII

Results of Coronary Angiography in Asymptomatic Aircrewmen with only Abnormal Maximal Treadmill Tests Studied at USAFSAM from 1971 to 1974

#	111
Mean age (S.D.)	43 (7%)
Number without any angiographic CAD	60 (54.0%)
Number with significant angiographic lesion(s) 50%	34 (30.6%)

TABLE IX

Possible Causes of an Abnormal ST-Segment Response to Exercise Testing

1. Coronary atherosclerotic heart disease

2. Conditions and techniques causing abnormal responses not due to coronary artery disease

3. Hypothetical other causes

Normal variant	Coronary artery spasm
Cardiomyopathies	Cellular—membrane defect
Viral myocarditis	Small vessel disease
Neurogenic imbalance	Oxygen—hemoglobin dysfunction

TABLE X

Some of the Aspects and Limitations of the Use of
ECG Exercise Testing for the Diagnosis of CAD

1. Nonspecific nature of repolarization abnormalities (ST-TW)
   not only due to ischemia; ie, orthostatic,[41] hyperventilation,[42]
   eating,[43] drugs,[44] abnormal depolarization [45]

2. Repolarization abnormalities secondary to relative ischemia
   hypertrophy,[46] valvular and congenital heart disease,[47]
   excessive double product,[28] sudden high workload [48]

3. Technical problems
   inadequate recording equipment,[49] improper lead system,[28]
   imprecise interpretation [50]

testing. Other conditions such as valvular and congenital heart disease can be detected in better ways. Poor testing techniques should be avoided. The other causes listed in Table IX are hypothetical including subclinical cardiomyopathies and subclinical myocarditis. These other possible causes do not pose as significant a threat to public health as does CAD.

Table X lists some of the aspects and limitations of the use of electro-

TABLE XI

Analysis of How Maximal Treadmill Testing (MTMT) Functioned
in 52 Patients Studied with Coronary Angiography Because of
Either a Probable Myocardial Infarct or Mild Angina Pectoris

%with Abnormal MTMT	% of Those with Significant Angiographic CAD who had Abnormal MTMT (Sensitivity)	Relative Risk of Having Angiographic CAD if MTMT Response is Abnormal vs Normal	% of Those with Abnormal MTMT who had Significant Angiographic CAD (Predictive Value)
65% $\left(\frac{34}{52}\right)$	78% $\left(\frac{25}{32}\right)$	1.9 ×	74% $\left(\frac{25}{34}\right)$

cardiographic exercise testing for the diagnosis of CAD.[41-50] ST-segment depression is "nonspecific"; that is, it is not only due to ischemia related to CAD. ST-segment depression can be secondary to conditions that cause relative ischemia. As with any type of testing, technical problems can affect the interpretation. These things partially explain why an abnormal test cannot be equated with CAD.

Relationship of Predictive Value to Prevalence

Clinical studies evaluating exercise testing in hospital or clinical populations have had fewer false-positives [51] than screening studies. Also, at USAFSAM fewer false-positives and a higher predictive value were found when exercise testing a separate group of patients more likely to have CAD. Table XI shows the angiographic results in 52 patients with mild angina and a history of probable myocardial infarction who were studied, regardless of the result of their exercise tests. Approximately 63% of them had significant angiographic CAD. The predictive value of 74% is much higher than the 31% found in the asymptomatic, apparently healthy men who only had abnormal treadmill tests.

How is this difference in test performance possible? The predictive value of an abnormal test is the percentage of those with an abnormal test who have the disease. The false-positive rate is equal to the predictive value subtracted from 100%. Neither the predictive value nor the false-positive rate can be determined directly from the specificity and sensitivity of a test. Predictive value is dependent upon the prevalence of disease in the population tested. This can be easily demonstrated by a series of simple calculations.

Table XII demonstrates how a test with a sensitivity of 60% and a specificity of 90% performs in a population with a 5% prevalence of disease. As previously demonstrated these values approximate the sensitivity and specificity of maximal or near maximal exercise testing. Since 1% of the 10,000 men have

TABLE XII

Performance of a Test with a 60% Sensitivity and a 90%
Specificity in a Population with a 5% Prevalence of Disease

Subjects	# with Abnormal Test		# with Normal Test	
500 Diseased	300	(TP) (Sensitivity)	200	(FN)
9,500 Nondiseased	950	(FP) (Specificity)	8,550	(TN)
Total	1,250		8,750	

Predictive value of an abnormal test $= \dfrac{TP}{TP + FP} = \dfrac{300}{1,250} = 24\%$

False-positive rate $= 100 - 24 = 76\%$
Relative risk $= 10.4$

disease, 100 men have disease. In the middle column are the number of men with abnormal tests and in the far right column are the number with normal tests. Since the test is 60% sensitive, 60% of those with disease have abnormal tests and are true positives. The remaining 40% have normal tests and are false-negatives. Since the test is 90% specific, 90% of the 9,900 without disease are true negatives while the remainder are false-positives. To calculate the predictive value, the true positives are divided by all those with an abnormal test. Table XIII shows the performance of the test with the same 60% sensitivity and

TABLE XIII

Performance of a Test with a 60% Sensitivity and a 90%
Specificity in a Population with a 50% Prevalence of Disease

Subjects	# with Abnormal Test		# with Normal Test	
5,000 Diseased	3,000	(TP) (Sensitivity)	2,000	(FN)
5,000 Nondiseased	500	(FP) (Specificity)	4,500	(TN)
Total	3,500		6,500	

Predictive value of an abnormal test $= \dfrac{TP}{TP + FP} = \dfrac{3,000}{3,500} = 85.7\%$

False-positive rate $= 100 - 85.7 = 14.3\%$
Relative risk $= 2.8$

TABLE XIV

The Effect of the Prevalence of a Disease on the Predictive
Value and False-positive Rate of an Abnormal Response to
a Test that has a 60% Sensitivity and 90% Specificity

Prevalence (%)	Predictive Value (%)	False-positive Rate (%)	Relative Risk
1.0	5.7	94.3	12.7
5.0	24	76	10.4
10.0	40	60	8.5
50.0	85.7	14.3	2.8

90% specificity in a population with a 50% prevalence of disease. After performing the same calculations, it is obvious that using the test in a population with a greater prevalence of disease reduces the false-positive rate and increases the predictive value. Interestingly, the risk ratio declines with increasing prevalence.

Table XIV shows the predictive value and the false-positive rate for an abnormal test with a 60% sensitivity and a 90% specificity when used in four populations of differing prevalences. The values were determined as calculated in the two previous figures. It is obvious that as the prevalence of disease increases, the predictive value increases and the false-positive rate decreases. Table XV shows how a test with a 95% specificity and a 95% sensitivity functions in populations with a spectrum of prevalences of disease. Such a test would be the near perfect test and presently there is no such screening or diagnostic technique available. However, the same relationship of disease prevalence to predictive value is demonstrated, confirming that this relationship is characteristic of all tests. This is consistent with Bayes theorem and the predictive model.[52-54]

Relationship of Sensitivity and Specificity

Another important relationship is the "trade-off" between sensitivity and specificity. The more specific a particular test is the less sensitive it is. This "trade-off" is altered by adjusting the criteria for abnormal according to the application of the test. In the USAFSAM follow-up study, when the criterion for an abnormal electrocardiographic response to exercise testing was altered to make it more specific for CAD, sensitivity was lessened. If the criterion for an abnormal response was changed from 0.1 mv to 0.2 mv of horizontal or downward sloping ST-segment depression, 54% of the true positives and 30% of the false-positives by the 0.1 mv criterion would still be abnormal. Thus, using 0.2 mv or more as criterion for an abnormal response decreased sensitivity from 61 to 30% while only increasing the predictive value from 20 to 30%. This same

TABLE XV

The Effect of the Prevalence of a Disease on the Predictive
Value and False-positive Rate of an Abnormal Response to
the Nearly "Perfect" Test (95% Sensitivity, 95% Specificity)

Prevalence (%)	Predictive Value (%)	False-positive Rate (%)
0.1	2	98
1.0	16	84
2.0	28	72
5.0	50	50
10.0	68	32
50.0	95	5

type of analysis was done in the 111 men with angiographic end points. Forty-seven percent of the true positives and 33% of the false-positives had 0.2 mv or more of horizontal or downward sloping ST-segment depression. Thus, in this group as well, sensitivity was decreased by half. In contrast, computer criteria for an abnormal response such as ST integral and ST index have been designed to increase sensitivity, but it is not certain how these new criteria affect specificity.[55-57]

Time Patterns of ST Depression

Table XVI shows an analysis of the time patterns of ST-segment depression. In the USAFSAM follow-up study the relative risk for only exercise-induced

TABLE XVI

An Analysis of the Time Occurrence Patterns of ST-Segment
Depression in the Two USAFSAM Studies Screening Asymptomatic Men for Latent CAD with Maximal Treadmill Testing

Occurrence Time	140 Asymptomatic Men with Abnormal Treadmill Response in Follow-up Study		111 Asymptomatic Men with Abnormal Treadmill Response in Angiographic Study	
	Occurrence Rate (%)	Predictive Value (%)	Occurrence Rate (%)	Predictive Value (%)
Exercise only	9	23	11	8
Recovery only	36	12	42	28
Exercise and recovery	55	25	47	39
All abnormal responders	100	20	100	30.6

TABLE XVII

Analysis of Age and the Age-adjusted Risk Factors and Physiological Parameters in the 111 Asymptomatic Men with Abnormal Treadmill Response Studied with Coronary Angiography with Probability Levels of the Differences Between the Two Groups. The Risk Factors and Physiological Parameters were Analyzed by Analysis of Covariance

	Mean Age (S.D.)	Cholesterol (mg%)	Triglycerides (mg%)	Resting Blood Pressure	$\dot{V}O_2$ $\left(\dfrac{ccO_2}{kg\text{-}min}\right)$	Maximal Heart Rate
False-positive responders (n = 77)	42 (7)	228	128	131/83	35	182
	p < .001	p < .001	p < .06	p < .02	NSD	p < .06
True positive responders (n = 34)	48 (5)	262	156	139/90	34	178

abnormal ST-segment depression was 7.4, for recovery only, 4, and when occurring both during exercise and recovery, 12. Until more experience is gathered with the time patterns of ST-segment depression it must be concluded that the occurrence of ST-segment depression at any time puts an individual at increased risk for CAD. It is interesting to note the frequent occurrence of abnormal ST-segment depression at 5 minutes recovery. Approximately 80% of our abnormal responders have had abnormal ST depression at this time alone or in addition to other times.[13] This pattern occurs more often when patients are monitored in the supine position postexercise rather than in the sitting position. It is probable that the supine position postexercise increases the sensitivity of exercise testing in accordance with Laplace's law, which can be related to increased myocardial oxygen demand with increased heart volume.

Other Risk Factors

The analysis of other risk factors and treadmill performance has shown some differences between the true positives and the false-positives in the angiographic study (Table XVII). A multiple logistic probability equation has been developed using the Duncan-Walker technique[58] based on the results of coronary angiography in 325 aircrewmen.[40] This may enable the prediction of the probability of having angiographic CAD in the USAF population. Initially, the cardinal risk factors were used but additional data including the resting ECG, functional performance and arrhythmia prevalence could be used later.

Computer Application

The application of computer techniques to the ECG and exercise ECG can certainly facilitate their analysis as well as enable measurements to be made more accurately.[59] Standard visual interpretive techniques have been demonstrated to be inconsistent.[50] However the impact of computer techniques upon sensitivity and specificity are uncertain and need to be demonstrated. It is also obvious that pre-exercise resting repolarization parameters must be considered when the repolarization response to exercise is to be optimally analyzed.[60] The higher incidence of angiographic CAD in patients with both resting ST-segment depression and an abnormal treadmill test compared to those with normal resting ECG's and abnormal treadmill tests has demonstrated the importance of accurately measuring the ST segment at rest and in response to exercise.[13] Initial studies have suggested that computerized ECG analysis require new ST-segment criteria for an abnormal response.[18] The new criteria will most likely have to be defined after considering resting repolarization parameters, sex, whether measurements were taken during exercise or recovery, R-wave height, and the heart rate.

The use of additional data obtained during treadmill testing has been stressed by other investigators. This data includes maximal heart rate and blood pressure, functional aerobic capacity and the heart rate and blood pressure response to submaximal work loads.[61-63] However, the criteria for abnormality and the sensitivity and specificity of the limits set on these measurements have not been adequately determined.[64]

Summary

In summary, near maximal or maximal exercise electrocardiographic testing has a sensitivity of approximately 60% and a specificity of approximately 90% for CAD. When screening asymptomatic men with exercise testing, an abnormal response identifies a group of men at very high risk for CAD. However, the predictive value limitations are obvious and the false-positive problem must be realized. Currently, there is not a second line of noninvasive studies that can separate a false-positive exercise test from a true positive one with certainty. The consideration of risk factors may help separate them. The development of myocardial isotope scanning techniques is also promising in this regard. Also, the sensitivity limitations of exercise testing must be considered when evaluating people at high risk for CAD.

An abnormal test does not absolutely predict the presence of CAD and a normal response does not rule out CAD. In appropriate instances where coronary angiography and left ventriculography can be performed at minimal risk and when it is justified for reasons of public safety or individual well-being, these procedures can give a relatively definitive diagnosis to the apparently healthy person with an abnormal exercise test. However, at other times an individual with an abnormal exercise test should be screened for other possible risk factors for CAD, counselled in changing his lifestyle, and followed serially. Iatrogenic "cardiac cripples" can be the most common complication of screening test and should be avoided. Good clinical judgment needs to be used in conjunction with exercise testing, especially when screening for latent CAD.

References

1. Intersociety commission for heart disease. Primary prevention of the atherosclerotic diseases (abstract). *Circulation* 42:55-67, 1970.
2. Stamler J: Acute myocardial infarction—progress in primary prevention. *Brit Heart J* 33 (suppl): 145-153, 1971.
3. Froelicher VF: The dietary prevention of atherosclerosis. *Amer Fam Physician* 7:79-85, 1973.
4. Kannel WB: Some lessons in cardiovascular epidemiology from Framingham. *Amer J Cardiol* 37:269-277, 1976.
5. Keys A: Coronary heart disease—the global picture. *Atherosclerosis* 22:149-192, 1975.
6. Froelicher VF: The detection of asymptomatic coronary artery disease. Ann Rev Med 28:1-12, 1977.
7. Froelicher VF: The application of electrocardiographic screening and exercise testing to preventive cardiology. *Prev Med* 2:592-599, 1973.
8. Carruthers M: Maintaining the cardiovascular fitness of pilots. *Lancet* I:1048-1050, 1973.
9. Froelicher VF: "Does Physical Exercise Delay the Progression of Myocardial Ischemia?" in Brest A et al (Eds): *Cardiovascular Clinics*, vol 8, no 1, pp 11-31, Philadelphia: F.A. Davis, 1976.
10. Shephard RJ: Sudden death—a significant hazard of exercise? *Brit J Sports Med* 8:101-110, 1974.
11. Abelmann WH: Cardiologic manpower resources and their distribution: a challenge for the future. *Amer J Cardiol* 36:550-554, 1975.
12. Froelicher VF, Thomas M, Pillow C, et al: An epidemiological study of asymptomatic men screened by maximal treadmill testing for latent coronary artery disease. *Amer J Cardiol* 34:770-775, 1974.
13. Froelicher VF, Thompson AJ, Longo MR, et al: The value of exercise testing for screening asymptomatic men for latent coronary artery disease. *Progr Cardiovasc Dis* 18:265-272, 1976.
14. Balke B, Ware RW: An experimental study of physical fitness of Air Force personnel. *U.S. Armed Forces Med J* 10:675-688, 1959.
15. Froelicher VF, Brammell H, Davis G, et al: A comparison of the reproducibility and physiological response to three maximal treadmill protocols. *Chest* 65:512-517, 1974.
16. Froelicher VF, Thompson AJ: Letter to the Editor. *Amer Heart J* 88:534, 1974.
17. Froelicher VF, Thompson AJ, Davis G, et al: Prediction of maximal oxygen consumption: Comparison of the Bruce and Balke treadmill protocols. *Chest* 68:331-336, 1975.
18. Froelicher VF, Wolthuis R, Keiser N, et al: Two bipolar exercise ECG leads compared to V_5. *Chest* 70:530-536, 1976.
19. Pipberger HV, Carter TN: Analysis of the normal and abnormal vectorcardiogram in its own reference frame. *Circulation* 25:827-840, 1962.
20. Froelicher VF, Thompson AJ, Yanowitz F, et al: Treadmill exercise testing at the USAFSAM: physiological responses in aircrewmen and the detection of latent coronary artery disease. AGARDOGRAPH No. 210. NASA, Langley Field, Virginia 23365, 1975.
21. Epstein FH: Predicting coronary heart disease. *JAMA* 201:795-800, 1967.
22. Taylor CB, Hass GM, Ho K: Risk factors in the pathogenesis of atherosclerotic heart disease and generalized atherosclerosis. *Ann Clin Lab Sci* 2:239-243, 1972.
23. Neufeld HN: Precursors of coronary arteriosclerosis in the pediatric and young adult age groups. *Mod Conc Cardiovasc Dis* 43:93-97, 1974.
24. Bruce RA, McDonough JR: Stress testing in screening for cardiovascular disease. *Bull NY Acad Med* 45:1288-1295, 1969.
25. Aronow WS, Cassidy J: Five-year follow-up of double Master's test, maximal treadmill stress test, and resting and post exercise apexcardiogram in asymptomatic persons. *Circulation* 52:616-618, 1975.
26. Cumming GR, Samm J, Borysyk L, et al: Electrocardiographic changes during exercise in asymptomatic men: 3-year follow-up. *Canad Med Ass J* 112:578-581, 1975.
27. Doyle JT, Kinch SH: The prognosis of an abnormal electrocardiographic stress test. *Circulation* 41:545-553, 1970.

28. Bruce RA: "Exercise Electrocardiography," in Hurst JW (Ed): *The Heart*, ed 3, New York: McGraw-Hill, 1974.

29. Thompson AJ, Froelicher VF, Longo MR, et al: Normal coronary angiography in an aircrewman with serial exercise test changes. *Aviat Space Environ Med* 46(1):69-73, 1975.

30. Mason RE, Likar I, Biern RO, et al: Multiple lead exercise electrocardiography. Experience in 107 normal subjects and 67 patients with angina pectoris, and comparison with coronary cinearteriography in 84 patients. *Circulation* 36:517-522, 1967.

31. Kasselbaum DG, Sutherland KI, Judkins MP: A comparison of hypoxemia and exercise electrocardiography in CAD. *Amer Heart J* 75:759-774, 1969.

32. Roitman D, Jones WB, Sheffield LT: Comparison of submaximal exercise ECG test with coronary cineangiocardiogram. *Ann Intern Med* 72:641-647, 1970.

33. Ascoop CA, Simoons ML, Egmond WG, et al: Exercise test, history, and serum lipid levels in patients with chest pain and normal electrocardiogram at rest: comparison to findings at coronary arteriography. *Amer Heart J* 82:609-617, 1971.

34. McHenry PL, Phillips JF, Knoebel SB: Correlation of computer-quantitated treadmill exercise electrocardiogram with arteriographic location of coronary artery disease. *Amer J Cardiol* 30:747-752, 1972.

35. Bartel AG, Behar VS, Peter RH, et al: Graded exercise stress tests in angiographically documented coronary artery disease. *Circulation* 49:348-356, 1974.

36. Borer JS, Brensike JF, Redwood DR, et al: Limitation of the electrocardiographic response to exercise in predicting coronary artery disease. *New Eng J Med* 293:367-372, 1975.

37. Lintgen AB: Death from myocardial infarction after exercise test with normal result. *JAMA* 235:837-839, 1976.

38. Bruce RA, Hornstein T, Blackman J: Myocardial infarction after normal response to exercise. *Circulation* 38:552-555, 1968.

39. Froelicher VF, Yanowitz F, Thompson AJ, et al: The correlation of coronary angiography and the ECG response to maximal treadmill testing in 76 asymptomatic men. *Circulation* 48:597-604, 1973.

40. Froelicher VF, Thompson AJ, Wolthuis R, et al: Angiographic findings in asymptomatic aircrewmen with electrocardiographic abnormalities. *Amer J Cardiol* 39:32-38, 1977.

41. Friesinger G, Biern R, Likar I, et al: Exercise ECG and vasoregulatory abnormalities. *Amer J Cardiol* 30:733-738, 1972.

42. Lary D, Goldschlager N: Electrocardiographic changes during hyperventilation resembling myocardial ischemia in patients with normal coronary arteriograms. *Amer Heart J* 37:383-390, 1974.

43. Simonson E, Keys A: The effect of an ordinary meal on the electrocardiogram. *Circulation* 1:1000-1005, 1950.

44. Bruce RA: The effects of digoxin on fatiguing static and dynamic exercise in man. *Clin Sci* 34:29-33, 1968.

45. Whinnery JE, Froelicher VF, Stewart A, et al: The electrocardiographic response of asymptomatic men with left bundle branch block to maximal treadmill exercise. *Chest* 71:335-340, 1977.

46. Harris C, Aronow W, Parker D, et al: Treadmill stress test in left ventricular hypertrophy. *Chest* 63:353-357, 1973.

47. Hellerstein H, Brozan G, Liebow I, et al: Two-step exercise test as a test of cardiac function and chronic rheumatic heart disease and arteriosclerotic heart disease with old myocardial infarction. *Amer J Cardiol* 7:234-242, 1961.

48. Barnard R, MacAlpin R, Kattus A, et al: Ischemic response to sudden strenuous exercise in healthy men. *Circulation* 48:936-942, 1973.

49. Berson AS, Pipberger HV: Electrocardiographic distortions caused by inadequate high frequency response of direct-writing electrocardiographs. *Amer Heart J* 74:208-212, 1967.

50. Blackburn H: The technical group on exercise electrocardiography. The exercise electrocardiogram: differences in interpretation. *Amer J Cardiol* 21:871-882, 1968.

51. Blomqvist CG: Use of exercise testing for diagnostic and functional evaluation of patients with arteriosclerotic heart disease. *Circulation* 44:1120-1136, 1971.

52. Vecchio TJ: Predictive value of a single diagnostic test in unselected populations. *New Eng J Med* 274:1171-1176, 1966.

53. Jelliffe RW: Quantitative aspects of clinical judgment. *Amer J Med* 55:431-437, 1973.

54. Galen RS, Gambino SR: *Beyond Normality*, New York: Wiley & Sons, 1975.

55. McHenry PL, Stowe DE, Lancaster MC: Computer quantitation of the ST-segment response during maximal treadmill exercise. *Circulation* 38:691-697, 1968.
56. McHenry PL, Phillips JF, Knoebel SB: Correlation of computer-quantitated treadmill exercise electrocardiogram with arteriographic location of coronary artery disease. *Amer J Cardiol* 30:747-752, 1972.
57. Sheffield LT, Holt JH, Lester FM, et al: On-line analysis of the exercise ECG. *Circulation* 60:935-955, 1969.
58. Walker SH, Duncan DB: Estimation of probability of an event as a function of several independent variables. *Biometrika* 54:167-179, 1967.
59. Rautaharju PM, Wolff HB: "Computer Interpretation and Classification of Exercise ECG's; VCG Aspects," in Hoffman I (Ed): *Proceedings XI International ECG Symposium*, p 223, Amsterdam: North-Holland, 1971.
60. Villadiego RB, Dagenais GR, Rautaharju PM: Characteristics of frank lead ST and T waveforms in ischemic heart disease. *Circulation* 52 (abstract suppl):II-48, 1975.
61. Bruce RA: Values and limitations of exercise electrocardiography (editorial). *Circulation* 50:1-4, 1974.
62. Bruce RA, Fisher LD, Cooper MN, et al: Separation of effects of cardiovascular disease and age on ventricular function with maximal exercise. *Amer J Cardiol* 34:757-763, 1974.
63. Ellestad MH, Wan MKC: Predictive implications of stress testing. *Circulation* 51:363-369, 1975.
64. Wolthuis R, Froelicher VF, Fischer J, et al: The response of healthy men to treadmill exercise. *Circulation* 55:153-157, 1977.

14

Disturbances of Cardiac Rhythm and Conduction Induced by Exercise: Diagnostic, Prognostic and Therapeutic Implications

Anthony N. DeMaria, MD
Zakauddin Vera, MD
Ezra A. Amsterdam, MD
Dean T. Mason, MD

Disturbances of cardiac rhythm and conduction are commonly observed during exercise stress testing and may provide important clinical information on cardiovascular status. Thus, exertion-induced ectopic ventricular rhythms may be of diagnostic,[1, 2] prognostic [3] and therapeutic [4] significance in coronary artery disease. In addition, exercise stress testing has been utilized to evaluate the role of arrhythmias in patients with syncopal episodes and to assess the efficacy of antiarrhythmic therapy.[5] In this chapter we will review current knowledge of the electrophysiologic response of the heart to physical exertion and examine directions for future investigation.

Electrophysiologic Effects of Exercise

Exercise is capable of inducing a number of alterations in the electrical activity of the myocardium, the net result of which may be either enhancement or inhibition of ectopic rhythms and abnormal conduction. Derangement of cardiac electrophysiology as a response to exercise is unpredictable in an individual subject, and cardiac rhythm and conduction may vary as a function of the level of exer-

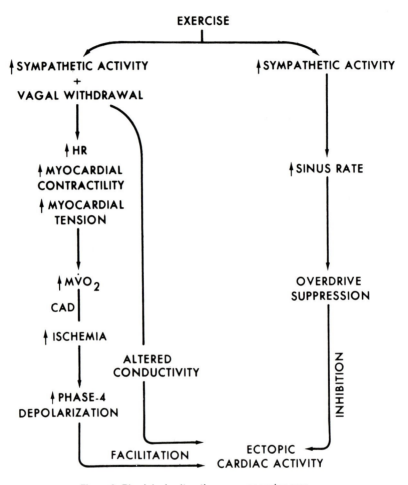

Figure 1. Physiologic alterations accompanying exercise. ↑ = increased; ↓ = decreased; → = unchanged.

tion or stress. Figure 1 illustrates physiologic alterations accompanying exercise and their possible sequelae.

Pathophysiologic Basis for Arrhythmias During Exercise—The stress of exertion frequently results in the appearance of arrhythmias not present in the resting state. The production of such arrhythmias by exercise has been attributed to heightened sympathetic tone, increased myocardial oxygen demand, or a combination of these factors. Augmented sympathetic drive to the myocardium may provoke ectopic Purkinje pacemaker activity by accelerating the rate of phase 4 depolarization at this site, enhancing its spontaneous discharge and thereby increasing automaticity.[6, 7] Increased myocardial oxygen demand, when not matched by oxygen supply, results in local tissue hypoxia. Myocardial hypoxia produces temporal dispersion of depolarization and repolarization as well as alterations in conduction velocity and thereby provides an ideal substrate for the appearance of arrhythmias related to both automaticity and reentry.[8] Thus, myocardial ischemia may act as the stimulus for the appearance of abnormalities of rhythm and conduction during stress testing.

Myocardial ischemia is a common response to exercise stress in the presence of coronary artery disease. Myocardial oxygen consumption ($M\dot{V}O_2$) is determined by heart rate, contractility and intramyocardial tension.[9] The effect of exercise upon these factors augments $M\dot{V}O_2$ and thus may result in myocardial ischemia if oxygen demand exceeds supply. This disparity is usually a consequence of the restricted flow reserve of the coronary circulation in coronary atherosclerotic disease. Such an imbalance may be related not only to elevated levels of exercise stress, but also to events in the immediate postexercise period. At this time, peripheral arteriolar dilatation induced by exercise, and reduced cardiac output resulting from diminished venous return secondary to the abrupt cessation of muscular activity, may combine to produce a reduction in blood pressure and decreased coronary perfusion while the heart rate is still increased. Thus, a pathophysiologic basis for the occurrence of arrhythmias at various points during exercise stress is indicated.

Abolition of Arrhythmias by Exercise—Although the precipitation of arrhythmias by exercise is widely recognized, abolition during exercise of ectopic cardiac activity present at rest is a less appreciated phenomenon. The ability of exercise to abolish arrhythmias present in the resting state has generally been attributed to two mechanisms, both of which are related to the sinus tachycardia resulting from vagal withdrawal and increased sympathetic stimulation accompanying exercise. Thus, sinus tachycardia may inhibit an ectopic focus before its intrinsic discharge reaches threshold potential, an example of overdrive suppression. In addition, there is evidence that rapid stimulation may result in decreased automaticity of Purkinje tissue and thus sinus tachycardia may inhibit automaticity of an ectopic focus.[10]

Spectrum of Exercise-Induced Alterations of Rhythm and Conduction

Supraventricular Arrhythmias—A wide variety of supraventricular arrhythmias may be noted in the process of stress testing. Wandering or ectopic atrial pacemakers and sinus arrhythmias are particularly common after exercise.[5] However, although 3 to 5 beat episodes of paroxysmal atrial and junctional tachyarrhythmias occurred frequently during exertion in 3,000 patients studied by Gooch,[5] sustained bouts lasting more than 15 seconds occurred in only 5 patients. Several investigators [2-5] have noted that atrial fibrillation and flutter are only rarely induced by exertion and, when they do occur, revert spontaneously. Indeed, observation of the response of ventricular rate to various levels of activity has provided an excellent method of assessing adequacy of digitalization in patients with atrial fibrillation.[11] This response could not be predicted from the resting heart rate. Finally, rare episodes of sinoatrial block and sinus arrest have been noted during stress testing, usually after termination of exercise.[5]

Conduction Defects—Alterations of cardiac conduction involving both the atrioventricular (AV) node and bundle branches may occur during the course of exercise testing. AV conduction is accelerated during exertion under normal circumstances [12] and absence of such shortening has been regarded as an abnormal response indicative of AV junctional block. In addition, the appearance of frank first degree heart block or its progression to more advanced block has also been noted in association with exercise.[2-5] Conversely, preexisting block of the AV node has been noted to decrease in this setting, a phenomenon that may be related to enhanced conduction velocity due to increased sympathetic stimulation.

Abnormalities of ventricular conduction consisting of intraventricular conduction defects and bundle branch block involving either the left or right bundle branch were observed in 8 of 733 patients undergoing stress testing.[5] Seven of these eight patients had clinical evidence of heart disease. Sandberg [2] reported on a small group of patients who manifested bundle branch block during exertion and in whom the appearance of the defect with mild effort was associated with clinical evidence of cardiac disease. In both of the latter studies the abnormalities of conduction were usually preceded by evidence of incomplete block in the resting electrocardiogram, and they appeared during exercise and disappeared after termination of the stress.

Ventricular Arrhythmias—Ectopic beats and tachyarrhythmias of ventricular origin have been frequently described during exercise testing.[13-18] Thus, ventricular arrhythmias with exertion were noted in 39% of patients by Kosowsky et al,[16] in 31 to 49% by McHenry et al,[14] in 20% by Goldschlager et al [13] and in 30% by Blackburn et al.[15] Ectopic ventricular beats were observed most commonly in the postexercise period in all but one study [15] and frequently occurred late in the recovery period. Thus, two thirds of the arrhythmias in one report [1] occurred within 2 minutes of cessation of exercise and the single death reported in a large group of patients with coronary disease occurred suddenly 4 minutes after completion of the exercise test.[13] Salvos of ventricular tachycardia were preceded by single ectopic beats in the vast majority of cases. Premature ventricular contractions occurred with increased frequency with advancing age [14] and higher levels of effort [14, 15] of the patients evaluated.

Diagnostic Significance of Ventricular Arrhythmias Precipitated by Exercise

Considerable interest has been stimulated in the diagnostic and prognostic implications of ventricular arrhythmias occurring during graded bicycle or treadmill exercise testing. Although the significance of these rhythm disturbances has not been firmly established, certain patterns seem evident on the basis of the information currently available.

Debate continues on the significance of exercise-induced ventricular extrasystoles as indicators of the presence of organic heart disease. Several early investigations [19-22] demonstrated the occurrence of ventricular arrhythmias in apparently normal persons and failed to find a correlation between ventricular ectopic beats elicited during effort and clinical evidence of cardiac disease. Sandberg [2] found that the subset of patients who demonstrated ventricular arrhythmias after light effort also manifested clinical heart disease, and Gooch and McConnell [1] related bursts of ventricular tachycardia to the presence of cardiac abnormalities. These conclusions were supported by McHenry and associates [14] who, while observing ventricular ectopy in more than one-third of apparently normal subjects, noted an even greater frequency of ventricular arrhythmias in patients with clinically evident or suspected cardiac disease. In the patients manifesting these abnormalities, ventricular ectopic beats were provoked by lighter exertion and at lower heart rates and had a greater tendency to be frequent, multifocal or repetitive. In all these studies the criteria for heart disease were based upon clinical evidence; thus, subclinical cardiac abnormalities may well have been present and undetected in the "normal" group.

Zaret et al [23] evaluated exercise-induced ventricular irritability in a group of patients undergoing coronary arteriography and found coronary atherosclerosis in 72%. Multiple vessel disease was significantly more common than in matched patients without arrhythmias. Goldschlager et al [13] compared a group of patients with ventricular arrhythmias elicited by exertion with a group of patients without such disturbances who had undergone cardiac catheterization and coronary arteriography. These investigators found significant coronary stenosis in 89% of patients with exercise-precipitated ventricular extrasystoles. In addition, they observed a significantly greater prevalence of double and triple vessel coronary artery disease and abnormal left ventricular motion in this group than in patients with coronary heart disease without arrhythmias. Provoked arrhythmias occurred more frequently during the recovery period in this study. A striking finding was the disappearance of ectopic beats during exercise stress in a high percentage of patients with significant coronary disease.

The relationship between exercise and ventricular arrhythmias in patients with coronary heart disease was also investigated by Helfant et al.[18] They observed that ventricular extrasystoles appeared or were increased in frequency with exercise in 22 of 38 patients with coronary atherosclerosis; the vast majority of these patients manifested multivessel coronary disease and ventricular dyssynergy. Importantly, 20 of the 22 patients in this study who exhibited exercise-related arrhythmias also manifested evidence of myocardial ischemia by virtue of the development of 2 mm or greater ST-segment depression on ECG. However, other investigators have not observed a similar relationship between exercise-induced arrhythmias and ST-segment depression.[17]

Although there is no question that ventricular arrhythmias may occur in the absence of organic heart disease, certain conclusions appear justified from the findings cited: (1) Ventricular arrhythmias provoked by exertion occur significantly more frequently in patients who have cardiac disease than in normal subjects; (2) Ventricular ectopic beats that occur with minor increases in heart rate, or demonstrate high frequency, multifocal pattern or repetitive firing are particularly suggestive of cardiac disease; (3) Patients with coronary atherosclerosis who have ventricular rhythm disorders induced by stress testing have a greater frequency of multiple vessel disease and abnormalities of wall motion; (4) The termination of ventricular ectopy during exertion does not indicate the absence of flow-limiting coronary atherosclerosis.

Prognostic Significance of Exercise-Induced Ventricular Arrhythmias

Of major interest is the prognostic significance of exercise-induced ventricular arrhythmias. Premature ventricular contractions manifested in a resting electrocardiogram [24, 25] or during activities [26] have been associated with an increased incidence of coronary atherosclerosis, subsequent mortality and sudden death.[15] This risk is especially prominent in patients with known cardiovascular abnormalities.[27] However, the resting electrocardiogram has a substantially lower yield than exercise electrocardiography in the detection of ectopic ventricular rhythms.[16] It would seem reasonable that ectopic ventricular beats evoked during exertion might carry serious prognostic implications and thus be of major importance in the issue of sudden death.[28] Long-term epidemiologic studies will be required to provide a definitive answer to this question. However, exercise-elicited ventricular extrasystoles have already been correlated with the coronary risk factors of hypertension and glucose intolerance as well as with ischemic electrocardiographic abnormalities and enlargement of the cardiac silhouette on roentgenographic study.[3] Indeed, in this study population, sudden death occurred in two patients with exertional ventricular irritability. That such potential disasters may be amenable to therapy is suggested by Bryson et al,[4] who reported in three patients exertional ventricular tachycardia and fibrillation which prompted coronary arteriography, revealing significant coronary atherosclerosis. Subsequently these arrhythmias were abolished by coronary artery bypass graft surgery.

Usefulness of Holter Monitoring vs. Exercise Stress in the Detection of Arrhythmias

Premature ventricular beats elicited by exertion can be evaluated either by prolonged ambulatory monitoring, a costly and time consuming procedure, or by graded exercise testing. Kosowsky et al [16] compared the sensitivity of ambulatory electrocardiographic monitoring and treadmill exercise testing in revealing ectopic ventricular activity in 81 patients with and without coronary artery disease. Of 66 patients with a normal resting electrocardiogram, prolonged monitoring was positive for arrhythmias in 27%, whereas exercise was positive in 39%. Exercise also revealed serious rhythm abnormalities that would not have been suspected by use of monitoring alone. A subsequent study from this same laboratory however, reported that ambulatory monitoring detected ventricular extrasystoles in 88% of coronary patients as compared with exercise which provoked rhythm disturbance in 56% of these patients.[17] This later study employed 24-hour as opposed to 12-hour monitoring as well as advanced techniques of analysis. However, this study revealed that ambulatory monitoring detected ventricular tachycardia in only four of seven patients who exhibited this arrhythmia in response to exercise. Accordingly, Ryan et al [17] suggested that the results of monitoring and exercise electrocardiography might reflect different electrophysiologic aspects of the myocardium. In this regard, Blackburn et al [15] demonstrated a 35% increase in the yield of premature ventricular complexes and of multiform and repetitive ventricular ectopic beats during maximal as opposed to submaximal exercise testing. Obviously, these additional arrhythmias would be detected by portable monitoring only if the patient performed activities requiring maximal exertion.

We have been impressed with the capacity of both exercise stress testing and prolonged portable electrocardiographic monitoring as means of detecting ventricular ectopic rhythms. Of 22 patients with angiographically documented coronary artery disease, 5 (23%) manifested ventricular ectopic beats on the resting electrocardiogram. Ventricular premature beats developed in 59% during exercise and were detected in 82% of the group by 10 to 12-hour portable monitoring during normal activity.[29]

Effects of Physical Conditioning on the Frequency of Premature Ventricular Complexes

The effect of physical conditioning on ectopic ventricular beats has not been definitely established. Blackburn et al [15] evaluated the response of ectopic ventricular beats to physical conditioning in 196 middle-aged, "high risk" men free of clinically manifest heart disease. These previously sedentary subjects were evaluated before and 18 months after a program of progressive exercise conditioning. Among subjects adhering well to the program there was inconclusive but suggestive evidence that the work threshold for ventricular ectopic activity was increased. This finding certainly merits further investigation.

Ventricular Irritability and Termination of Exercise Testing

In light of these data, certain practices have evolved in our laboratory concerning ventricular irritability and the performance of exercise stress testing. Thus, the presence of ectopic ventricular beats in a patient whose condition is otherwise stable immediately before study is not considered a contraindication to exercise testing. Exercise is begun slowly at low work loads and is terminated on occurrence of significant increase in frequency of ectopic beats or dangerous ventricular arrhythmias such as frequent multifocal extrasystoles, R on T phenomenon, coupled ventricular beats or runs of ventricular tachycardia. In our experience exercise testing has infrequently required interruption because of ventricular arrhythmias. Upon completion of exercise the patient is seated with legs elevated to increase venous return, and the electrocardiogram is carefully monitored for at least 6 minutes.

Summary

Alterations of cardiac rhythm and conduction occur frequently during exercise stress testing and may provide significant information regarding cardiovascular status. Exertion may induce arrhythmias as a result of sympathetically enhanced phase 4 depolarization of ectopic foci or the induction of myocardial ischemia secondary to increased myocardial oxygen demand. Exercise may abolish arrhythmias present in the resting state, an effect attributed to overdrive suppression and inhibition related to sinus tachycardia. Although a wide spectrum of electrophysiologic changes may be elicited by stress testing, ventricular arrhythmias are of primary importance. Premature ventricular contractions that are frequent, multifocal, repetitive or associated with light work loads have been particularly indicative of coronary artery disease. Exertional ventricular irritability has been observed more frequently in patients with coronary atherosclerosis involving two or more coronary vessels and accompanied by abnormalities of left ventricular wall motion. Exercise testing may have advantages over portable monitoring in the detection of ventricular arrhythmias. The mere presence of ventricular ectopic beats at rest does not preclude carefully performed graduated stress testing nor does their disappearance during effort exclude the presence of coronary artery disease.

This study was supported by Research Program Project Grant HL-14780 from the National Heart and Lung Institute, National Institutes of Health, Bethesda, Maryland.

References

1. Gooch AS, McConnell D: Analysis of transient arrhythmias and conduction disturbances occurring during submaximal treadmill exercise testing. Prog Cardiovasc Dis 13:293-307, 1970.
2. Sandberg L: The significance of ventricular premature beats or runs of ventricular tachycardia developing during exercise tests. Acta Med Scand 169:1-117, 1961.
3. Vedin JA, Wilhelmsson CE, Wilhelmsson L, et al: Relations of resting and exercise-induced ectopic beats to other ischemic manifestations and to coronary risk factors. Men born in 1913. Amer J Cardiol 30:25-31, 1972.
4. Bryson AL, Parisi AF, Schecter E, et al: Life threatening arrhythmias induced by exercise: cessation after coronary bypass surgery. Amer J Cardiol 32:995-999, 1973.
5. Gooch AS: Exercise testing for detecting changes in cardiac rhythm and conduction. Amer J Cardiol 30:741-746, 1972.
6. Vassalle M, Levine MJ, Stuckey JH: Sympathetic control of ventricular automaticity: the effects of stellate ganglion stimulation. Circ Res 23:249-258, 1968.
7. Vassalle M, Stuckey JH, Levine MJ: Sympathetic control of ventricular automaticity: role of the adrenal medulla. Amer J Physiol 217:930-937, 1969.
8. Rosen MR, Hoffman BF: Mechanisms of action of antiarrhythmic drugs. Circ Res 32:1-8, 1973.

9. Sonnenblick EH, Skelton CL: Oxygen consumption of the heart: physiologic principles and clinical implications. *Mod Concepts Cardiovasc Dis* 40:9-16, 1971.
10. Alanis J, Benitez D: The decrease in the automatism of the Purkinje pacemaker fibers provoked by high frequencies of stimulation. *Jap J Physiol* 17:556-571, 1967.
11. Gooch AS, Natarajan G, Goldberg H: Influence of exercise on arrhythmias induced by digitalis-diuretic therapy in patients with atrial fibrillation. *Amer J Cardiol* 33:230-237, 1974.
12. Lister JW, Stein E, Kosowsky BD, et al: Atrioventricular conduction in man. Effect of rate, exercise, isoproterenol and atropine on the P-R interval. *Amer J Cardiol* 16:516-523, 1966.
13. Goldschlager N, Cake D, Cohn K: Exercise-induced ventricular arrhythmias in patients with coronary artery disease. Their relation to angiographic findings. *Amer J Cardiol* 31:434-440, 1973.
14. McHenry PL, Fisch G, Jordan JW, et al: Cardiac arrhythmias observed during maximal exercise testing in clinically normal men. *Amer J Cardiol* 29:331-336, 1972.
15. Blackburn H, Taylor HL, Burtram H, et al: Premature ventricular complexes induced by stress testing. Their frequency and response to physical conditioning. *Amer J Cardiol* 31:441-449, 1973.
16. Kosowsky BD, Lown B, Whiting R, et al: The occurrence of ventricular arrhythmias with exercise as compared to monitoring. *Circulation* 44:826-832, 1971.
17. Ryan M, Lown B, Horn H: Comparison of ventricular ectopic activity during 24-hour monitoring and exercise testing in patients with coronary heart disease. *New Eng J Med* 292:224-229, 1975.
18. Helfant R, Pine R, Kabde V, Banka V: Exercise-related ventricular premature complexes in coronary heart disease. *Ann Intern Med* 80:589-592, 1974.
19. Lamb LE, Burcheil HB: Premature ventricular contractions and exercise. *Proc Staff Meet Mayo Clin* 27:383-389, 1952.
20. Master AM, Rosenfelt I: Two-step exercise test: current status after twenty-five years. *Mod Concepts Cardiovasc Dis* 36:19-24, 1967.
21. Mattingly TW: The postexercise electrocardiogram. *Amer J Cardiol* 9:395-409, 1962.
22. Sheffield LT, Holt JH, Reeves TJ: Exercise graded by heart rate in electrocardiographic testing for angina pectoris. *Circulation* 32:622-629, 1965.
23. Zaret BL, Conti CR Jr: Exercise-induced ventricular irritability: hemodynamic and angiographic correlation (abstract). *Amer J Cardiol* 29:298, 1972.
24. Chiang BM, Perlman LV, Ostrander LD Jr, et al: Relation of premature systoles to coronary heart disease and sudden death in the Tecumseh epidemiologic study. *Ann Intern Med* 70:1159-1166, 1969.
25. Blackburn H, Taylor HL, Keyes A: The electrocardiogram in prediction of five-year coronary heart disease incidence among men aged forty through fifty-nine. *Circulation* 41 (suppl I): 154-161, 1970.
26. Hinkle LE Jr, Carver ST, Stevens M: The frequency of asymptomatic disturbances of cardiac rhythm and conduction in middle-aged men. *Amer J Cardiol* 24:629-650, 1969.
27. Rodstein M, Wollock L, Guber R: Mortality study of the significance of extrasystoles in an insured population. *Circulation* 44:617-625, 1971.
28. Lown B, Wolf M: Approaches to sudden death from coronary heart disease. *Circulation* 44:130-142, 1971.
29. Amsterdam EA, DeMaria AN, Vismara LA, et al: "Lethal Arrhythmias in the Pathogenesis of Pre-hospital Sudden Death," in Gensini G (Ed): *Concepts on the Mechanisms and Treatment of Arrhythmias*, pp 29-37, Mt. Kisko, New York: Futura, 1974.

15

Exercise Testing in the Indirect Assessment of Myocardial Oxygen Consumption: Application for Evaluation of Mechanisms and Therapy of Angina Pectoris

Ezra A. Amsterdam, MD
James E. Price, MD
Daniel Berman, MD
James L. Hughes, III, MD
Kay Riggs, BS
Anthony N. DeMaria, MD
Richard R. Miller, MD
Dean T. Mason, MD

Appreciation of the pathophysiology of angina pectoris has provided a rational approach to the diagnosis and treatment of this disorder. The systematic application of exercise in evaluation of angina has played a significant role in advancing physiologic understanding of the syndrome. Exercise has been utilized not only in diagnosis but also as an objective means of assessing clinical severity and investigating the circulatory dynamics associated with angina. Relation of the latter alterations to cardiac energetics in terms of myocardial oxygen consumption ($M\dot{V}O_2$) has been of major importance in elucidating the mechanisms of angina, quantifying functional impairment and clarifying modes of therapy in this syndrome.

218

Value of Exercise Testing in Assessment of Angina

Although the symptom of ischemic cardiac pain is the most overt manifestation of the anginal syndrome, assessment of symptomatology is of limited reliability in estimating severity of the disease because of the subjective nature of the symptom and the variability of provoking factors. Use of exercise testing to determine functional status has significantly extended clinical evaluation of the patient with angina. Measurement of exercise capacity provides a reliable, quantitative index of functional impairment in angina not attainable by clinical appraisal alone. Thus, systematic assessment of exercise capacity under controlled conditions in patients with angina yields reproducible results in terms of duration of exertion required to provoke the pain of myocardial ischemia.[1] However, underlying cardiac functional capacity is of primary concern in relation to severity of the disease in angina. Although exercise ability provides a functional index in patients with angina, it does not necessarily reflect cardiac capacity. In the response of the body to external work, the relation between skeletal muscle performance and the load sustained by the heart is not always direct,[2] thereby rendering this method of limited value as a precise indicator of cardiac performance. These qualifications also pertain to maximal total body oxygen consumption ($\dot{V}O_2$ max), traditionally considered the most reliable extracardiac index of overall cardiovascular functional capacity.[3,4] This quantity, like external exercise capacity, may also vary under certain conditions in its relation to cardiac performance during exertional stress.[5,6]

Extracardiac Factors Modifying Response to Exercise—It is now appreciated that many factors can modify the cardiac response to any given physical stress and thereby alter angina-limited exercise ability without changing cardiac functional capacity.[2] Among these are reduced environmental temperature,[2] emotional stress,[7] the postprandial state[2] and the acute effects of cigarette smoking,[8] which can, in themselves, augment myocardial mechanical effort and diminish exercise capacity.

In addition, of course, conditions such as musculoskeletal or peripheral circulatory diseases that impair the function of organ systems other than the heart may significantly reduce exercise capacity. It is therefore apparent that exercise performance may be determined not only by the work load directly imposed on the skeletal muscles, but also by other ambient variables influencing the myocardium. This is exemplified by the reduction in exercise performance (decreased time to onset of angina) that accompanies reduced environmental temperature. In this setting, in which intrinsic cardiac functional capacity may be unchanged, decreased exercise performance is related to the augmented cardiac work load, indicated by the increased heart rate and blood pressure, associated with reduced temperature.[2] Similarly, the fasting state may be associated with enhanced exercise capacity in relation to onset of angina compared with exercise capacity in the postprandial state. Again, the altered performance is unassociated with change in cardiac function and is a result of the reduced work load on the heart, as determined by the circulatory response to a given physical stress, in the fasting state compared with that in the period after a meal.[2] Appropriate interpretation of the preceding results would be obscured if exercise capacity were assessed only in terms of duration of exercise before onset of angina. Thus, to the extent that extrinsic influences alter exertional capacity when anginal pain is the limiting factor, the value of this measure as a means of assessing cardiac performance is diminished.

Relation of M$\dot{V}O_2$ to Evaluation of Angina

It is apparent that an approach more closely reflecting the performance of the heart is required for meaningful evaluation of cardiac function in angina. It must encompass the distinction between external work, as entailed by the activity of the musculoskeletal system, and internal work, represented by the mechanical performance of the heart. The latter can be assessed in terms of cardiac energy utilization which, by virtue of the obligatory aerobic nature of myocardial metabolism,[9] is directly related to the oxygen consumption of the heart (M$\dot{V}O_2$).[10]

Peak M$\dot{V}O_2$—Angina is the result of an imbalance between myocardial oxygen demand and supply that is typically related to a restricted coronary circulation consequent to coronary atherosclerosis.[11] Coronary circulatory reserve is compromised and, in response to increases in M$\dot{V}O_2$, coronary blood flow, and thereby oxygen delivery, cannot be augmented beyond a limit fixed by the degree of arterial obstruction. The level of M$\dot{V}O_2$ at which the disparity between myocardial oxygen supply and demand occurs represents the internal or cardiac threshold for angina. Thus, peak M$\dot{V}O_2$ at the point of angina (hereafter referred to as peak M$\dot{V}O_2$) is an index of maximal tolerated cardiac stress, which is directly related to cardiac functional capacity in angina and may be independent of external work load as determined by the influence of extrinsic factors on the heart. In the absence of alterations in delivery capacity of the coronary circulation, as may occur with progression of coronary artery disease, M$\dot{V}O_2$ at the point of angina is constant for a given patient. Peak M$\dot{V}O_2$ also provides a relative measure of maximal attainable coronary blood flow since coronary blood flow follows M$\dot{V}O_2$ *pari passu*, as demonstrated both experimentally [12, 13] and in man.[6] This relationship is a result of the exclusively aerobic pattern of cardiac metabolism, requiring near maximal oxygen extraction by the myocardium even under basal conditions, thereby precluding use of this mechanism for increasing oxygen supply. Alterations in M$\dot{V}O_2$ are therefore effected by changes in coronary blood flow.[14]

M$\dot{V}O_2$ at Angina vs. M$\dot{V}O_2$ at Given External Work Load—In addition to providing a measure of cardiac performance through peak M$\dot{V}O_2$, the foregoing relationships afford insight into mechanisms of therapeutic interventions and other factors that may alter exercise capacity in patients with angina. Therapy in angina is based on restoration of a favorable balance between myocardial oxygen demand and supply, thereby alleviating myocardial ischemia. This balance can be achieved by increasing oxygen supply or reducing demand.[15] An increase in peak tolerated $M\dot{V}O_2$ after an intervention is consistent with increased blood flow and oxygen supply to ischemic areas of myocardium. A decrease in peak $M\dot{V}O_2$ implies diminished myocardial perfusion and increased ischemia, and thus a lower level of maximal tolerated cardiac stress.

Interventions that enhance physical performance in patients with angina by reducing myocardial oxygen requirements are associated with no change in peak tolerated $M\dot{V}O_2$. However, myocardial mechanical effort at any given level of external work is decreased by these interventions and attainment of angina-limiting $M\dot{V}O_2$ is thereby delayed, allowing work of greater intensity and duration. Thus, valid interpretation of the mechanism of action of an intervention that alters angina-limited exercise capacity requires knowledge of $M\dot{V}O_2$ both at angina and at a given external work load.[16] Reduction of myocardial oxygen requirements is achieved by attenuating the response to external stress of the hemodynamic variables upon which $M\dot{V}O_2$ is dependent. These include heart rate, intramyocardial tension (directly related to ventricular pressure and volume), myocardial contractility and certain minor factors (Table I, Chapter 2).[10] The rationale for this therapeutic approach is consistent with the demonstration of hemodynamic alterations indicative of increased $M\dot{V}O_2$ in association with angina that has been provoked by exercise,[17] catecholamine stimulation [18] or pacing-induced tachycardia,[19] or has occurred spontaneously.[20]

Indirect Indices of $M\dot{V}O_2$ (Heart Rate–Blood Pressure Product)—$M\dot{V}O_2$ can be directly determined as the product of myocardial arteriovenous oxygen difference and coronary blood flow, but since both of these measurements require cardiac catheterization, this technique is not feasible for general application. However, indirect approaches to assessment of $M\dot{V}O_2$ have been rewarding as practical means of estimating this quantity. Consistent with their importance as major determinants of myocardial oxygen utilization, derived indices comprising blood pressure and heart rate have provided a reasonable approximation of relative $M\dot{V}O_2$. These have included the product of mean aortic pressure and heart rate,[13] the tension-time index [21] (product of the integral of left ventricular pressure during systole and heart rate), the triple product of heart rate, systolic blood pressure and systolic ejection period [7] and the double product of heart rate and systolic blood pressure.[6, 22-24]

These indirect indices of $M\dot{V}O_2$, although affording ease of assessment, also involve inherent limitations. Thus, they fail to include ventricular volume and the contractile state of the myocardium, two major determinants of $M\dot{V}O_2$. Whereas heart rate and blood pressure are readily determined, measurement of volume and contractility is complex and thus inconsistent with pursuit of a widely applicable approach to $M\dot{V}O_2$. Further, the significance of the duration of ventricular ejection (systolic ejection period) in influencing $M\dot{V}O_2$, and thus the relative advantages of the triple or double product has been unclear. However, experimental [23] and recent clinical [6, 22-24] studies have suggested that duration of ejection, initially considered a significant determinant of $M\dot{V}O_2$,[21] is relatively unimportant.

Despite these theoretical limitations, the utility of indirect assessment of $M\dot{V}O_2$ has been supported by a series of investigations demonstrating a close correlation between directly measured $M\dot{V}O_2$ and the heart rate–blood pressure product during exercise in normal young men [6, 22, 23] and in patients with coronary artery disease.[24] In normal individuals studied during upright bicycle exercise [6, 22] there was a high degree of correlation between $M\dot{V}O_2$ and the product of (1) heart rate $\times$ peak systolic aortic pressure (r = 0.90), (2) heart rate $\times$ mean systolic aortic pressure (r = 0.90) and (3) heart rate $\times$ mean aortic pressure (r = 0.80). Heart rate alone also correlated closely with $M\dot{V}O_2$ (r = 0.88). The relationship between measured coronary blood flow and the preceding indices was similarly close. Tension-time index and the triple product of heart rate, pressure and systolic ejection period correlated less well with $M\dot{V}O_2$, indicating that systolic ejection time, which is included in the tension-time index and triple product but is absent in the heart rate–blood pressure product, is not a major determinant of $M\dot{V}O_2$. Further, total body oxygen consumption ($\dot{V}O_2$) was a poor predictor of $M\dot{V}O_2$, demonstrating that there may be a significant disparity between external work and that performed by the heart. In a further study of bicycle and isometric exercise separately and simultaneously in normal subjects, $M\dot{V}O_2$ was well reflected by heart rate (r = 0.80) and heart rate $\times$ aortic systolic blood pressure (r = 0.88).[23] Again, the correlation with $M\dot{V}O_2$ was diminished by utilization of systolic ejection time to calculate tension-time index (r = 0.67) and the triple product (r = 0.75).

Studies of the usefulness of indirect indices of $M\dot{V}O_2$ in patients with coronary artery disease have yielded findings similar to those in normal subjects. $M\dot{V}O_2$ correlated well with heart rate $\times$ blood pressure (r = 0.83) and slightly less closely with tension time index (r = 0.80).[24] The effect on these relationships of propranolol, an agent that can alter myocardial contractility and prolong the systolic ejection period,[25] was assessed in normal individuals.[22] As in previous studies, heart rate $\times$ blood pressure was well correlated with $M\dot{V}O_2$ (r = 0.85) and the tension-time index, which was significantly increased by the lengthened systolic ejection period, was not as accurate in predicting $M\dot{V}O_2$ (r = 0.68). The foregoing findings indicate that changes in $M\dot{V}O_2$ may be indirectly assessed with reasonable reliability from the readily available hemodynamic variables, heart rate and blood pressure. Further, the close relationship between $M\dot{V}O_2$ and heart rate $\times$ blood pressure pertains in patients with coronary artery disease as well as in normal individuals, and in initial studies it has been unaffected by drug-induced alterations in myocardial contractility and systolic ejection time.

Application of Indirect Indices of $M\dot{V}O_2$ to Angina

Although the importance of heart rate in the precipitation of angina was recognized more than three decades ago,[26] this relation was subsequently ques-

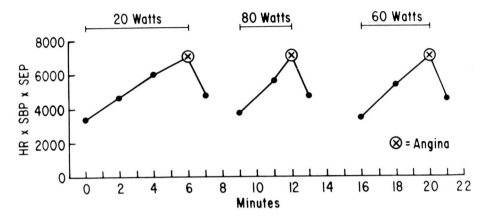

Figure 1. Relation of onset of angina to duration and intensity of exercise on the bicycle ergometer and the triple product of heart rate (HR), intra-arterial systolic blood pressure (SBP) and systolic ejection period (SEP). Duration of exercise is inversely related to the work load but angina occurs at a constant triple product.

tioned,[27] and blood pressure was discounted as a significant factor in the production of angina in these early studies.[26, 27] These findings may be related to limitations in methodology since they were derived from indirect, cuff blood pressure measurements [26, 27] and data obtained after termination of exercise.[26] Recent reevaluation of the relation of heart rate and blood pressure to the occurrence of angina has confirmed the significance of both variables and upheld the applicability of indirect indices of $M\dot{V}O_2$ to evaluation of angina. Thus, it has been demonstrated that for the individual patient, precipitation of angina occurs at a constant value for the triple product of heart rate, intra-arterial systolic pressure and systolic ejection period.[7] This relationship is consistent and independent of variations in the type, intensity and duration of exercise (Figure 1).[7] Thus, external exertional capacity, as indicated by intensity and duration of exercise, varies as a function of the imposed load. However, provocation of angina is related to attainment of a critical triple product that reflects the stress on the myocardium, the essential factor in the production of angina. These findings provide indirect support for the concept, discussed earlier, that each patient experiences angina at a critical or peak level of $M\dot{V}O_2$, which can be approximated by the triple product or double product of heart rate × blood pressure and is determined by the delivery capacity of the coronary circulation to the region of lowest threshold for imbalance between oxygen supply and demand.

Since heart rate–blood pressure indices of $M\dot{V}O_2$ are constant at the point of angina for a given individual despite their failure to account for several principal determinants of $M\dot{V}O_2$, it is reasonable to conclude that under the conditions of study, the omitted factors either are constant or are in a manner that causes their effects on $M\dot{V}O_2$ to be canceled. In such instances, $M\dot{V}O_2$ would, in effect, vary as a function of the readily measurable hemodynamic variables, blood pressure and heart rate, as suggested by the previously cited studies in normal subjects [6, 22, 23] and in patients with coronary artery disease.[24]

Application of Rate-Pressure Product to Interpretation of Pathophysiology of Angina—With use of derived indices of heart rate and blood pressure to estimate $M\dot{V}O_2$, it is possible to clarify mechanisms of angina occurring under various circumstances. Thus, exercise in the postprandial state has been accompanied by an elevated triple product at any given level of external work in comparison to the response in the fasting state, and angina occurs earlier. However, the triple product at the point of angina was the same in the two states.[2] These data suggest that the diminished exercise capacity after a meal is the result of an augmented circulatory response, *ie*, more rapid increase in heart rate and blood pressure, to exercise associated with this condition and is not related to changes intrinsic to the myocardium and coronary circulation. The unaltered triple product at angina is consistent with the latter conclusion. Likewise, the diminished exertional ability and earlier provocation of angina during exercise after smoking a cigarette is associated with an increased rate-pressure product above that occurring in the control exercise state.[8] An augmented circulatory response to physical exertion at low ambient temperature is similarly productive of angina after less exercise.[2] These studies, which implicate extramyocardial mechanisms in the alteration of exercise capacity under the conditions cited, demonstrate the application of indirect indices of $M\dot{V}O_2$ to interpretation of the pathophysiology of angina.

Use of Indirect Blood Pressure Measurement—The studies described previously, while providing a simplified approach to assessment of $M\dot{V}O_2$, involve measurement of intra-arterial pressure and are therefore not widely applicable. A noninvasive means of obtaining this information would be of obvious clinical advantage. Although current data vary, several studies suggest that indirectly measured brachial artery pressure may be useful in obtaining indirect indices of $M\dot{V}O_2$. Nelson et al,[23] in their study correlating $M\dot{V}O_2$ with heart rate × blood pressure during upright bicycle exercise, demonstrated that the relationship applied whether the pressure was determined by a catheter in the central aorta (r = 0.88) or by blood pressure cuff over the brachial artery (r = 0.85). Excellent correlation was demonstrated by Karlefors et al [28] between direct and indirect measurements of systolic blood pressure during upright bicycle exercise at varying intensities of workload. Group mean differences in systolic pressure between the two methods were less than 4 mm Hg during mild through heavy exercise. In a recent study comparison of cuff and intra-arterial blood pressure to calculate heart rate–blood pressure product during bicycle exercise revealed no difference in results for the two methods.[25] By contrast, during a treadmill exercise study in which direct radial artery pressure was compared to indirect brachial artery pressure, group mean systolic pressure by the two techniques differed by up to 15 mm Hg.[29] However, the wider divergence between direct and indirect pressures in this investigation

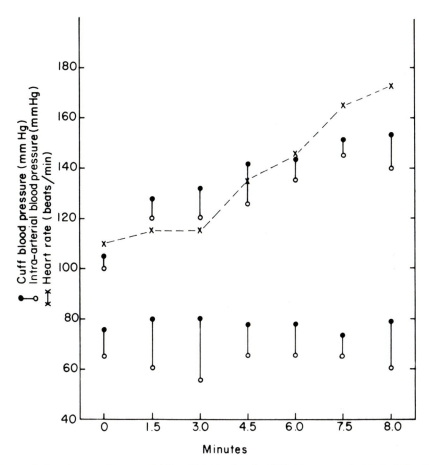

Figure 2. Simultaneous intra-arterial (brachial artery) and cuff blood pressure during graded, multi-stage treadmill exercise in a patient with coronary heart disease and angina. The open and closed circles between 100 and 160 mm Hg indicate simultaneous intra-arterial and cuff systolic blood pressures, respectively. The lower pairs of open and closed circles indicate diastolic blood pressures.

than in those previously cited is not surprising since the pressures compared were obtained from different sites.

The reproducibility of indirectly measured blood pressure during exercise is an important issue in the use of this method in determination of serial data to assess the effects of an intervention on indices of $M\dot{V}O_2$. Of significance in this regard are findings indicating comparable reproducibility at the anginal threshold for the heart rate–blood pressure product derived from cuff or directly measured blood pressure.[30] Consistency of indirectly measured blood pressure has also been demonstrated during bicycle exercise tests performed weekly.[31]

Our initial experience comparing simultaneously measured brachial artery pressure by intra-arterial catheter and cuff during treadmill exercise indicates

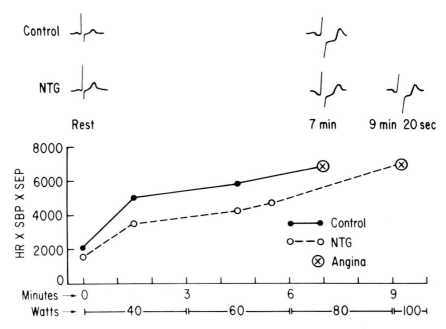

Figure 3. Exercise performance on the bicycle ergometer in a patient with coronary heart disease, before and after sublingual administration of nitroglycerin (NTG). The triple product (HR × SBP × SEP) is reduced after administration of nitroglycerin, resulting in increased exercise capacity. However, the triple product at angina is unchanged. Ischemic ST-segment depression (lead V_5) is delayed after administration of nitroglycerin until greater exercise performance has been achieved. Abbreviations as in Figure 1.

reliable correlations in directional changes but variable agreement in absolute values (Figure 2). It would appear at present that during bicycle exercise and with careful attention to technique, sphygmomanometric measurement of blood pressure may be valid for use in the indirect assessment of M$\dot{V}O_2$. Determination of the precise utility for this purpose of indirect blood pressure during treadmill exercise, with its associated motion artifacts, requires further evaluation.

Evaluation of Therapeutic Mechanisms in Angina by Indirect Assessment of M$\dot{V}O_2$

It has generally been concluded that medical therapy is beneficial in angina pectoris by attenuating the circulatory response to physical or emotional stress.[15] Thus, the nitrates and beta adrenergic blocking agents are associated with a reduced rate-pressure product and a delay in attainment of angina threshold. The beneficial effects of the hemodynamic actions of these drugs thereby result in enhanced exertional capacity.

Effect of Nitrates in Angina—The effects of nitroglycerin on exercise perform-

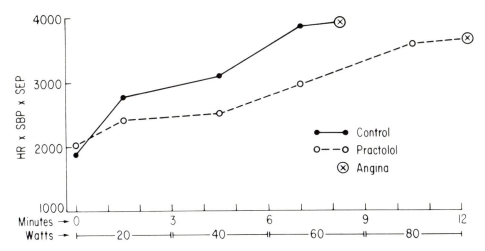

Figure 4. Exercise performance (bicycle ergometer) in a patient with coronary heart disease before and after cardioselective beta adrenergic blockade with intravenously administered practolol. The response to exercise of the triple product (HR × SBP × SEP) is attenuated after administration of the drug, resulting in increased duration and intensity of exercise before the onset of angina. Angina occurs at similar triple product before and after administration of the drug. Abbreviations as in Figure 1.

ance, the triple product and the exercise electrocardiogram in a patient with ischemic heart disease are demonstrated in Figure 3. After nitroglycerin, ability to perform more exercise is related to a lower triple product at levels of work comparable to those imposed before nitroglycerin. Angina occurs at the same triple product as before administration of the drug but its onset is delayed. Similar findings result with utilization of the double product. These data, which are consistent with a primary therapeutic action on the hemodynamic determinants of $M\dot{V}O_2$ rather than improvement in myocardial perfusion, have been demonstrated by others for nitroglycerin [32, 33] and sublingually administered isosorbide dinitrate.[33] Further, direct measurement of coronary blood flow at the point of exercise-induced angina before and after nitroglycerin demonstrated no change in peak coronary flow [34] associated with enhanced exercise capacity and intracoronary injection of nitroglycerin was ineffective on exercise capacity while the sublingually administered drug which produced hemodynamic alterations resulted in enhanced exercise capacity.[35] These findings are in accord with the results obtained utilizing indirect indices of $M\dot{V}O_2$.

Although these indirect indices are useful, their limitations must be appreciated in considering the effects of the nitrates in angina. Thus, the major hemodynamic action of the nitrates in decreasing $M\dot{V}O_2$ is reduction of ventricular volume,[36] the effects of which are not accounted for by the indirect methods. Further, the double product of heart rate and blood pressure is increased at angina after administration of the nitrates, which could be attributable to decreased ventricular volume or increased perfusion of ischemic myocardium. In this regard, it has been suggested that a separate effect of enhanced myocardial perfusion may play a role in the beneficial actions of the nitrates.[15] If such an effect were minor in relation to reduced myocardial oxygen demand, it would not be discernible by indirect assessment of $M\dot{V}O_2$, since the latter methods reflect the resultant of the separate actions of any intervention on $M\dot{V}O_2$.

Effects of Beta Adrenergic Blockade in Angina—Improvement in effort tolerance by beta adrenergic blockade is consistent with a reduction in $M\dot{V}O_2$ in man during exercise.[15] As shown in Figure 4, the triple product is reduced for a given level of stress and angina is delayed. Although the triple product at angina after beta adrenergic blockade is similar to that of the control study in the example displayed, this finding is uncommon and our data [37] and those of others [38] generally demonstrate a reduction in triple product or rate-pressure product at angina after administration of beta adrenergic blocking drugs. Diminished myocardial oxygen requirement in response to a given level of exercise after propranolol has been confirmed in man by direct measurement of $M\dot{V}O_2$.[22] This may be related to a possible increase in ventricular size due to the depressant effect of these agents on myocardial contractility or to reduction in coronary blood flow. On the other hand, it has been suggested that propranolol may favorably redistribute coronary blood flow [39] and enhance release of oxygen from red blood cells to the myocardium.[40] These latter factors cannot be specifically delineated by indirect methods but the reduction of the rate-pressure product at angina after beta adrenergic blockade suggests that increased myocardial oxygen supply is not a major factor in the beneficial effects of these agents. The salutory effects of carotid sinus nerve stimulation in improving functional status in angina were also the result of reduced $M\dot{V}O_2$, as indicated by increased exercise ability without change in the triple product and reduction of the triple product at submaximal loads of exercise.[41] There has usually been no increase in heart rate–blood pressure product at angina after a training program, suggesting no increase in perfusion of ischemic myocardium.[30, 42]

Physical Training in Angina—Physical training, which may augment exertional ability in patients with angina, also appears to act by attenuating the response of the heart to physical stress.[5, 30, 42, 43] Thus, the heart rate–blood pressure product is lower at a given external work load after a training program.[30, 42] However, neither heart rate–blood pressure product [30] nor measured $M\dot{V}O_2$[42] at angina was altered by training. The increase in triple product at angina in some trained patients has been interpreted as a possible indication of enhanced myocardial perfusion.[5] However, this could be related to changes in other factors not reflected in the triple product, among them attenuated adrenergic response to exercise stress after a conditioning program,[43] which would reduce $M\dot{V}O_2$ by reducing myocardial contractility while simultaneously allowing attainment of a higher triple product.

Aortocoronary Bypass Graft—The effects of aortocoronary saphenous vein bypass graft on indirect indices of $M\dot{V}O_2$ differ from those of other therapeutic modalities previously considered in this discussion and suggest a fundamental-

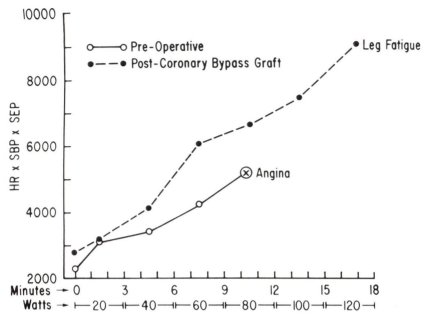

Figure 5. Exercise performance (bicycle ergometer) in a patient with coronary heart disease, before and after aortocoronary bypass graft surgery. Surgical therapy is associated with increased exercise capacity, abolition of exercise-induced angina and elevated triple product. Abbreviations as in Figure 1.

ly different mechanism of action. Thus, we have evaluated the triple product during exercise in patients with angina before and after coronary bypass graft surgery. Our findings in patients with patent grafts are exemplified in Figure 5. There has been no consistent effect on the triple product during exercise at given work loads before and after operation. However, the triple product at angina before surgery has been exceeded in association with patent bypass grafts and angina has occurred at a markedly greater triple or double product or exercise capacity has been augmented to the point of volitional fatigue without angina,[44, 45] as depicted in Figure 5. Similar improvement in the rate-pressure product calculated from cuff blood pressure has been reported after aortocoronary bypass graft surgery.[46] We have investigated the utility of indirect blood pressure measurement for this purpose and our initial studies of the effect of coronary bypass graft on peak double product have yielded comparable results with directly measured and cuff blood pressure (Figure 6). That an increased triple product with or without angina postsurgery correlates with enhanced myocardial oxygen delivery is supported by the associated normalization or improvement of exercise-induced ischemic ST alterations following myocardial revascularization[45] (Figure 7).

It has been suggested that improved clinical status and exercise capacity fol-

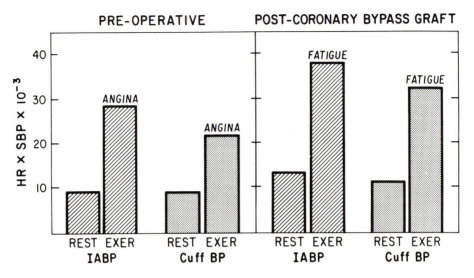

Figure 6. Double product of heart rate (HR) and systolic blood pressure (SBP), obtained by intra-arterial (IABP) and cuff measurement. The pre- and postoperative comparisons of the two methods yield similar results.

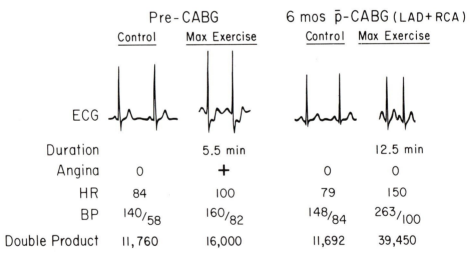

Figure 7. Pre- and postoperative treadmill exercise tests in a patient with coronary heart disease who received coronary bypass grafts to the left anterior descending and right coronary arteries. Blood pressure was measured by brachial artery catheter.

lowing aortocoronary bypass graft surgery may be related not only to graft patency, but also to intraoperative infarction of ischemic myocardium.[16, 47] In a study in which this question was evaluated,[46] the great majority of patients with intraoperative infarction did not show clear improvement in exercise capacity as assessed by rate-pressure product and ST-segment changes during exercise, although a few manifested enhanced function. The outcome in terms of cardiac capacity in such situations would appear to be the result of the interplay between the functional effects of the graft and the infarction, when the latter occurs.

Summary

Exercise testing is an important means of evaluating the patient with angina pectoris, providing objective data not available from clinical assessment. In utilizing exercise to determine functional impairment in angina, it is essential to distinguish between external stress, or the load on the skeletal muscles, and internal or cardiac stress. Evaluation of external exercise capacity alone is limited as a measure of cardiac performance since the relationship between external function and cardiac performance is not necessarily a direct one. A readily applicable approach to determination of cardiac capacity in angina is afforded by indirect assessment of myocardial oxygen consumption ($M\dot{V}O_2$). This is achieved through derived indices utilizing heart rate and blood pressure, two major determinants of $M\dot{V}O_2$, in the form of the product of heart rate and systolic blood pressure. Although this approach does not encompass all the major determinants of $M\dot{V}O_2$, changes in the heart rate–blood pressure product bear a close correlation to alterations in directly measured $M\dot{V}O_2$. Within limits and employed with caution, indirect assessment of $M\dot{V}O_2$ is useful in elucidating mechanisms of action of extracardiac and intrinsic myocardial factors in the provocation and therapy of angina.

Acknowledgment—Technical assistance was given by Ms. Elizabeth Matthews, Ms. Martha Wood and Ms. Denise Salmon.

This study was supported by Research Program Project Grant HL-14780 from the National Institutes of Health, Bethesda, Maryland.

References

1. Redwood DR, Rosing DR, Goldstein RE, et al: Importance of the design of an exercise protocol in the evaluation of patients with angina pectoris. *Circulation* 43:618-628, 1971.
2. Epstein SE, Redwood DR, Goldstein RE: Angina pectoris: pathophysiology, evaluation, and treatment. *Ann Intern Med* 75:263-296, 1971.
3. Mitchell JH, Blomquist G: Maximal oxygen uptake. *New Eng J Med* 284:1018-1022, 1971.
4. Simonson E: Evaluation of cardiac performance in exercise. *Amer J Cardiol* 30:722-726, 1972.
5. Redwood DR, Rosing DR, Epstein SE: Circulatory and symptomatic effects of physical training in patients with coronary artery disease and angina pectoris. *New Eng J Med* 286:959-965, 1972.
6. Kitamura K, Jorgensen CR, Gobel F, et al: Hemodynamic correlates of myocardial oxygen consumption during upright exercise. *J Appl Physiol* 32:516-522, 1972.
7. Robinson BF: Relation of heart rate and systolic blood pressure to the onset of pain in angina pectoris. *Circulation* 35:1073-1083, 1967.
8. Aronow WS, Kaplan MA, Jacob D: Tobacco: a precipitating factor in angina pectoris. *Ann Intern Med* 69:529-536, 1968.
9. Amsterdam EA: Function of the hypoxic myocardium. *Amer J Cardiol* 32:461-471, 1973.
10. Sonnenblick EH, Skelton CL: Oxygen consumption of the heart: physiological principles and

clinical implications. *Mod Con Cardiovasc Dis* 40:9-16, 1971.

11. Amsterdam EA, Zelis R, Miller RR, et al: "Pathophysiology of Angina Pectoris," in Likoff W, Moyer JH, Segal BL (Eds): *Atherosclerosis and Coronary Heart Disease*, pp 178-189, New York: Grune & Stratton, 1972.
12. Eckenhoff JE, Hafkenschiel JH, Landmesser CM, et al: Cardiac oxygen metabolism and control of the coronary circulation. *Amer J Physiol* 149:634-649, 1947.
13. Katz LN, Feinberg H: The relation of cardiac effort to myocardial oxygen consumption and coronary flow. *Circ Res* 6:656-669, 1958.
14. Berne RM: Regulation of coronary blood flow. *Physiol Rev* 44:1-29, 1964.
15. Amsterdam EA, Hughes JL, Miller RR, et al: "Physiologic approach to the medical and surgical treatment of angina pectoris," in Hellerstein HK, Naughton J (Eds): *Exercise Testing and Exercise Training in Coronary Heart Disease*, pp 103-117, New York: Academic Press, 1973.
16. Goldstein RE, Epstein SE: The use of indirect indices of myocardial oxygen consumption in evaluating angina pectoris. *Chest* 63:302-306, 1973.
17. Parker JE, West RO, Case RB, et al: Temporal relationships of myocardial lactate metabolism, left ventricular function, and S-T segment depression during angina precipitated by exercise. *Circulation* 40:97-111, 1969.
18. Cohen LS, Elliott WC, Rolett EL, et al: Hemodynamic studies during angina pectoris. *Circulation* 31:409-416, 1965.
19. Parker JE, Chiong MA, West RO, et al: Sequential alterations in myocardial lactate metabolism. S-T segments, and left ventricular function during angina induced by atrial pacing. *Circulation* 40:112-131, 1969.
20. Amsterdam EA, Manchester JH, Kemp HG, et al: Spontaneous angina pectoris (SAP): hemodynamic and metabolic changes (abstract). *Clin Res* 17:225, 1969.
21. Sarnoff SJ, Braunwald E, Welch GH Jr, et al: Hemodynamic determinants of oxygen consumption of the heart with special reference to the tension-time index. *Amer J Physiol* 192:148-156, 1958.
22. Jorgensen CR, Wang K, Gobel FL, et al: Effect of propranolol on myocardial oxygen consumption and its hemodynamic correlates during upright exercise. *Circulation* 48:1173-1182, 1973.
23. Nelson RR, Gobel FL, Jorgensen CR, et al: Hemodynamic predictors of myocardial oxygen consumption during static and dynamic exercise. *Circulation* 50:1179-1189, 1974.
24. Gobel FL, Nordstrom LA, Nelson RR, et al: The rate-pressure product as an index of myocardial oxygen consumption during exercise in patients with angina pectoris. Unpublished data.
25. Wolfson S, Gorlin R: Cardiovascular pharmacology of propranolol in man. *Circulation* 40:501-511, 1969.
26. Wayne EJ, Lapiace LB: Observations in angina of effort. *Clin Sci* 1:103-129, 1933.
27. Riseman JEF: Relation of the systolic blood pressure and heart rate to attacks of angina pectoris precipitated by effort. *Amer Heart J* 12:53-69, 1936.
28. Karlefors T, Nilsen R, Westling H: On the accuracy of indirect ausculatory blood pressure measurements during exercise. *Acta Med Scand* 449 (suppl):81-87, 1968.
29. Henschel A, de la Vega F, Taylor HL: Simultaneous direct and indirect blood pressure measurements in man at rest and work. *J Appl Physiol* 6:506-508, 1954.
30. Clausen JP, Trap-Jensen J: Heart rate and arterial blood pressure during exercise in patients with angina pectoris. Effects of training and of nitroglycerin. *Circulation* 53:436-442, 1976.
31. Sime WE, Whipple IR, Berkson DM, et al: Reproducibility of systolic and diastolic blood pressure at rest and in response to submaximal bicycle ergometer tests in middle-aged men. *Human Biol* 47:483-492, 1975.
32. Robinson BF: Mode of action of nitroglycerin in angina pectoris. *Brit Heart J* 30:295-301, 1968.
33. Goldstein RE, Rosing DR, Redwood DR, et al: Clinical and circulatory effects of isosorbide dinitrate. *Circulation* 43:629-640, 1971.
34. Parker JO, West RO, DiGiorgi S: The effect of nitroglycerin on coronary blood flow and the hemodynamic response to exercise in coronary artery disease. *Amer J Cardiol* 27:59-65, 1971.
35. Ganz E, Marcus HS: Failure of intracoronary nitroglycerin to alleviate pacing-induced angina. *Circulation* 46:880-889, 1972.
36. Mason DT, Zelis R, Amsterdam EA: Actions of the nitrites on the peripheral circulation and myocardial oxygen consumption: significance in the relief of angina pectoris. *Chest* 59:296-305, 1971.
37. Amsterdam EA, Hughes JL, Mansour E, et al: Circulatory effects of practolol: selective cardiac beta adrenergic blockade in arrhythmias and angina pectoris (abstract). *Clin Res* 19:109, 1971.

38. Robin E, Cowans C, Puri P: A comparative study of nitroglycerin and propranolol. *Circulation* 36:175-186, 1967.
39. Becker LC, Fortuin NJ, Pitt B: Effect of ischemia and antianginal drugs on the distribution of radioactive microspheres in the canine left ventricle. *Circ Res* 28:263-269, 1971.
40. Oski FA, Miller LD, Delicoria-Papadopoulos M, et al: Oxygen affinity in red cells: changes induced *in vivo* by propranolol. *Science* 175:1372-1373, 1972.
41. Epstein SE, Beiser GD, Goldstein RE, et al: Treatment of angina pectoris by electrical stimulation of the carotid sinus nerves. *New Eng J Med* 280:971-978, 1969.
42. Wolfson S, Acosta AE, Rose LI, et al: Effects of conditioning on plasma catecholamine levels during exercise in patients with coronary artery disease (abstract). *Amer J Cardiol* 29:297, 1972.
43. Sim DN, Neill WA: Investigation of the physiological basis for increased exercise threshold for angina pectoris after physical conditioning. *J Clin Invest* 54:763-770, 1974.
44. Amsterdam EA, Iben A, Hurley EJ, et al: Saphenous vein bypass graft for refractory angina pectoris: physiologic evidence for enhanced blood flow to the ischemic myocardium (abstract). *Amer J Cardiol* 26:623, 1970.
45. Grehl T, Amsterdam EA, Matthews E, et al: Evaluation of coronary bypass graft surgery by exercise testing: objective assessment by effect on ischemic ST depression, heart rate-blood pressure product and correlation with postoperative angiography (abstract). *Amer J Cardiol* 39:268, 1977.
46. Guiney TE, Rubinstein JJ, Sanders CA, et al: Functional evaluation of coronary bypass surgery by exercise testing and oxygen consumption. *Circulation* 47, 48 (suppl III):141-145, 1973.
47. Griffith LSC, Achuff SC, Conti CR, et al: Changes in intrinsic coronary circulation and segmental ventricular motion after saphenous vein coronary bypass graft surgery. *New Eng J Med* 288:589-595, 1973.

16

Exercise Testing in Patients with Valvular Heart Disease

Fred Harris, MD
Anthony N. DeMaria, MD
Ezra A. Amsterdam, MD
Garrett Lee, MD
Richard R. Miller, MD
Najam Awan, MD
Dean T. Mason, MD

The primary application of exercise testing in the evaluation of the patient with cardiac disease has thus far been determination of the presence or absence of myocardial ischemia in the setting of chest pain of unknown etiology. However, since exertional capacity is primarily determined by cardiocirculatory dynamics in the absence of extracardiac factors limiting oxygen transport,[1] exercise testing should provide a suitable modality for quantitation of functional impairment in cardiac performance induced by the presence of valvular heart disease. Despite this potential application, relatively little data are available concerning the use of exercise testing to evaluate the hemodynamic severity of valvular heart disease. This chapter will review the available information regarding this question and summarize our preliminary studies comparing exercise capacity with multiple parameters of cardiac performance obtained by cardiac catheterization in patients with valvular heart disease.

Physiologic Response to Exercise

The ability to exercise involves a complex interaction between metabolic, neural, ventilatory and hemodynamic responses.[2-9] During exercise a redistribution of regional blood flow occurs, causing an increase in coronary perfusion and blood flow to active skeletal musculature, while blood flow to inactive skeletal muscles and the splanchnic circulation is reduced.[10] Neither the diffusion of oxygen through the lungs nor the oxygen-carrying capacity of blood is a significant factor affecting exercise performance in normal subjects. However, during exercise there is augmentation and redistribution of cardiac output as well as increased extraction of oxygen from blood by involved tissues, resulting in greater oxygen transport and utilization. The exercise-induced increase in cardiac output is accomplished by augmentation of heart rate, myocardial contractility and stroke volume, and is associated with a rise in arterial blood pressure and, when large muscle groups such as those of the legs are involved, a fall in total peripheral vascular resistance. The increase in cardiac output with exercise bears a linear relationship to total body oxygen consumption and appears to be the primary determinant of exertional performance in normal subjects. Exercise performance, as represented by total body oxygen consumption, is a reflection of overall myocardial pump function in the absence of extracardiac factors such as pulmonary disease, anemia and peripheral vascular disease, which interfere with oxygen transport.

It is not an uncommon phenomenon for patients with heart disease to manifest relatively normal cardiac function at rest and to demonstrate abnormalities only during exercise. Hemodynamic measurements during exercise have been utilized to expose latent cardiac dysfunction as indicated by diminution of cardiac reserve. The hemodynamic response to exercise is dependent upon the type of exertion performed and the body position utilized. Therefore, at a given oxygen intake, heart rate and arteriovenous oxygen difference are less and cardiac output and stroke volume greater during exercise in the supine as compared with the upright position.[11] Attention must be given to the exercise protocol applied in the evaluation of cardiac function.

Hemodynamic Function and Oxygen Consumption During Exercise

Supine Exercise—Exercise has been applied in the evaluation of the functional consequences of valvular heart disease during direct invasive examination. The circulatory response to exercise in patients with valvular heart disease was initially evaluated during supine exercise. Wade and Bishop [12] performed supine exercise in patients with mitral stenosis and observed a decreased cardiac output at rest with a subnormal increase in output with exercise for any level of oxygen intake. However, during exercise evaluation there was a poor correlation between hemodynamic response and impairment in exercise tolerance in individual patients.

Bache et al [13] evaluated 20 patients with isolated aortic stenosis during supine exercise and observed no significant change in left ventricular end-diastolic pressure in relation to increasing degree of aortic valvular obstruction. Further,

TABLE I

New York Heart Association
Functional Classification

Class	Symptoms
I	None
II	With ordinary activity
III	With less than ordinary activity
IV	At rest

there was no difference in exercise factor between individuals with normal and those with depressed resting cardiac indices.

Ross et al [14] studied seven normal patients and 19 patients with significant mitral or aortic stenosis during supine exercise. Multiple hemodynamic parameters of cardiac performance were found to be insensitive in the detection of cardiac dysfunction. Maximal oxygen uptake assessed during supine exercise correlated in general with the degree of functional impairment in aortic stenosis patients, but not in those with mitral stenosis. Maximal oxygen uptake was more depressed in valvular patients than in normal subjects, but this difference was not significant. Thus, from these studies it would appear that supine exercise is of limited value in the assessment of cardiac function in patients with valvular heart disease.

Upright Exercise—Moderate and intense upright exercise was utilized by Epstein et al [15] to assess cardiac performance in six normal subjects, 19 patients with various valvular lesions and two patients with cardiomyopathy during right heart catheterization. The patients studied were functional Class I, II and III by The New York Heart Association Classification (Table I). Stroke volume and pulmonary artery pressure consistently differed between the normal subjects and cardiac patients at mild and intense levels of upright exercise. In all normal subjects stroke volume was noted to increase on transition from sitting rest to mild upright treadmill exercise, and was augmented further at maximal levels of exertion in five of these subjects. The majority of valvular patients was also able to increase stroke volume from rest to mild exercise but, in contrast to normals, this parameter either did not change or actually fell as the intensity of exercise increased. In addition, patients with the most depressed cardiac function demonstrated a fall in stroke volume even on transition from rest to the lowest level of exertion. At a level of upright exercise at which pulmonary artery oxygen saturation fell to 30%, cardiac index was significantly lower in patients with valvular disease compared to normals. Thus, this study demonstrated the value of upright exercise in the identification of impaired cardiac function in patients with valvular heart disease.

Upright exercise was also utilized by Bruce et al [16] to evaluate cardiac function in 14 patients with valvular heart disease, seven of whom had multiple valvular involvement. Stroke index fell and arteriovenous oxygen difference widened significantly with change in position from supine to sitting upright in these patients. With upright treadmill exertion heart rate, cardiac output and mean arterial pressure increased. Although stroke index also increased with exertion, it did not exceed the resting supine value. These workers confirmed the findings of Epstein et al [15] regarding the inappropriate response of stroke volume to exercise in patients with valvular heart disease. Further, maximal oxygen uptake was more depressed in the functional Class III than in the Class II patients. In another study, of 24 patients with aortic and mitral valvular lesions, the majority of which were stenotic, Bruce et al [17] observed that severe valvular disease can result in exertional hypotension. In ten of their patients with aortic or mitral stenosis, hypotension was noted during treadmill exercise. These patients had slightly increased levels of peripheral resistance and lower cardiac index while sitting at rest than the group without exertional hypotension.

Blackmon et al [18] also found upright exercise beneficial in the functional classification of patients with valvular heart disease. They evaluated seven patients with mitral stenosis by upright treadmill exercise and noted that a decreased maximal oxygen uptake was correlated closely with a decreased stroke volume.

In summary, exercise is a valuable adjunct in assessing the functional limitation of cardiac performance consequent to valvular heart disease during direct pressure and flow measurements. It has been found that upright exercise is preferable to supine exertion in this regard. The most valuable index of cardiac dysfunction would appear to be a reduction of stroke volume at progressively more strenuous levels of exertion.

Exercise Testing and Functional Classification

The primary use of the exercise test in valvular heart disease at present is to determine functional classification. Maximal oxygen uptake obtained by exercise testing affords an objective means of categorizing individuals with valvular heart disease in terms of physical capacity, just as the more commonly employed functional classification of the New York Heart Association (N.Y.H.A.) (Table I) provides a convenient, subjective means of assessing exertional ability.[19] The subjective assessment of functional classification and the results of maximal exercise tolerance have been found to correlate well in groups of patients, but are commonly different in individual cases. Kellermann et al,[20] utilizing multistage spiro-ergometry, studied 135 patients with rheumatic valvular heart disease who were functional Class I, II or III by history. Ninety-four patients had mitral valvular disease, 22 had aortic valvular disease and 19 had combined aortic and mitral lesions. Functional classification by the N.Y.H.A. criteria vs. spiro-ergometry was identical in 54% of patients. The N.Y.H.A. classification was one class lower in 11% of patients and one class higher in 35%, compared with the results of spiro-ergometry. Thus, these two methods of exercise tolerance are frequently similar, but may differ significantly in any given individual.

Maximal oxygen uptake determined on exercise may also be utilized in predicting hemodynamic function as well as functional classification in valvular heart disease. The most comprehensive investigation concerning the relationship between exertional capacity and hemodynamic function was performed by Patterson et al.[21] These workers studied 43 patients with congenital or valvular heart disease who underwent maximal or near maximal multistage exercise tests. The patients were divided into four groups (Class I to IV) based on maximal oxygen consumption during exercise. Class I patients had an oxygen consumption greater than 22 ml/kg/min, while Class IV patients had an oxygen consumption less than 10 ml/kg/min. Cardiac catheterization was performed in all patients and was compared with exercise test results. Good agreement was observed between functional classification determined by treadmill exercise and functional classification assessed historically according to the criteria proposed by the N.Y.H.A. in 74% (32/43) of patients. Peak oxygen consumption achieved during exercise testing correlated well with left ventricular end-diastolic pressure and manifested a progressive decrease with increases in this hemodynamic factor. Cardiac index and stroke volume index were also shown to decrease significantly in proportion to a progressive decrease in oxygen consumption. It was concluded from the above data that patients with cardiac disease begin to experience activity-limiting symptoms when peak oxygen consumption is less than 22 ml/kg/min. Further, these results indicated that subjective assessment of functional class correlates closely in the majority of instances with functional classification based on exercise testing. Finally, it was also suggested that a direct correlation existed between decreasing maximal oxygen consumption and increasing hemodynamic dysfunction, although the patients evaluated were not solely afflicted by valvular disease, and no intraclass relationships could be estimated due to the limited number of patients included in the study.

In another study, Ashley et al [22] performed exercise tests in 17 patients with valvular heart disease. The etiology of the disease was primarily rheumatic, although one patient had idiopathic hypertrophic subaortic stenosis, and two patients had idiopathic cardiomyopathy. All patients had a catheter positioned in the pulmonary artery at the time of exercise testing and the treadmill exercise protocol was designed to increase oxygen consumption by a multiple of the resting value for each progressive level of work. Heart rate, pulmonary artery pressure and arterial pressure were determined at each workload. Heart rate and arterial pressure increased as expected with exercise, but no significant difference was observed between N.Y.H.A. functional Class II and III individuals in regard to pulmonary arterial systolic or diastolic pressure. Pulmonary arterial oxygen saturation decreased progressively with exercise and proved to be the best determinant for the separation of Class II and III patients. This study, although including a small number of patients and providing limited analysis of ventricular function, again suggested the possibility of analyzing hemodynamic performance by means of exercise testing.

In an earlier study, Lee et al [23] evaluated 34 patients with isolated aortic stenosis. The patients were divided into three groups according to the calculated aortic valve area index, as determined by cardiac catheterization. Group I patients had an aortic valve area index of greater than 0.8 cm²/M² while the value for Group III patients was less than 0.5 cm²/M². The maximal oxygen uptake attained by these individuals on upright bicycle ergometry correlated with cardiac dysfunction as determined by hemodynamic parameters and the degree of valvular stenosis as indicated by the calculated valve area index. In Group I patients cardiac output, stroke volume, pulmonary vascular resistance and work capacity were not significantly impaired. These parameters, however, were significantly affected in Group III individuals who had severe valvular stenosis. Cardiac output and stroke volume were significantly reduced and pulmonary vascular resistance and left ventricular end-diastolic pressure were increased in these individuals. In addition to the greater degree of cardiac dysfunction in Group III patients, their maximal oxygen uptake was observed to be markedly depressed secondary to angina or dyspnea associated with markedly elevated left ventricular end-diastolic pressures. In this investigation, depression of maximal oxygen uptake correlated well with severity of orifice reduction and impaired left ventricular function in the setting of severe aortic stenosis.

Relation of Treadmill Evaluation to Cardiac Catheterization

Stimulated by these data and the desirability of noninvasively quantitating hemodynamic function, we studied 100 patients with valvular heart disease who underwent cardiac catheterization as well as graded treadmill exercise tests. All patients had normal coronary arteriograms and isolated stenosis or regurgitation of a single valve. Initially, we evaluated patients with isolated valvular stenosis. All exercise tests were performed to maximal exertion, and oxygen consumption was estimated from established values at our institution relating workload to oxygen intake. The estimated mean maximal oxygen consumption observed in 23 patients with mitral stenosis and 18 patients with aortic stenosis was 15 and 18 cc/kg/min, respectively. No correlation was found between maximal oxygen consumption and catheterization determined pulmonary wedge pressure, cardiac index or left ventricular ejection fraction in the mitral or aortic stenosis patients. Importantly, although there was a general correlation between diminution of exercise capacity and increasingly severe valvular stenosis, the group mean calculated valve area in mitral stenosis patients classified I and II by exercise testing was similar to that in patients classified III and IV. Further, calculated valve area was also identical in the group of patients with aortic stenosis determined to be Class I or II by exercise test and those categorized as Class III and IV. Thus, these data indicate that exertional capacity is limited in ability to reflect the severity of obstruction of the valve orifice in patients with mitral or aortic stenosis.

We also evaluated 30 patients with aortic regurgitation and 28 patients with mitral regurgitation. Maximal oxygen consumption was 17 and 18 cc/kg/min, respectively, and again it did not correlate with mean pulmonary wedge pressure, cardiac index or ejection fraction. Further, the degree of regurgitation assessed by angiography (graded 1+ to 4+) was similar for patients with Class I and II exercise tests and those with Class III and IV tests.

Comparison of estimated maximal oxygen consumption with the severity of valvular stenosis by calculated valve area and degree of valvular insufficiency by angiographically graded regurgitation revealed that oxygen consumption was significantly less for mitral stenosis patients with a valve area less than 1 cm^2 than for those patients with a valve area greater than 1 cm^2; it was also lower in patients with Grade 3 and 4 aortic regurgitation compared to those with Grade 1 and 2. However, this type of analysis did not separate patients with more severe from those with lesser degrees of either mitral regurgitation or aortic stenosis.

The results of our studies would indicate that significant limitations exist in the use of exercise testing to predict hemodynamic abnormalities in valvular heart disease. However, it would appear that in patients with mitral stenosis and aortic regurgitation there is a useful correlation between decreased maximal oxygen consumption and severity of the valvular lesion. The application of exercise testing to predict hemodynamic impairment in patients with valvular heart disease could be of value in this select group of patients.

In summary, the determination of maximal oxygen uptake with multistage upright exercise appears to be the most sensitive method for separation and functional classification of patients with valvular heart disease. If this form of exercise is combined with hemodynamic measurements, the sensitivity of detecting abnormal cardiac function in valvular heart disease is increased.

Congenital Heart Disease

Exercise testing for detection of cardiac dysfunction has also been utilized in evaluating patients with congenital heart disease. In ten asymptomatic individuals who had had previous complete surgical correction of tetralogy of Fallot, resting hemodynamics were essentially normal except for small residual right ventricular outflow tract gradients.[24] However, during upright exercise of sufficient intensity to lower pulmonary arterial oxygen saturation to 30%, the increased cardiac output was less than that attained by normal subjects in eight of the ten patients. Right ventricular outflow tract gradients measured in six subjects during exertion increased in each patient, with right ventricular systolic pressures reaching levels of 75 to 106 mm Hg in four patients. The long-term significance of these findings remains to be determined, but it would appear that residual cardiac dysfunction persists in this setting despite corrective surgery. Subsequently, James et al [25] studied 43 asymptomatic patients by upright exercise one to 14 years after total correction of tetralogy of Fallot. Maximal heart rates and physical working capacity were lower in these patients compared to age-matched controls. In addition, an inverse relationship was observed between maximal working capacity and age at the time of surgery in both male and female patients. Impaired cardiac performance again was evident after corrective surgery for this cardiac lesion and exercise performance as quantified by maximal working capacity was reduced compared to normal subjects. These data suggest that earlier surgical treatment should be a consideration in this entity.

Exercise Electrocardiogram

The exercise electrocardiogram has been used to evaluate valvular heart disease in terms of stress-related electrocardiographic alterations. The Master "2-step" exercise test was the first exercise protocol to be applied in the assessment of valvular heart disease. Hellerstein et al [26] studied 92 patients with rheumatic valvular disease, 48 of whom had an abnormal ST-segment response to exercise utilizing the Master "2-step" exercise test. Of 50 patients not taking digitalis, 23 had abnormal ST-segment responses to exercise. In this study patients with a greater impairment of exercise tolerance and poorer functional class and those with a greater degree of cardiac enlargement were more likely to have a positive Master "2-step" exercise test. Although coronary anatomy was not defined, the authors concluded that electrocardiographic alterations occurring after exercise in patients with valvular heart disease were not diagnostic of coronary artery disease or due to decreased myocardial blood supply.

Ramsey and Beedle [27] evaluated the exercise electrocardiograms of 40 patients with isolated mitral stenosis who were functional Class I, II and III. Of 26 patients not taking digitalis, 18 manifested electrocardiographic ST-segment depression during the Master "2-step" exercise test. These authors concluded that the electrocardiographic changes observed were related to myocardial ischemia. These observations were extended by Datey et al [28] in 60 patients with rheumatic valvular disease, of whom 45% had abnormal Master "2-step" exercise tests. An increased incidence of positive responses was observed in individuals with greater degrees of functional limitation. In this study it was concluded that the electrocardiographic changes were not related to coronary atherosclerosis, but to the effects of the valvular disease itself.

The foregoing reports are difficult to interpret because of lack of angiographic documentation of coronary anatomy. Therefore, the prevalence of positive Master "2-step" exercise tests in the absence of coronary artery disease ("false"-positives) in these patients could not be determined. Subsequently, Aronow et al [29] performed submaximal treadmill exercise tests in 34 patients with mitral and aortic stenosis, all of whom had normal coronary arteries demonstrated by coronary arteriography and no electrocardiographic evidence of left ventricular hypertrophy. Seven of 19 patients (37%) with significant aortic valve gradients had one or more mm of ST-segment depression during exercise, while three of 15 patients (20%) with significant mitral valve gradients also had this finding. These abnormal exercise electrocardiograms in the absence of drugs or coronary disease suggested the production of an unfavorable balance between myocardial oxygen demand and supply by exertional stress, thereby producing myocardial ischemia. Thus, a significant number of positive exercise tests may be observed with valvular heart disease in the absence of coronary disease with or without left ventricular hypertrophy.

Exercise electrocardiography has also been applied to the pediatric age group in congenital valvular disease. Chandramouli et al [30] evaluated 44 patients between the age of five and nineteen with congenital aortic stenosis by graded treadmill exercise testing and cardiac catheterization. Twelve subjects with peak aortic valvular gradients of 54 mm Hg or more had ST-segment depression of 1 mm or more during exercise, while 32 individuals with aortic valve gradients of 10 to 48 mm Hg had less than 1 mm or no ST-segment depression with exertion. The conclusions of these investigators were that exercise testing could be used in congenital aortic stenosis to aid in selecting those individuals who should undergo cardiac catheterization, and that 1 mm or more ST-segment depression with exertion is suggestive of severe left ventricular outflow tract obstruction. Although coronary arteriography was not performed in this study, it may reasonably be presumed that there was no coronary artery disease in this group.

In patients with stenosis of a cardiac valve, the consequences of the valvular disease alone may produce ischemic electrocardiographic alterations during exertional stress. Stenotic valvular disease may produce cardiac hypertrophy. This can occur in the presence of normal coronary arteries and may be the result of an imbalance between oxygen supply and demand. Myocardial oxygen requirements may be increased in these patients by cardiac hypertrophy and dilatation and elevated intraventricular pressure, while oxygen delivery can be diminished by restriction to left ventricular outflow.

Exercise Training

Exercise training has been attempted in patients with valvular heart disease. Compared to ischemic heart disease, few data are available regarding the effects of physical training in patients with valvular heart disease. Seven women with multiple rheumatic valvular lesions were evaluated by Auchincloss and Gilbert [31] before and after physical training over a two-week period. These workers utilized a progressively increasing workload exercise protocol via a treadmill and exercise periods of 30 to 60 minutes once or twice daily. All seven patients in this study demonstrated an increase in exercise tolerance but in only two was this increase judged significant. The augmented exercise tolerance was not due to increased myocardial efficiency since a lower maximal oxygen uptake at the same level of activity was not achieved; nor was it due to increased physical fitness as a lower heart rate at the same level of oxygen consumption was not attained. These authors concluded that the improved exercise tolerance was most probably secondary to increased familiarity with the testing procedure. Unfortunately, the evaluation was limited to only a two-week period of training. With more prolonged training, a conditioning effect might be attainable in patients with valvular heart disease, but further investigation of this question is required.

Summary

Exercise has been applied in both the evaluation and therapy of patients with valvular heart disease. Since, in the absence of extracardiac conditions limiting oxygen transport, exertional capacity is primarily dependent upon cardiac performance, exercise testing has been utilized to quantify the extent of hemodynamic impairment consequent to valvular heart disease. Although alterations in direct measurements of cardiac function in response to supine exertion have been inconsistent, upright exercise has been found to be of value in exposing cardiac dysfunction. Several studies have demonstrated the inability of patients with valvular heart disease to appropriately increase cardiac index and stroke volume in response to upright exercise. Thus, the direct measurement of cardiac pressures and blood flow during upright exercise has been of value in defining the level of cardiac dysfunction in patients with valvular heart disease. Determination of exertional capacity has also been utilized in an attempt to quantify the severity of cardiac valvular lesions. However, data regarding the magnitude of valvular stenosis or regurgitation and its relation to work capacity have been inconclusive. Accordingly, further data are required before exercise testing can be relied upon to precisely predict the severity of valvular heart disease. In regard to the appearance of ST-segment abnormalities during or after exercise, such electrocardiographic changes have been observed in patients with valvular heart disease even in the absence of concomitant coronary atherosclerosis. These ST changes may be related to an imbalance between myocardial oxygen supply and demand induced by cardiac anatomical and functional alterations resulting from the valve lesion. In patients with congenital aortic stenosis, the appearance of ST-segment depression during exercise correlated well with the presence of a major transvalvular pressure gradient. Although it would seem feasible, at present data are not available to document that exercise training can induce benefits upon functional capacity in patients with valvular heart disease.

References

1. Rosing DR, Reichek N, Perloff JK: The exercise test as a diagnostic and therapeutic aid. *Amer Heart J* 87:584-596, 1974.
2. Åstrand PO, Cuddy TE, Saltin B, et al: Cardiac output during submaximal and maximal work. *J Appl Physiol* 19:268-274, 1964.
3. Mitchell JH, Blomqvist G: Maximal oxygen uptake. *New Eng J Med* 284:1018-1022, 1971.
4. Bevegard BS, Shepherd JT: Regulation of the circulation during exercise in man. *Physiol Rev* 47:178-213, 1967.
5. Skinner ND Jr, Powell WH: Regulation of skeletal muscle blood flow during exercise. *Circ Res* 20 (suppl 1): 59-69, 1967.
6. Robinson BF, Epstein SE, Beiser GD, et al: Control of heart rate by the autonomic nervous system. *Circ Res* 19:400-411, 1966.
7. Huckabee WE: The role of anaerobic metabolism in the performance of mild muscular work. II: The effect of asymptomatic heart disease. *J Clin Invest* 37:1593-1602, 1958.

8. Braunwald E, Sonnenblick EH, Ross J, et al: An analysis of the cardiac response to exercise. *Circ Res* 20 (suppl 1): 44-58, 1967.
9. Margaria R, Cerretelli P: "The Respiratory System and Exercise," in Falls HB (Ed): *Exercise Physiology*, New York: Academic Press, 1968.
10. Lange Anderson K: "The Cardiovascular System in Exercise," in Falls HB (Ed): *Exercise Physiology*, New York: Academic Press, 1968.
11. Bevegard S, Holmgren A, Jonsson B: The effect of body position on the circulation at rest and during exercise, with special reference to the influence on the stroke volume. *Acta Physiol Scand* 49:279-298, 1960.
12. Wade DL, Bishop JM: *Cardiac Output and Regional Blood Flow*, Oxford: Blackwell Scientific, 1962.
13. Bache RJ, Wang Y, Jorgensen CR: Hemodynamic effects of exercise in isolated valvular aortic stenosis. *Circulation* 44: 1003-1013, 1971.
14. Ross J Jr, Gault JH, Mason DT, et al: Left ventricular performance during muscular exercise in patients with and without cardiac dysfunction. *Circulation* 34:597-608, 1966.
15. Epstein SE, Beiser GD, Stampfer M, et al: Characterization of the circulatory response to maximal upright exercise in normal subjects and patients with heart disease. *Circulation* 35:1049-1062, 1967.
16. Bruce RA, Cobb LA, Morledge JH, et al: Effects of posture, upright exercise, and myocardial stimulation on cardiac output in patients with diseases affecting diastolic filling and effective systolic ejection of the left ventricle. *Amer Heart J* 61:476-484, 1961.
17. Bruce RA, Cobb LA, Katsura S, et al: Exertional hypotension in cardiac patients. *Circulation* 19:543-551, 1959.
18. Blackmon JR, Rowell LB, Kennedy JW, et al: Physiological significance of maximal oxygen intake in "pure" mitral stenosis. *Circulation* 36:497-510, 1967.
19. Hurst JW, Logue B: *The Heart*, p. 468, New York: McGraw-Hill, 1974.
20. Kellermann JJ, Mann A, Lederman P, et al: Functional evaluation of cardiac work capacity by spiroergometry in patients with rheumatic heart disease. *Arch Phys Med* 50:189-193, 1969.
21. Patterson JA, Naughton J, Pietras RJ, et al: Treadmill exercise in assessment of the functional capacity of patients with cardiac disease. *Amer J Cardiol* 30:757-762, 1972.
22. Ashley WW, Bhaduri U, Pietras RJ, et al: Pulmonary arterial oxygen saturation during treadmill exercise. A discriminative index of functional class. *Amer Heart J* 90:463-471, 1975.
23. Lee SJ, Jonsson B, Bevegäro S, et al: Hemodynamic changes at rest and during exercise in patients with aortic stenosis of varying severity. *Amer Heart J* 79:318-331, 1970.
24. Epstein SE, Beiser GD, Goldstein RE, et al: Hemodynamic abnormalities in response to mild and intense upright exercise following operative correction of an atrial septal defect or tetralogy of Fallot. *Circulation* 47:1065-1075, 1973.
25. James FW, Kaplan S, Schwartz DC, et al: Response to exercise in patients after total surgical correction of tetralogy of Fallot. *Circulation* 54:671-679, 1976.
26. Hellerstein HK, Prozan GB, Liebow IM, et al: Two step exercise test as a test of cardiac function in chronic rheumatic heart disease and in arteriosclerotic heart disease with old myocardial infarction. *Amer J Cardiol* 7:234-252, 1961.
27. Ramsey LH, Beedle J: Electrocardiographic response to exercise in patients with mitral stenosis. *Circulation* 19:424-429, 1959.
28. Datey KK, Misra SN: The evaluation of two-step exercise test in patients with heart disease of different etiologies. *Dis Chest* 53:294-300, 1968.
29. Aronow WS, Harris CN: Treadmill exercise test in aortic stenosis and mitral stenosis. *Chest* 68:507-509, 1975.
30. Chandramouli B, Famice DA, Lauer BM: Exercise induced electrocardiographic changes in children with congenital aortic stenosis. *J Pediat* 87:725-730, 1975.
31. Auchincloss JH Jr, Gilbert R: Short-term physical training in patients with rheumatic heart disease. *Chest* 64:163-169, 1973.

17

Detection of Myocardial Ischemia by Rest and Exercise Thallium-201 Scintigraphy

Daniel S. Berman, MD
Ezra A. Amsterdam, MD
Dean T. Mason, MD

The high prevalence of coronary heart disease in our society and the progress in its management have resulted in the increasing importance of early identification of patients with this entity. To this end, a diagnostic technique which is noninvasive and therefore both widely applicable and of low risk would be of obvious advantage. The resting electrocardiogram is an insensitive tool for the detection of coronary heart disease in the absence of evidence of transmural myocardial infarction. As noted in previous chapters, exercise electrocardiography has greatly enhanced the sensitivity of the electrocardiographic detection of coronary artery disease, but this approach also has important limitations in both sensitivity and specificity. The recent development of a technique which combines exercise stress testing with assessment of regional myocardial perfusion by radioisotopic scintigraphy has significantly advanced the noninvasive detection of myocardial ischemia.[1-4] In this chapter the techniques, results and clinical applications of combined stress electrocardiography and myocardial scintigraphy are described.

The technique of rest and exercise scintigraphy provides assessment of relative regional myocardial perfusion through the use of radionuclides which are distributed to the myocardium in proportion to regional myocardial blood flow. It thereby offers an indirect means of detecting a profusion deficit in the myocardium and, by inference, the possibility of obstructive coronary artery disease.

Radiopharmaceuticals

The radioisotopic materials used for analysis of regional myocardial perfusion have been termed cold-spot agents because areas of decreased myocardial perfusion are identified by a decrease in regional radioactivity or a cold-spot. There are three major groups of cold-spot agents: (1) Radioactive potassium and potassium analogues, (2) Radioisotopic iodinated fatty acids, and (3) Radioactive particles. Of these, the potassium analogues have proven the most satisfactory for noninvasive assessment of regional myocardial blood flow.[5] Fatty acids currently under evaluation appear to be too rapidly metabolized for imaging purposes, and the particulate agents require intracoronary injection.[5] Potassium-43 has been utilized for rest and exercise imaging [1]; however, the beta emissions of this radionuclide lead to a relatively high patient radiation dose, and high gamma ray energies make this agent less than ideal for conventional scintillation camera imaging. Although rubidium-81 ([81]Rb) is a potassium analogue with no beta emissions, and therefore, improved radiation dosimetry compared to potassium-43, the high energies of the radioactive emissions of rubidium-81 also render this agent less than ideal for scintillation camera imaging.[5] However, if a pinhole collimator with a special lead shield to stop the penetration of the high energy emissions is used, rubidium-81 can be successfully employed for rest and exercise myocardial scintigraphy with the scintillation camera.[3, 6] Cesium, another potassium analogue, is neither rapidly nor efficiently extracted by the myocardium, and is therefore not useful in the assessment of transient ischemia.[7] ^{13}N-ammonium has a 20-minute half-life and positron emissions, and is therefore impractical for rest and exercise scintigraphy with current instrumentation.

The potassium analogue which has proven best suited to scintillation camera imaging of the myocardium at rest and after exercise is thallium-201 (^{201}Tl).[5] The radiation dosimetry is favorable, and most importantly there are no high energy gamma emissions. Therefore, for scintillation camera imaging with this agent, conventional collimators can be used, thereby simplifying the performance of the rest and exercise studies. In practice, the 68 to 80 kiloelectron volt (keV) X-ray emissions of a mercury daughter of thallium-201 are utilized during the imaging procedure.[4]

Physiologic Basis of Myocardial Scintigraphy with Potassium Analogues

Potassium and related cations are avidly extracted by all muscle including the myocardium.[7] Following intravenous injection, high proportions of potassium, rubidium and thallium are extracted during the initial circulation of radioactivity through the myocardial capillary bed.[7] Therefore, the relative amount of radioactivity in each region of the myocardium is principally determined by regional myocardial blood flow.[8] In the presence of normal blood flow, there is homogeneous distribution of radioactivity throughout the myocardium at rest.[3] With maximal exercise, blood flow is uniformly increased throughout all portions of the myocardium, and following the injection of radioactivity at peak exercise, there will again be uniform distribution of radioactivity throughout

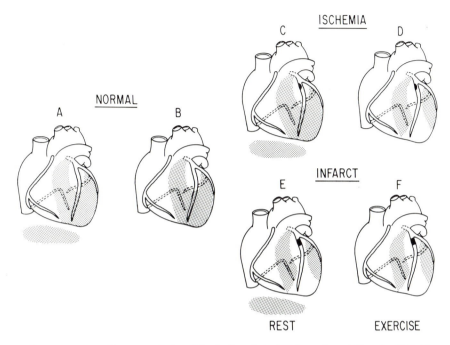

Figure 1. Schematic representation of the findings in rest and exercise scintigraphy. Panel A and B: patient without obstructive coronary lesions. Uniform distribution of radioactivity throughout left ventricular myocardium constitutes a normal study. Panel C and D: patient with a critical stenosis of left anterior descending coronary artery but without myocardial infarction. At rest (C) study is normal; after exercise (D) decreased activity is noted in the regions supplied by the stenotic coronary artery. This pattern of a defect after exercise not seen at rest is the pattern of reversible ischemia. Panel E and F: patient with a 100% occlusion of left anterior descending coronary artery and a prior myocardial infarction. Other coronary arteries are normal. Decrease in radioactivity in the apex at rest is unchanged after exercise. This is the pattern of prior myocardial infarction. The shaded area beneath the resting images represents hepatic and gastric background radioactivity which is decreased after maximal exertion, and therefore, not seen in the exercise images.

the myocardium.[3] This pattern of homogeneous distribution of radioactivity at rest and after maximal exercise constitutes a normal study (Figure 1a and 1b). When stenosis of a major coronary artery is present at a stage of the disease prior to infarction, blood flow through the stenotic vessel appears to be normal at rest. In this regard, it has been demonstrated in the experimental animal, that up to 85% stenosis of a coronary artery is associated with normal resting blood flow.[9, 10] With exercise, however, there is an appropriate increase in blood flow to regions of the myocardium supplied by normal vessels, but little or no increase in flow in the area supplied by a vessel with a fixed, severe stenosis. This imbalance in blood flow leads to decreased radioactivity in the region supplied by the stenotic vessel compared to that supplied by the normal vessels (Figure 1).[3] Therefore, the pattern of the normal scintigram at rest with an area of decreased activity after stress constitutes the pattern of exercise-induced myocardial ischemia (Figure 1c and 1d). When infarction has occurred, whether old or new, there is decreased radioactivity at rest in the region of infarction. This is because there is reduced perfusion to areas of myocardial fibrosis. With exercise, if there is no peri-infarction ischemia, the size of the defect remains unchanged although there may be greater contrast between the abnormal and normal regions. Thus, a defect at rest that does not change in size with exercise represents the pattern of myocardial infarction (Figure 1e and 1f).[3] It can be seen, then, that the analysis of rest and exercise scintigrams allows the assessment of both the presence and location of prior myocardial infarction as well as the presence and location of regional exercise-induced ischemia.

Technique

The technique utilized in our laboratory for rest and exercise thallium-201 scintigraphy is outlined in Figure 2. Following a 10-hour fast, maximal treadmill exercise is performed using the Bruce protocol,[11] and is carried to the onset of angina or major fatigue. Ischemic ST-segment depression alone constitutes the end point only when severe (>2 mm). Prior to cessation of exercise, an intravenous injection of 2 millicuries (mCi) of ^{201}Tl or 4 mCi ^{81}Rb is made through an indwelling intravenous line. Exercise is continued for an additional 30 to 60 seconds. Immediately following exercise, multiple views of the myocardium are obtained on the scintillation camera. It is important that imaging be initiated immediately after exercise, in order to avoid false-negative findings that might result from imaging after equilibration of the radioactivity has taken place. If the exercise scintigram is normal, a resting scintigram need not be performed. However, if there is an exercise-induced abnormality, a resting study is performed 2 to 4 days following the exercise test with a separate intravenous injection of radioactivity. The temporal delay is required in order to allow for radioisotopic decay of the first injection. The resting images are obtained in the same views as the exercise images (anterior, 40° left anterior oblique, 60° left anterior oblique and left lateral).

Recently an alternative to a separate resting examination was proposed.[12] It may be possible to image the patient 4 hours after exercise without reinjecting the radionuclide. The pattern of radioactivity on the 4-hour images appears to reflect an equilibrium state in which regional activity is distributed in proportion to cellular mass, whereas the initial postexercise images reflect regional myocardial blood flow. Initial results have suggested that the exercise and equilibrium method provides the same results as the exercise and rest approach, saving the cost of an additional injection of radionuclide, and several days' time which is required before resting imaging can be performed.[12]

Results

Considerable data are now available regarding the sensitivity and specificity of the scintigraphic myocardial perfusion technique.[1-4, 13-16] For illustrative pur-

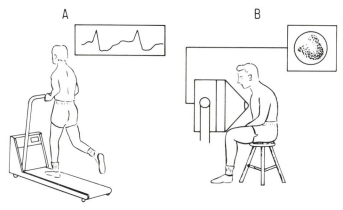

EXERCISE
    BRUCE PROTOCOL TO ANGINA, MAX HEART RATE, OR SEVERE FATIGUE
    INTRAVENOUS INJECTION OF 4mCi Rb-8I
    MULTIPLE VIEW SCINTIGRAPHIC IMAGING

REST
    2-DAY HIATUS
    REPEAT Rb-8I INJECTION AND IMAGING

Figure 2. Rest and exercise protocol for ^{81}Rb or ^{201}Tl scintigraphy. Panel A: tread-mill stress evaluation with exercise ECG showing ischemic ST changes. The radio-nuclide is injected at peak stress. Panel B: patient in front of the scintillation camera with the resultant myocardial image displayed at top right.

poses, we will describe in some detail a series of patients that we studied with rubidium-81 and a specially shielded scintillation camera.[3] The radionuclidic imaging was performed at rest and after exercise on 63 adults with known or suspected coronary artery disease. The results of the scintigraphic examination and of the treadmill stress electrocardiography were compared with the results of selective coronary arteriography in each patient (Table I). If both rest and

TABLE I

Results of Scintigraphy and Stress Electrocardiography Compared with Coronary Angiographic Findings in 63 Patients

	Coronary Arteriography		
	Significant Stenosis 33 patients	Borderline Stenosis 2 patients	No Significant Stenosis 12 patients
Rest/exercise ^{81}Rb scintigraphy			
Positive	43	0	0
Negative	6	2	12
Stress electrocardiography			
Positive	30	0	3
Negative	19	2	9

stress scintigrams demonstrated homogeneous distribution of radioactivity, they were interpreted as normal. Studies demonstrating decreased radioactivity in regions that normally have homogeneous uptake were considered abnormal. Studies in which a focal defect was present at rest were interpreted as suggestive of previous infarction. When a focal area of decreased activity was demonstrated after stress, and was either absent or smaller on the resting study, the scintigraphy was considered indicative of regional ischemia. The stress electrocardiograms were interpreted as positive if there was development of horizontal or down-sloping ST-segment depression of 1 mm (0.1 mV) or greater during or immediately following exercise in a lead which had an isoelectric ST segment in the control tracing. The coronary arteriograms were considered abnormal if there was stenosis of 75% or more in one or more of the three major coronary arteries. The results of this comparative electrocardiographic and scintigraphic study are depicted in Table I. Forty-nine of the 63 patients had greater than 75% stenosis of at least one of the three major coronary arteries. In two of the patients the coronary arteriograms were considered intermediate because lesions of only 50 to 75% narrowing were present. The remaining 12 patients either had normal coronary arteriograms or less than 50% narrowing of a major coronary artery.

The results of the stress electrocardiography in this group of 63 patients were similar to those reported in other series.[17, 18] Of the 49 patients with greater than 75% stenosis of at least one of the major coronary arteries, 30 (61%) had positive treadmill electrocardiograms, and in 19 of the 49 (39%) stress electrocardiography was negative. Furthermore, in the 12 patients with no significant coronary narrowing, stress electrocardiography was negative in nine (75%) but was positive in three patients (25%) with the syndrome of chest pain and normal coronary arteriograms.

The rest and exercise rubidium-81 scintigraphy was both more sensitive and more specific than treadmill electrocardiography. Of the 49 patients with significant coronary stenosis, 43 (88%) had positive exercise scintigrams; only six of the 49 (12%) were negative on the scintigraphic test. Therefore, of the patients with coronary artery stenosis, 88% were detected by the scintigraphic technique, whereas only 61% were detected by the stress electrocardiogram.[3] Of the 12 patients with no significant coronary stenosis, all were negative on exercise scintigraphy. Thus, there were no false-positive scintigrams compared to a 25% false-positive rate with the stress electrocardiogram. These data demonstrated greater accuracy in the detection of coronary artery disease with stress scintigraphy than stress electrocardiography.[3]

The combination of scintigraphy with stress electrocardiography was more sensitive in detecting coronary artery stenosis than either procedure alone. Of the 49 patients with greater than 75% stenosis of at least one of the three major coronary arteries, either scintigraphy or stress electrocardiography was positive in 45 (92%), whereas scintigraphy alone was positive in 88%, and stress electrocardiography alone was positive in 61%.[3]

TABLE II

Results of Rest and Exercise Imaging with Potassium Analogues

Study	Agent	# Patients	Sensitivity (%)	Specificity (%)
Zaret, 1973 [1]	^{43}K	31	84	100
Berman, 1975 [3]	^{81}Rb	61	88	100
Botvinick, 1977 [13]	^{81}Rb	56	91	91
Shames, 1976 [14]	^{201}Tl	53	95	93
Hamilton, 1977 [15]	^{201}Tl	101	78	96
Ritchie, 1977 [16]	^{201}Tl	176	81	86

Table II is a summary of reports by various other investigators of rest and exercise scintigraphy, utilizing potassium or potassium analogues. In general, the results are similar to that of our rubidium-81 scintigraphic study described above. The technique has a relatively high sensitivity and great specificity, which appears to exceed that of treadmill electrocardiography. Of particular interest is the last study listed on Table II. This was a multi-center cooperative study in which we participated with four other institutions to test the sensitivity and specificity of the ^{201}Tl scintigraphic technique compared with stress electrocardiography in assessing significant coronary disease as determined by coronary arteriography. Despite factors such as the multiplicity of investigators, differences in instrumentation (four types of scintillation cameras were used) and individual interpretive differences, the high sensitivity and specificity of the rest and exercise scintigraphic technique in detecting coronary disease were confirmed in this large study.[16]

Scintigraphic Patterns

Normal rest and exercise images obtained with the shielded scintillation camera using ^{81}Rb are shown in Figure 3. Of the cardiac structures, the left ventricular myocardium is visualized best due to its relatively large mass and blood flow. On the anterior view, the apex, inferior wall and lateral wall are well delineated. On the left anterior oblique view, the left ventricle is seen from the apex, optimally displaying the interventricular septum and the posterior wall. In most cases the faint outline of the right ventricular wall is also visualized in the left anterior oblique view. The left lateral view best defines the inferior left ventricular wall. Examples of patterns considered indicative of ischemia and infarction on comparative rest and exercise ^{81}Rb scintigraphic images are shown in Figure 4. Two classic patterns are shown. First, a prominent defect is seen posteriorly both at rest and without change after exercise corresponding to a well documented posterior myocardial infarction associated with occluded right and circumflex coronary arteries; and second, a defect is seen in

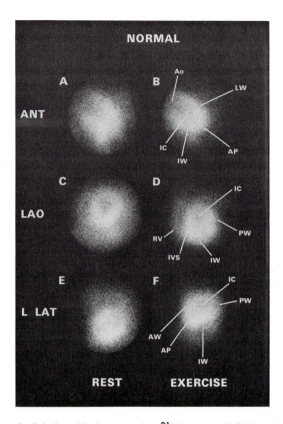

Figure 3. Scintigraphic images using ^{81}Rb at rest (A,C,E) and after exercise (B,D,F) in a patient with normal coronary arteriograms. The central area of decreased radioactivity seen most prominently on the LAO represents the left ventricular chamber (IC). On the anterior view, decrease in activity is seen in upper left representing the aortic outflow tract (Ao). Homogeneous distribution of radioactivity throughout the left ventricular myocardium at rest and after exercise constitutes a normal study. ANT = anterior view; LAO = left anterior oblique view; L. LAT = left lateral view; LW = lateral wall; AP = apex; IW = inferior wall; IVS = interventricular septum; PW = posterior wall; AW = anterior wall; RV = right ventricular wall. Reproduced by permission of The American Heart Association, Inc. from Berman DS et al: Noninvasive detection of regional myocardial ischemia using rubidium-81 and the scintillation camera. *Circulation* 52:619-628, 1975.

the apex after exercise that is not seen at rest. The latter defect is indicative of ischemia in the distribution of the left anterior descending coronary artery and correlated with 90% proximal stenosis of this vessel on angiography.

Clinical Applications

Combined scintigraphic and electrocardiographic rest and exercise evaluations have a number of clinical applications. Many series have demonstrated

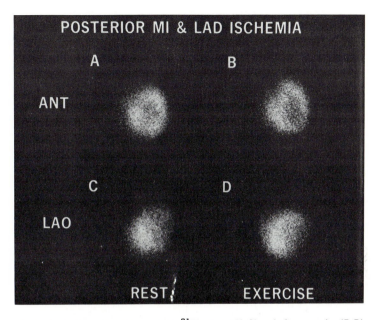

Figure 4. Scintigraphic images using [81]Rb at rest (A,C) and after exercise (B,D) in a patient with old posterior myocardial infarction and left anterior descending coronary artery (LAD) ischemia. The prominent posterior defect on the LAO both at rest (C) and after exercise (B) corresponds to the previous myocardial infarction. The striking defect in the apex after exercise (B) and not at rest (A) corresponds to a region of ischemia. Coronary arteriography revealed occluded right coronary and right circumflex coronary arteries, and a 90% stenosis of the LAD. Reproduced by permission of The American Heart Association, Inc. from Berman DS et al: Noninvasive detection of regional myocardial ischemia using rubidium-81 and the scintillation camera. *Circulation* 52:619-628, 1975.

the validity of this approach as a noninvasive screening test for significant coronary stenosis.[1-4, 13-16] In a select group of patients in whom coronary disease is considered unlikely, negative rest and exercise scintigraphy combined with negative stress electrocardiography may provide sufficient evidence of the absence of coronary artery disease to obviate cardiac catheterization. There are a number of clinical settings in which such a consideration arises. A major clinical problem is that of the syndrome of chest pain associated with normal coronary arteriograms. In a recent series, of 24 patients with this syndrome, we found that none had positive stress scintigrams (Figure 3).[19] It may, therefore, be possible in selected clinical settings where this syndrome is suspected, to avoid coronary arteriography on the basis of the information provided by this noninvasive evaluation. A similar problem is noted by patients with mitral valve prolapse syndrome. It has recently been demonstrated in a group of these patients that despite the presence of chest pain or positive stress electrocardiograms, the stress scintigraphic evaluation is uniformly negative.[20] Therefore, in these patients in whom clinical assessment deems the presence of coro-

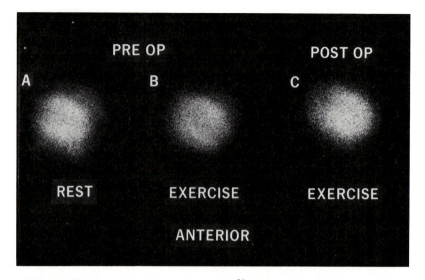

Figure 5. Anterior scintigraphic images using [81]Rb preoperatively (A,B) and post-operatively (C) in a patient with chronic angina pectoris and no evidence of myocardial infarction. Preoperative resting scintigram (A) is normal. Preoperative exercise scintigram (B) demonstrates an apical defect, corresponding to a 90% proximal stenosis of the LAD found at coronary arteriography. Arteriography also revealed a 90% stenosis of the left circumflex coronary artery and a 75% stenosis of the right coronary artery. The postoperative exercise scintigram (C) is normal, despite the patient's having exercised to a 60% greater workload then preoperatively before injection of radio-activity. The scintigraphic study, therefore, documents the efficacy of the patient's bypass surgery. Reproduced by permission of The American Heart Association, Inc. from Berman DS et al: Noninvasive detection of regional myocardial ischemia using rubidium-81 and the scintillation camera. *Circulation* 52:619-628, 1975.

nary disease unlikely, the negative stress scintigram may provide sufficient supportive information to exclude cardiac catheterization.

A particularly important use of the method arises in patients in whom the ischemia cannot be meaningfully interpreted on the stress electrocardiogram. This situation occurs when the resting electrocardiogram and ST segments are abnormal, as in left ventricular hypertrophy, left bundle branch block, digitalis administration and electrolyte imbalance. In these patients in whom the stress electrocardiogram is rendered questionable in detecting exercise-induced ischemia, the stress scintigraphic examination has particular clinical utility.

Response of subjective symptoms of angina to coronary artery bypass surgery does not provide a reliable mean of assessing the physiologic results of this procedure. The combination of stress electrocardiography and stress scintigraphy has been most useful in this regard (Figure 5). Preoperatively, ischemia was shown by a normal resting scintigram and an abnormal exercise image with a defect in the apex corresponding to a 95% stenosis of the left anterior descending coronary artery. The postcoronary bypass exercise scintigraphy, in which the perfusion pattern had returned to normal, objectively documented the effi-

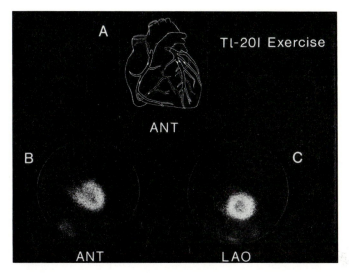

Figure 6. Coronary anteriograms (A) and rest and exercise scintigrams (B and C) performed with ^{201}Tl in a patient with 60% narrowing of the left anterior descending coronary artery and other lesions of less than 50% narrowing. The rest and exercise scintigrams were entirely normal, as was the treadmill electrocardiogram. Therefore, the patient had neither electrocardiographic nor scintigraphic evidence of myocardial ischemia.

cacy of surgical myocardial revascularization in this patient.[21] In a group of 15 patients undergoing coronary artery bypass surgery and evaluated by preoperative and postoperative rest and exercise myocardial scintigraphy, we demonstrated a high degree of correlation between symptomatic relief of angina and objective evidence of improvement in both the exercise electrocardiogram and stress scintigram.[21]

A further application of the scintigraphic technique is in assessing patients whose coronary lesions are of questionable significance. The patient depicted in Figure 6 had a 60% narrowing of the left anterior descending coronary artery. With this lesion of borderline angiographic significance, it was difficult to determine whether the patient had hemodynamically significant coronary obstruction. The treadmill electrocardiogram was entirely within normal limits, despite the fact that the patient reached peak predicted heart rate prior to cessation of the examination. Further supporting evidence of the absence of myocardial ischemia was gained from the normal stress scintigrams shown in Figure 6. There was uniform distribution of thallium-201 throughout all portions of the left ventricular wall. Therefore, the patient had neither electrocardiographic nor stress scintigraphic evidence of myocardial ischemia. This patient was not selected for coronary bypass surgery. Hypothetically, on the other hand, if major ischemic changes had been visualized on the thallium-201 scintigram, hemodynamic significance of the questionable narrowing would

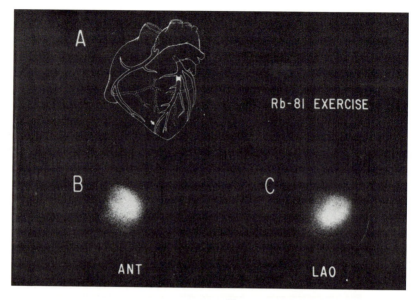

Figure 7. Coronary arteriograms (A) and [81]Rb exercise myocardial scintigrams (B and C). Coronary arteriograms demonstrated 100% occlusion
of the left anterior descending coronary artery, but excellent collateral
filling of the distal LAD from the right coronary artery. The left ventricular cineangiogram was normal, as was the resting electrocardiogram,
consistent with the absence of prior myocardial infarction. Normal exercise [81]Rb scintigrams are seen, which in conjunction with the normal
exercise electrocardiogram and the absence of exertional chest pain
documented the functional significance of the coronary collaterals.

have been demonstrated, and the patient could have been rationally chosen as a
candidate for bypass surgery.

The question of the functional significance of coronary collateral vessels remains incompletely answered despite a great deal of investigative work in this
area. Angiographic evaluation of coronary collaterals does not provide quantitative information with respect to myocardial blood flow through these vessels. The stress scintigram can be utilized to determine whether collaterals visualized at the time of angiography are hemodynamically adequate in an individual patient.[22] The patient in Figure 7 had a 100% occlusion of the left
anterior descending coronary artery in its proximal portion. Excellent collateral
filling of the distal left anterior descending coronary artery was noted at the
time of angiography after injection of the right coronary artery. Figure 7 demonstrates entirely normal stress scintigrams in this patient with the occluded left
anterior descending artery. Therefore, in this patient, with neither exercise-induced chest pain, positive exercise treadmill electrocardiogram, nor positive
stress myocardial scintigram, there was evidence that the collateral vessel was
protecting the patient from the development of exercise-induced ischemia. Con-

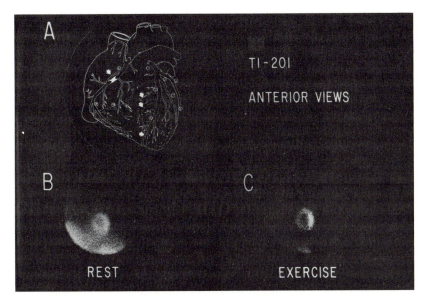

Figure 8. Coronary arteriograms (A) and rest and exercise ^{201}Tl myocardial scintigrams (B and C). Coronary arteriography demonstrated a 100% occlusion of the proximal right coronary artery with excellent collateral filling of the distal right coronary artery by collaterals from the left coronary system. The left ventricular cineangiogram, resting electrocardiogram, and resting myocardial scintigram are all normal, documenting the absence of prior myocardial infarction. The stress scintigram demonstrated striking decrease in radioactivity along the inferior wall of the left ventricle (C), indicating the presence of exercise-induced myocardial ischemia despite the presence of the high-grade collateral vessels. Therefore, in this more typical patient with coronary collaterals, there was no evidence of protection against exercise-induced ischemia by the collateral vessels.

servative management was selected for this patient.

In contrast to the unusual findings in the previous patient, the patient in Figure 8 had a more typical scintigraphic pattern. Coronary arteriography demonstrated an occluded right coronary artery in its proximal portion. Excellent collateral filling of the distal right coronary artery was seen after injection of the left coronary system. This patient also did not have exercise-induced chest pain or a positive treadmill electrocardiogram. The resting scintigram was normal (Figure 8b). However, the stress scintigram (Figure 8c) demonstrated striking decrease in radioactivity along the inferior wall of the left ventricle, the region supplied by the right coronary artery. Therefore, in this patient who also had apparently adequate collateral vessels by angiography, there was evidence of stress-induced ischemia on the scintigraphic examination. In a large number of patients matched for extent of coronary disease and for the quality of the the collateral vessels, myocardial ischemia after maximal exercise was as prevalent in the group with "good" collaterals, assessed by angiography, as in the group of patients without such collaterals.[22] However, in isolated patients such

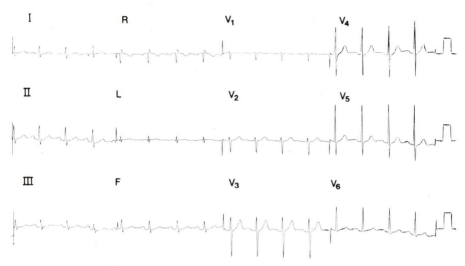

Figure 9. 12-Lead electrocardiogram in a 47-year-old man.
Resting electrocardiogram is normal. See Figure 10 and 11.

as the one described in Figure 7, "good" collateral vessels appeared to protect against the development of exercise-induced ischemia.

Screening of Asymptomatic Patients

Recently an increasing number of asymptomatic patients have been undergoing stress electrocardiography. These individuals represent an entirely different subset of patients from those with suspected coronary disease in whom stress electrocardiography is applied. In the latter patients, the rate of false-positive stress electrocardiograms is approximately 10%.[17] However, in asymptomatic patients, the prevalence of coronary disease is much less than that in the group with clinically suspected coronary disease (Chapter 13). Therefore, with the wider application of treadmill electrocardiography in asymptomatic groups, the proportion of patients with false-positive stress electrocardiograms can be anticipated to increase dramatically. Clinicians will then be faced with the decision of management of the asymptomatic individual who has a positive treadmill electrocardiogram. In this setting, the results of rest and stress thallium-201 scintigraphy are particularly important. Our initial findings in these patients have demonstrated that the scintigraphic technique offers an excellent tool for separating patients with asymptomatic positive treadmill tests into two groups, those with positive scintigrams and those with negative scintigrams. Due to the very high specificity of the scintigraphic technique, a positive scintigram is associated with a very high probability of the presence of coronary artery disease. Therefore, an asymptomatic patient with a positive treadmill electrocardiogram accompanied by a positive thallium-201 scintigram may be rationally considered for further study with coronary arteriog-

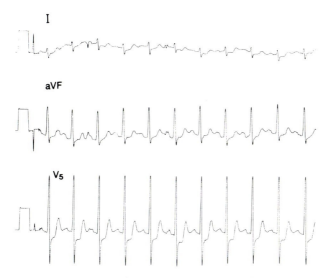

Figure 10. Representative samples from the stress electro-cardiogram of an asymptomatic patient (see Figure 9 and 11). Three millimeters of horizontal ST depression is seen in the V_5, despite the absence of pain. Leads I, aVF and V_5 are shown.

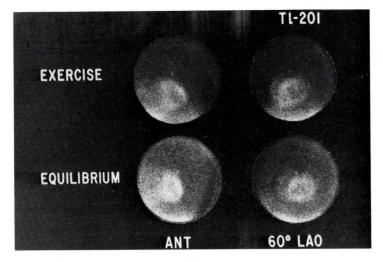

Figure 11. Exercise and equilibrium ^{201}Tl scintigrams in same asymptomatic patient as in Figure 9 and 10. Upper panel: exercise scintigrams; lower panel: equilibrium scintigrams. After exercise, a marked defect is seen in the region of the apex (upper left) that is not seen at equilibrium (lower left), indicating revers-ible apical myocardial ischemia. The exercise LAO image (upper right) demon-strates a defect in the posterior wall of the left ventricle which is not seen at equilibrium (lower right), indicating reversible posterior wall ischemia. Cardiac catheterization with coronary arteriography revealed 90% stenoses of all three of the major coronary arteries, with no evidence of prior myocardial infarction.

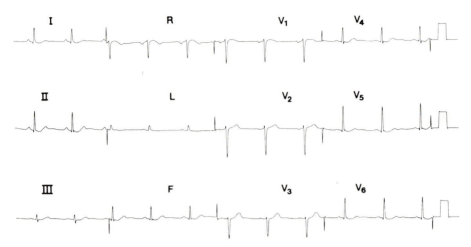

Figure 12. Resting electrocardiogram in a 50-year-old man with no exertional chest pain. Note minor ST-T–wave abnormalities and poor R-wave progression In V_1 through V_3. See Figure 13 and 14.

raphy if indicated by other findings in his case. On the other hand, owing to the relatively high sensitivity of the scintigraphic technique, asymptomatic patients with positive stress electrocardiograms but negative stress scintigrams are less likely to have coronary artery disease. In this latter group, if the risk factor profile as well as the stress scintigrams are negative, it may be rational to select these patients for conservative management rather than for coronary arteriography (Figure 9 to 14). The patient in Figure 9 through 11 was a 47-year-old male jogger with no exertional chest pain. He had had a syncopal episode when jogging at peak capacity on a hot day with ambient temperature 105°F. A resting electrocardiogram was normal (Figure 9). The treadmill electrocardiogram (Figure 10) demonstrated 3 mm of horizontal ST depression in V_5, with the abnormality first arising at heart rate 120 beats/min. There was no exertional chest pain. Exercise and equilibrium scintigrams are demonstrated in Figure 11. There is a marked defect in the region of the apex and inferior wall of the left ventricle after exercise that has resolved by the time of the equilibrium image 4 hours after injection. Therefore, in this asymptomatic patient, stress scintigraphy demonstrates the presence of regional myocardial ischemia. Subsequent arteriograms revealed 90% stenosis of the left anterior descending, left circumflex and right coronary arteries. There was no evidence of prior myocardial infarction.

The patient in Figures 12 through 14 also had no exertional chest pain. In this 50-year-old man with no known risk factors for coronary artery disease, treadmill electrocardiography was performed in evaluation for a jogging program. The patient was on no cardiac medications. The resting electrocardiogram demonstrated minimal ST-T–wave abnormalities (Figure 12). The exercise electrocardiogram became abnormal at a heart rate of 100 beats/min. At peak heart rate 3.5 mm of down-sloping ST-segment depression was noted in lead V_5, with ST-

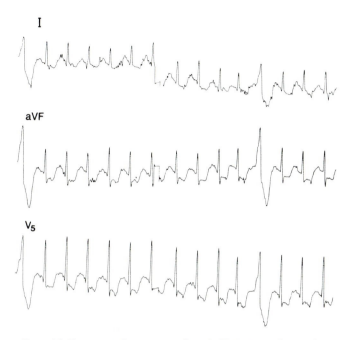

Figure 13. Representative segment of treadmill electrocardiogram in an asymptomatic patient (see Figure 12 and 14). Three and one-half millimeters of down-sloping ST depression is noted in V_5 with ST depression also in aVF. In addition, frequent PVC's are noted.

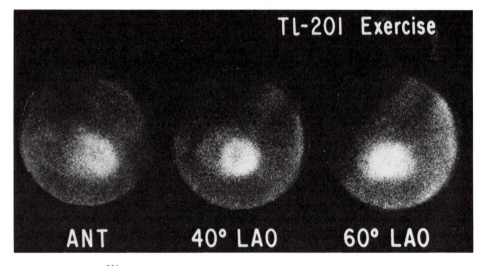

Figure 14. Exercise ^{201}Tl myocardial scintigrams in same asymptomatic patient as in Figure 12 and 13. Uniform distribution of radioactivity throughout the left ventricular myocardium is consistent with the absence of regional myocardial ischemia. Cardiac catheterization with coronary arteriography demonstrated entirely normal coronary arteriograms and normal left ventricular cineangiogram.

segment depression also noted in aVF (Figure 13). In addition frequent PVC's were seen with exercise (Figure 13). The exercise scintigrams (Figure 14) in this patient were entirely normal. There was uniform distribution of radioactivity throughout all portions of the left ventricle. Subsequent arteriography revealed normal coronary arteries with no evidence of luminal narrowing. The left ventriculogram and hemodynamic measurements were also entirely normal. Therefore, the scintigraphic tests in this patient had provided further evidence that coronary disease was not present. In view of a negative risk factor profile and the absence of symptoms, the negative scintigraphic evaluation may well have provided sufficient evidence to avoid cardiac catheterization. Subsequent work in our laboratory with approximately 20 patients has demonstrated excellent separation by the scintigraphic technique of asymptomatic patients with positive treadmill electrocardiograms into those with and those without coronary disease.

Summary

Rest and exercise cold-spot myocardial scintigraphic imaging with intravenously injected rubidium-81 or thallium-201 and the scintillation camera provides an accurate, objective, noninvasive means for the assessment of relative left ventricular regional blood flow. In this chapter, the clinical value of this new technique has been shown in the improved detection of myocardial ischemia due to coronary stenosis. This atraumatic radioisotopic method has also been successful in evaluation of the efficacy and serial follow-up of surgical revascularization in coronary patients. In addition, examples have been shown demonstrating the usefulness of stress scintigraphy in evaluation of the asymptomatic patient with a positive treadmill electrocardiogram, patients in whom stress electrocardiography is difficult to interpret, patients with borderline lesions on coronary arteriography, and in assessment of the adequacy of coronary collateral vessels. With the additional risk of a small amount of radioactivity, the stress scintigram appears to significantly enhance the clinical utility of stress electrocardiography.

Acknowledgment—Jasie Loving and Kurt Newcomer provided technical assistance.

This study was supported in part by Research Program Project Grant HL-14780 from The National Heart, Lung and Blood Institutes of Health, Bethesda, Maryland and California Chapters of The American Heart Association, Dallas, Texas.

References

1. Zaret BL, Stenson RE, Martin ND, et al: Potassium-43 myocardial perfusion scanning for the noninvasive evaluation of patients with false-positive exercise tests. *Circulation* 48:1234-1241, 1973.
2. Martin ND, Zaret BL, McGowan RL, et al: Rubidium-81: a new myocardial scanning agent *Radiology* 111:651-656, 1974.
3. Berman DS, Salel AF, DeNardo GL, et al: Noninvasive detection of regional myocardial is-

chemia using rubidium-81 and the scintillation camera. *Circulation* 52:619-628, 1975.

4. Bailey IK, Griffith LFC, Rouleau J, et al: Thallium-201 myocardial perfusion at rest and during exercise. *Circulation* 55:79-87, 1977.

5. Poe ND: Rationale and radiopharmaceuticals for myocardial imaging. *Seminars Nucl Med* 7:7-14, 1977.

6. Berman DS, Salel AF, DeNardo GL: Comparison of Rb-81 and Tl-201 rest and exercise myocardial scintigraphy in the noninvasive detection of regional myocardial ischemia (abstract). *Clin Res* 25:87, 1977.

7. Love WD, Ishihara Y, Lyon LD, et al: Differences in the relationships between coronary blood flow and myocardial clearance of isotopes of potassium, rubidium and cesium. *Amer Heart J* 76:353-355, 1968.

8. Prokop EK, Strauss HW, Shaw J, et al: Comparison of regional myocardial perfusion determined by ionic potassium-43 to that determined by microspheres. *Circulation* 50:978-984, 1974.

9. Gould KL, Lipscomb K, Hamilton GW: Physiologic basis for assessing critical coronary stenosis. *Amer J Cardiol* 33:87-94, 1974.

10. Gould KL, Hamilton GW, Lipscomb K, et al: Method for assessing stress-induced regional malperfusion during coronary arteriography. Experimental validation and clinical application. *Amer J Cardiol* 34:557-564, 1974.

11. Bruce RA, Hornstein TR: Exercise stress testing in evaluation of patients with ischemic heart disease. *Prog Cardiovasc Dis* 12:371-390, 1969.

12. Pohost GM, Beller GA, McKusic KA, et al: Thallium-201 redistribution following transient myocardial ischemia (abstract). *J Nucl Med* 17:535, 1976.

13. Botvinick EH, Shames DM, Gershengorn KM, et al: Myocardial stress perfusion with Rb-81 versus stress electrocardiography. *Amer J Cardiol* 39:364-371, 1977.

14. Shames D, Taradash M, Botvinick E: Comparison of Tl-201 stress myocardial perfusion imaging to stress electrocardiography (abstract). *J Nucl Med* 17:522, 1976.

15. Hamilton GW, Trobaugh GB, Narahara KA, et al: Thallium-201 myocardial imaging at rest and maximal exercise for the detection of coronary artery disease (abstract). *Amer J Cardiol* 39:321, 1977.

16. Ritchie JL, Zaret BL, Strauss HW, et al: Myocardial imaging with thallium-201 at rest and exercise—a multicenter study: coronary angiographic and electrocardiographic correlation (abstract). *Amer J Cardiol* 39:321, 1977.

17. Bartel AG, Behar VS, Peter RH, et al: Graded exercise stress tests in angiographically documented coronary artery disease. *Circulation* 49:348-356, 1974.

18. Tonkon M, Miller RR, DeMaria AN, et al: Multifactor analyses of determinants of ischemic response to stress test in coronary disease: role of distal flow and severity and number of stenoses (abstract). *Amer J Cardiol* 35:173, 1975.

19. Berman DS, Salel AF, DeNardo GL, et al: Angina with normal coronary arteriograms: analysis of regional myocardial perfusion by rest and exercise Rb-81 scintigraphy (abstract). *Clin Res* 25:87, 1977.

20. Massie B, Taradash M, Werner J, et al: Advantage of Tl-201 myocardial perfusion imaging in evaluating chest pain in patients with click murmur syndrome (abstract). *Clin Res* 25:92, 1977.

21. Lurie AJ, Salel AF, Berman DS, et al: Determination of improved myocardial perfusion after aortocoronary bypass surgery by exercise rubidium-81 scintigraphy. *Circulation* 54(suppl III): 20-23, 1976.

22. Berman DS, Bogren H, Miller RR, et al: Evaluation of the effects of graded coronary collaterals by Rb-81 and Tl-201 regional myocardial perfusion scintigraphy at rest and after maximal exercise (abstract). *Clin Res* 25:87, 1977.

PART IV

Preventive Aspects of Coronary Heart Disease

18

Individualized Exercise Prescription

Jack H. Wilmore, PhD

It is becoming increasingly evident that regular exercise can be an essential part of one's lifestyle for developing and maintaining optimal health, performance and appearance. While the role of exercise in preventive medicine is equivocal at this time, interest in this area is high, as illustrated by the fact that three major symposia on exercise and coronary heart disease have been held during the past four years alone,[1-3] as well as the intensive study of the interaction between physical activity and obesity for a number of years.[4] In both coronary heart disease and obesity, the lack of physical activity appears to be a significant contributing factor.[4, 5] World renowned exercise physiologist and physician, Dr. Per-Olaf Åstrand of Stockholm, has managed to resolve this apparent dilemma to his own satisfaction. He stated: "It will take 100 years to determine the exact relationship between physical activity and premature death from coronary heart disease. Personally, I can't afford to wait that long to find out so I elect to exercise."[6]

With the importance of exercise coming more clearly into focus, exercise programs for adults are being initiated throughout the United States. While the majority of these programs are well organized and fundamentally sound, many of these programs do not take into account the many advances that have been made recently in the exercise and sport sciences. These advances have direct implications for the conduct of adult exercise programs. With this in mind, the American Heart Association published *Exercise Testing and Training of Apparently Healthy Individuals: A Handbook for Physicians* [7] in 1972, and the American College of Sports Medicine published *Guidelines for Graded Exercise Testing and Exercise Prescription* [8] in 1975. These publications are intended to educate medical and paramedical professionals relative to the state of the art in the areas of exercise testing, exercise prescription and exercise training. This hopefully will result in an upgrading of those programs presently in existence, and serve as a model for future programs.

In the introduction to a recent Symposium on Exercise and the Heart, Adams stated: "Exercise as a therapeutic tool to improve cardiac and physical performance should be recommended in all age groups provided the subjects are thoroughly evaluated and the exercise program individualized."[9]

What is a thorough evaluation and how can exercise be prescribed individually? What constitutes a good exercise program for adults and how are these programs organized? This chapter will attempt to answer these and other related questions.

Medical Clearance

Prior to entering an exercise program, it is important that the prospective participant schedule a medical examination with his family physician. The examination should include a thorough family and personal health history, a physical examination, a resting electrocardiogram and resting blood pressure determination, and an exercise electrocardiogram. The current American College of Sports Medicine guidelines [8] suggest that this examination be required of all individuals who are 35 years of age or older, or younger, if they are at high risk for coronary heart disease. For those under 35 years of age, the examination is suggested but not required.

Certain diseases or medical conditions contraindicate the prescription of exercise in some individuals. These are discussed in Chapter 23. There are also certain individuals who should be exercising only under the direct supervision of a qualified physician. This would include postmyocardial infarction and coronary by-pass graft patients, as well as those with angina pectoris and those who have exhibited electrocardiographic abnormalities during a graded exercise stress test. It is therefore important to identify any prospective participant who might fall into any one of these "abnormal" categories.

The importance of the exercise electrocardiogram in the medical screening profile should not be overlooked. After the age of 35, abnormal exercise electrocardiograms, suggesting the presence of coronary heart disease, are found with increasing frequency, reaching ~ 10% in certain age groups of normal, asymptomatic individuals.[7] It is recommended that the graded exercise test be taken to complete volitional fatigue, *ie*, until the subject is unwilling or unable to push himself any farther. A recent study by Cumming [10] reported that ~ 50% of the abnormal exercise electrocardiographic responses are missed if the test is stopped at 85% of the subject's predicted, age-adjusted maxmimal heart rate.

Exercise Prescription

An individualized exercise prescription provides a practical answer to several problems. Most individual exercise programs are self-designed, *ie*, a man or woman selects an activity and begins exercising. This is a potentially dangerous practice since most people do not recognize their limitations and are likely to exceed a safe level of exercise. Just as important, people are likely to initiate an activity program without proper medical evaluation. A substantial number of persons have potential symptoms of cardiovascular disease (eg, angina pectoris), make a self diagnosis, and with a fear of the physician confirming their diagnosis, embark on their own exercise program in an attempt to remedy the situation. Group programs also have associated problems. Although a medical examination may be required for participation in these programs, the exercise is usually prescribed on a mass basis and little or no recognition is given to individual differences. Everyone is expected to do exactly the same. The individualized prescription of exercise avoids these hazards. The participant receives medical clearance and his interests and physiologic capacity are individually determined, thus ensuring accurate prescription of an appropriate exercise regimen.

Once the individual has been medically cleared to participate in the exercise program, he must be provided with an exercise prescription. Four factors constitute the prescription: type of exercise, duration of the exercise session, frequency of participation each week and the intensity at which the participant is to exercise.[11] The activity should be of an endurance nature such as walking, jogging, running, swimming, bicycling or hiking. It is important to prescribe activities that the individual will enjoy and be willing to follow. The endurance conditioning aspect of a tennis program is not nearly as great as that found for jogging, but if the participant dislikes jogging and enjoys tennis, tennis is the activity that should be prescribed, even though it may take him longer to gain the same endurance benefits. Exercise must be looked on as a lifetime pursuit, not a 6 to 12-month endeavor. Therefore, attractive activities must be made available.

For those individuals who start an exercise program with a very low initial endurance capacity, it is advisable to prescribe an activity with a high endurance component such as jogging, for the first 3 to 6 months. Once the individual reaches the desired endurance level, he can then be placed on a maintenance program with activities such as tennis, handball, badminton, etc.

Pollock[12] recently summarized the existing research relative to the frequency, duration and intensity of the exercise program. It appears that 3 to 4 days a week at 20 to 40 minutes per day is an optimal frequency and duration. This is not to say that longer or more frequent exercise sessions would not result in greater improvement, for they will. It simply implies that to invest additional time above the suggested optimal time will produce less return relative to the time invested. With regard to the intensity of the exercise, it appears that there is a minimal threshold, below which a conditioning effect will not occur. This appears to be somewhere around 50% of the participant's endurance capacity, although there is a great deal of individual variation. A training intensity of 50 to 80% of one's endurance capacity appears to be optimal. This can be easily monitored by the participant, by determining the heart rate equivalent to the selected working intensity. He then monitors his pulse rate during exercise attempting to keep it at this training level. This is referred to as the training heart rate (THR).

Why is the heart rate a desirable variable for controlling the intensity of exercise? Intensity is the most critical factor in the exercise prescription. Individuals can get into trouble if they exert themselves beyond a safe and reasonable intensity. The heart rate represents a simple physiological parameter that can be easily monitored by the individual and which provides meaningful insight into the degree of metabolic and myocardial stress. The linear relationship between heart rate and oxygen consumption at submaximal levels of work allows heart rate to be used to estimate the metabolic cost of the work.[13] More importantly, there is a high correlation (r ~ 0.89) between heart rate and both myocardial blood flow and myocardial oxygen consumption.[14] By maintaining a constant THR, the work of the myocardium stays constant.

One other aspect of particular importance relative to the THR concept is that the heart rate, in its relationship to the work of the heart, is independent of the various environmental factors. If the exercising individual is suddenly confronted with hot, humid weather or takes a vacation at 8,000 feet altitude, the total workout will have to be reduced to maintain the THR. Thus, the work of the heart stays constant even though metabolic work has to be decreased. This is obviously desirable with regard to the degree of stress placed on the heart.

An additional advantage of using the heart rate to control the exercise intensity is that there is a natural progression in absolute work as training continues. Since the heart rate response to a standardized, submaximal bout of exercise decreases progressively with training, it will require more effort or work each day to reach the same THR.[15]

Training heart rate must be established individually. Use of a standard heart rate such as 150 beats/min for groups of persons of all ages is a questionable procedure. This heart rate represents 75% of the capacity of the 25-year-old subject but 98% of the capacity of the 65-year-old subject and is independent of training state.[12]

Education and Motivation

Appreciating the need for increased physical activity and translating this need into action are, unfortunately, unrelated events. Any successful exercise program must therefore accomplish two major goals: (1) Teach people why they should be physically active; and (2) Motivate them to follow through with a personal activity program. The majority of existing exercise programs are short on education.

People are told that they must exercise but are given little if any information on why they should exercise. The average person today has a relatively sophisticated knowledge of the basic biological sciences and medicine. If he thoroughly understands the reasons for following a routine program of physical activity, he will be more inclined to do so. Probably the most valuable contribution

TABLE I

Possible Physiological Alterations Resulting from Chronic Physical Activity

Heart
    Reduced resting heart rate
    Reduced heart rate for a standardized exercise bout
    Increased rate of heart rate recovery after a standardized exercise
    Increased blood volume pumped per heart beat (stroke volume)
    Increased size of heart muscle (myocardial hypertrophy)
    Increased blood supply to heart muscle
    Increased strength of cardiac contraction (contractibility)

Blood Vessels and Blood Chemistry
    Reduced resting systolic and diastolic arterial blood pressure, if originally elevated
    Reduced serum lipids or fats, *ie*, cholesterol, triglycerides
    Increased blood supply to muscles
    Increased blood volume
    More efficient exchange of O_2 and CO_2 in muscles

Lungs
    Increased functional capacity during exercise
    Increased blood supply
    Increased diffusion of respiratory gases
    Reduced nonfunctional volume of lung (residual volume)

Neural, Endocrine and Metabolic Function
    Increased glucose tolerance
    Reduced strain and nervous tension resulting from psychological stress
    Increased enzymatic function in muscle cells
    Reduced body fat content (adiposity)
    Increased muscle mass (lean body weight)
    Increased functional capacity during exercise (oxygen uptake capacity)

Adapted from unpublished material prepared by W. L. Haskell and J. H. Wilmore for the Preventive Medicine Center, Palo Alto, California.

made by Cooper [16] in his initial book, *Aerobics*, was to inform an educated audience specifically why exercise is essential to improving and maintaining health.

In addition to educating people, it is necessary to motivate them to act. Initially, much of this motivation can be in the form of external goals and rewards, but once a person has been actively exercising for several months or more, more subtle forms of internal motivation are needed. The individual man or woman must recognize that an exercise program is a lifetime pursuit.

Group programs provide excellent opportunities for motivation, teaching and interaction. The influence of the group and its leader or leaders has tremendous motivational significance. Unfortunately, group programs now involve a very small percent of our total adult population. Many people cannot or will not take advantage of existing programs, often for valid reasons. These people can be helped to develop their own personal exercise program.

TABLE II

Alterations in Endurance Capacity, Body Composition and Blood Lipid Levels in Middle-aged Men Consequent to a 3-Month and 6-Month Program of Prescribed Exercise

Variable	Initial		Final			
	Mean	σ	Mean	σ	Δ	$\% \Delta$
3-Month Program (n = 44)						
$\dot{V}O_2$ max (ml/kg · min)	28.2	6.2	32.4	6.3	4.2	14.9
Weight (kg)	81.4	10.6	78.5	10.2	-2.9	-3.6
Lean body weight (kg)	61.1	6.1	61.8	6.4	0.7	1.1
Fat weight (kg)	20.3	6.2	16.7	6.1	-3.6	-17.7
Relative fat (%)	24.5	5.2	20.9	4.9	-3.6	-14.7
Cholesterol (mg/100 ml)	246.2	41.6	227.3	41.5	-18.9	-7.7
Triglycerides (mg/100 ml)	145.8	85.7	94.1	40.3	-51.7	-35.5
6-Month Program (n = 32)						
$\dot{V}O_2$ max (ml/kg · min)	37.9	8.5	44.0	7.6	6.1	16.1
Weight (kg)	80.5	10.1	77.9	9.6	-2.6	-3.2
Lean body weight (kg)	61.9	6.7	62.9	6.5	1.0	1.6
Fat weight (kg)	18.5	6.7	15.0	6.1	-3.6	-19.4
Relative fat (%)	22.7	6.2	18.8	6.0	-3.9	-17.2
Cholesterol (mg/100 ml)	257.1	51.3	219.0	40.4	-38.1	-14.8
Triglycerides (mg/100 ml)	131.0	76.2	121.0	92.8	-10.0	-7.6

The medical and physiologic evaluation and consultation are used as educational experiences. The subject receives explanations of most of the testing procedures and both written and verbal interpretations of his own test results. In addition, he should receive educational materials during the consultation and at various times throughout the year. Participants should also be given specific goals to reach within a specified time period. For example, a subject may be asked to increase his maximal oxygen uptake from 24 to 31 mg/kg · min and decrease his relative fat from 27.5 to 22.5% within 6 months. Additional long-range goals are also provided. Participants should be encouraged to return after 6 to 12 months for reevaluation. This procedure, intended to assess the success of the prescription, is also a valuable motivational tool for maintaining participants in an exercise program for the intervening 6 to 12-month period.

Predicted Outcomes from Prescriptive Exercise Programs

The participant who follows the prescribed exercise program as outlined above can expect to see some rather dramatic changes as a result of his efforts within a relatively short 3 to 6-month period of time. The potential changes are outlined in Table I. Almost all of these changes have been documented in numerous studies cited in two recent review articles.[4, 12]

The results from two programs using this approach to exercise prescription are presented in Table II. The data in Table II represent changes after both a 3-month and a 6-month exercise program. In both cases, the changes are substantial and are all in the direction of improving the subjects' health profile. However, the changes in body composition and blood lipid levels cannot be attributed solely to the exercise program as many of the participants were also consuming modified diets prescribed by a dietician.

Summary

An individualized approach to the prescription of exercise has been shown to be both feasible and acceptable to the public. Programs based on this approach appear to provide meaningful changes in health. The two key factors in ensuring the success of an individualized program appear to be provision of adequate education and generation of the motivation needed to carry out the immediate program with an appreciation that exercise is a lifetime pursuit.

References

1. Adams CW (Ed): Symposium on exercise and the heart. *Amer J Cardiol* 30:713-756, 1972.
2. Naughton JP, Hellerstein HK (Eds): *Exercise Testing and Exercise Training in Coronary Heart Disease*, New York: Academic Press, 1973.
3. Amsterdam EA, Wilmore JH, DeMaria AN (Eds): Symposium on exercise in cardiovascular health and disease. *Amer J Cardiol* 33:713-790, 1974.
4. Oscai LB: "The Role of Exercise in Weight Control," in Wilmore JH (Ed): *Exercise and Sport Sciences Reviews*, vol I, New York: Academic Press, 1973.
5. Fox SM: "Relationship of Activity Habits to Coronary Disease," in Naughton JP, Hellerstein HK (Eds): *Exercise Testing and Exercise Training in Coronary Heart Disease*, New York: Academic Press, 1973.
6. Åstrand P-O: Talk presented at 1970 National Convention of the American Association of Health, Physical Education and Recreation, April 1970, Seattle, Washington.
7. American Heart Association: *Exercise Testing and Training of Apparently Healthy Individuals: A Handbook for Physicians*, New York, 1972.
8. American College of Sports Medicine: *Guidelines for Graded Exercise Testing and Exercise Prescription, and Behavioral Objectives for Physicians, Program Directors, Exercise Leaders and Exercise Technicians*, Philadelphia: Lea and Febiger, 1975.
9. Adams CW: Introduction. Symposium on exercise and the heart. *Amer J Cardiol* 30:713-715, 1972.
10. Cumming GR: Yield of ischemic exercise electrocardiograms in relation to exercise intensity in a normal population. *Brit Heart J* 34:919-923, 1972.
11. Wilmore JH: Individual exercise prescription. *Amer J Cardiol* 33:757-759, 1974.
12. Pollock ML: "The Quantification of Endurance Training Programs," in Wilmore JH (Ed): *Exercise and Sport Sciences Reviews*, vol I, New York: Academic Press, 1973.
13. Wilmore JH, Haskell WL: Use of the heart rate-energy expenditure relationship in the individual prescription of exercise. *Amer J Clin Nutr* 24:1186-1192, 1971.
14. Kitamura K, Jorgensen CR, Gobel FL, et al: Hemodynamic correlates of myocardial oxygen consumption during upright exercise. *J Appl Physiol* 32:516-521, 1972.
15. Wilmore JH: "Exercise Control, Heart Rate," in Wilson PK (Ed): *Adult Fitness and Cardiac Rehabilitation*, Baltimore: University Park Press, 1975.
16. Cooper KH: *Aerobics*, pp 1-182, New York: Bantam, 1968.

19

Coronary Risk Factor Modification by Chronic Physical Exercise

Joseph A. Bonanno, MD

Exercise conditioning programs have been widely recommended in both the medical literature and the lay press as a means of decreasing the incidence, prevalence, severity or mortality of coronary heart disease. These claims were initially based on epidemiologic studies [1-3] which suggested an inverse relationship between physical activity and coronary heart disease. Proponents of physical training grew in number and enthusiasm with the appearance of many reports which substantiated an improvement in cardiovascular functional capacity both in normal subjects and in patients with coronary heart disease following exercise programs.[4-10] However, a cause and effect relationship between physical inactivity and coronary heart disease has never been firmly demonstrated. Furthermore, there is as yet no conclusive proof that chronic physical exercise will in fact prevent this disease or reduce its mortality and morbidity.[11]

In the assessment of the effects of a regular exercise program on coronary heart disease there are two basic issues which need to be addressed: (1) What is the potential for primary prevention of coronary disease? and (2) What is the therapeutic or protective role in patients with manifest coronary disease? In this discussion attention will be focused on the potential role of chronic exercise in primary prevention. The physiological adaptations to exercise training and its potential therapeutic role in patients with overt coronary disease are discussed in Part II and Part V of this volume.

The etiology of coronary atherosclerosis has not yet been precisely defined but is generally accepted to be multifactoral. Thus, a number of factors have been repeatedly shown in epidemiologic investigations to be associated with clinical coronary heart disease in a frequency greater than in the general population. These are recognized as the "coronary risk factors." The most important coronary risk factors are hypertension, hyperlipidemia and cigarette smoking, as discussed in Chapter 1. Other factors which have been implicated in the genesis of coronary atherosclerosis include a family history of ischemic heart disease, diabetes, obesity, physical inactivity, emotional stress and symptomatic hyperuricemia. The high probability of unrecognized risk factors is an additional consideration. At present it is virtually impossible to assess the relative importance of any specific risk factor in an individual patient. Similarly, it would be equally difficult to demonstrate the impact of modification of a specific risk factor upon the incidence of coronary artery disease. However, the Framingham experience has shown that with increasing numbers of risk factors there is an exponential increase in the risk of a coronary event.[12] Accordingly, it is logical to assume that the elimination or reduction of one or more of these factors could lead to a corresponding decrease in the risk of developing coronary disease. Thus, if a regular exercise training program can favorably modify these risk factors, its potential for primary prevention of coronary disease is a reasonable possibility.

Hypertension

A number of investigators have observed a diminished blood pressure response to an acute bout of exercise as well as to sustained submaximal external workloads following physical conditioning.[13, 14] The reported effects of conditioning on the resting blood pressure, however, have been inconsistent. While some studies have reported an improvement in resting blood pressure in patients with hypertension following exercise training,[15, 16] other investigations have failed to demonstrate a significant change following conditioning.[17, 18] These apparent inconsistencies appear to be explained in part by the lack of adequate control groups, the failure to segregate normotensive from hypertensive subjects or the concomitant use of hypotensive medications. We recently evaluated the effects of exercise training as an isolated intervention in a controlled study [19] and were able to reconcile some of these differences.

Table I presents the resting blood pressure data for normotensive and hypertensive subjects in both the control and exercise groups before and after a training program. It is noteworthy that the normotensive exercise subjects had no significant change in the resting systolic blood pressure from their control values, a finding in accord with those previous reports which did not identify a hypotensive effect secondary to physical training. In addition, both normotensive and hypertensive subjects had a significant reduction of diastolic blood pressure at rest in the control as well as in the exercise groups. Therefore, the reduction in diastolic pressure cannot be attributed to physical training and may simply reflect a reduction of anxiety resulting from repeated examinations. This finding emphasized the need for caution in analyzing the design and effects of any study of blood pressure or program of treatment.

Systolic hypertension, however, was significantly reduced only in the exer-

TABLE I

Effects of Training on Blood Pressure
(means ± standard deviation)

	Mean Blood Pressure (mm Hg)	
	Systolic	Diastolic
Normotensive Subjects		
Control group (n = 4)		
Pre	135	87
Post	132	78
Δ	-3	-9*
Exercise group (n = 8)		
Pre	123	84
Post	126	78
Δ	+3	-6*
Hypertensive Subjects		
Control group (n = 15)		
Pre	150	101
Post	147	90
Δ	-3	-11*
Exercise group (n = 12)		
Pre	148	97
Post	135	83
Δ	-13*	-14*

*P < 0.01

cise subjects. The physiologic mechanisms responsible for this reduction are not known. Physical training has been shown to result in a decrease in exertional response of blood pressure, circulating norepinephrine levels, and peripheral vascular resistance in subjects undergoing acute exercise stress.[20-22] These findings suggest that conditioning results in a reduction in sympathetic tone during exercise, a condition that may also prevail at rest in physically fit individuals. Although the precise mechanisms for the diminished systolic blood pressure following exercise training are obscure, it is quite clear that chronic exercise can produce a substantial reduction of blood pressure independent of any other therapeutic modalities in hypertensive patients. This conclusion is also consistent with studies which have demonstrated an inverse relationship between physical fitness levels and systolic blood pressure.[23]

Hyperlipidemia

Triglycerides are an important energy source for acute exercise and the serum levels of these fats can be readily reduced with vigorous exertion. However, these changes are relatively short-lived and the triglyceride levels return to baseline values by 72 to 96 hours after exercise.[19] A chronic exercise program consisting of three sessions per week might therefore be beneficial for hypertriglyceridemia. The concomitant use of dietary fat restriction would be expected to have an additive effect and should also be employed in a therapeutic program of this type. Thus, a program of regular exercise is capable of making a substantial contribution to a reduction in serum triglycerides.

In contrast, the reported effects of exercise training on serum cholesterol have been inconsistent,[10, 24-26] with the majority of studies showing no appreciable change. A day to day variability exists in the level of serum cholesterol and therefore relatively dramatic changes are necessary before statistical significance can be attained. However, in a carefully controlled diet, when multiple determinations were obtained, there was no weight loss; exercise did not produce any significant effect on the serum cholesterol.[19]

Obesity

Obesity has long been implicated as a major contributing factor to coronary heart disease, hypertension and hyperlipidemia. However, there is little firm evidence to support this contention. When obesity per se is considered as an independent variable, it appears to be only a minor determinant of blood pressure or lipid level, and has little demonstrable effect on the development of coronary heart disease.[27] Nevertheless, the association between obesity and coronary heart disease has been too conspicuous to ignore.

The inverse relationship between excess body fat and physical activity [23] has prompted many investigators to examine the effects of training programs on body weight. Most reports of these studies have found minor weight loss or an increase in lean body mass, or both, in response to physical conditioning. However, when weight loss does occur with training it has generally been found to be associated with concomitant dietary restriction. Conversely, when dietary habits are not changed, there has been no appreciable weight loss or change in lean body mass with training.[19]

Psychological Profile

The psychological effects of chronic physical exercise programs and stress modification is discussed in Chapter 20. It is a fairly universal experience for exercising subjects to "feel better" and objective psychological improvement has been measured in some studies. However, for the most part these results have been obtained in short-term exercise studies. Permanent modifications in behavior are obviously the goal for heart disease prevention. The extent to which this goal can be achieved through chronic physical exercise remains speculative.

Summary

Chronic physical exercise, considered as an independent variable, has been demonstrated to favorably modify several major coronary risk factors: hypertension, hypertriglyceridemia and psychological stress. Thus, a program of regular exercise has been established as an adjunctive form of therapy for these risk factors. Although exercise training has not yet been unequivocally demonstrated to reduce the risk of developing coronary heart disease, the available data regarding coronary risk factors provide strong support for the potential value of exercise training in appropriate individuals.

References

1. Fox SM III, Haskel WL: Physical activity and the prevention of coronary heart disease. *Bull NY Acad Med* 44:950-967, 1968.
2. Zukel WJ, Lewis RH, Enterline PE, et al: A short-term community study of the epidemiology of coronary heart disease: a preliminary report of the North Dakota study. *Amer J Public Health* 49:1630-1639, 1959.
3. Frank CW, Weinblatt E, Shapiro S, et al: Myocardial infarction in men. *JAMA* 198:1241-1245, 1968.
4. Hellerstein HK: Exercise therapy in coronary disease. *Bull NY Acad Med* 44:1028-1047, 1968.
5. Hanson HS, Tabakin BS, Levy AM, et al: Long-term physical training and cardiovascular dynamics in middle-aged men. *Circulation* 38:783-797, 1968.
6. Detry J-MR, Rousseau M, Vandenbroucke G, et al: Increased arteriovenous oxygen difference after physical training in coronary heart disease. *Circulation* 44:109-117, 1971.
7. Clausen JP, Larsen OA, Trap-Jensen J: Physical training in the management of coronary artery disease. *Circulation* 40:143-153, 1969.
8. Frick MH, Katila M: Hemodynamic consequences of physical training after myocardial infarction. *Circulation* 37:192-201, 1968.
9. Siegel W, Blomqvist G, Mitchell JH: Effects of a quantitated physical training program on middle-aged sedentary men. *Circulation* 41:19-29, 1970.
10. Rechnitzer PA, Yuhasz MS, Paivio A, et al: Effects of a 24-week exercise programme on normal adults and patients with previous myocardial infarction. *Brit Med J* 1:734-735, 1967.
11. Fox SM III, Naughton JP, Gorman PA: Physical activity and cardiovascular health. *Mod Conc Cardiovasc Dis* 41(4):17-20, 1972.
12. Kannel W: The Framingham Heart Study: Habits and coronary heart disease. Public Health Service Publication No. 1515. U.S. Government Printing Office, 1966.
13. Tzankoff SP, Robinson S, Pyke FS, et al: Physiological adjustments to work in older men as effected by physical training. *J Appl Physiol* 33:346-350, 1972.
14. Mann GV, Garrett HL, Farhi A, et al: Exercise to prevent coronary heart disease. An experimental study of the effects of training on risk factors for coronary disease in men. *Amer J Med* 46:12-27, 1969.
15. Boyer JL, Kasch FW: Exercise therapy in hypertensive men. *JAMA* 211:1668-1671, 1970.
16. Rudd JL, Day WC: A physical fitness program for patients with hypertension. *J Amer Geriat Soc* 15:373-379, 1967.
17. Pyorala K, Karava R, Punsar S, et al: "A Controlled Study of the Effects of 18 Month's Physical Training in Sedentary Middle-aged Men with High Indexes of Risk Relative to Coronary Heart Disease," in Larson OA, Malmborg RO (Eds): *Coronary Heart Disease and Physical Fitness*, pp 261-265, Baltimore: University Park Press, 1971.
18. Taylor HL, Buskirk E, Balke B, et al: Relationship of adherence in a supervised physical activity program to change in CHD risk factors and work capacity. *Circulation* 46(suppl II): 12, 1972.
19. Bonanno JA, Lies JE: Effects of physical training on coronary risk factors. *Amer J Cardiol* 33:760-764, 1974.
20. Saltin B: "Central Circulation after Physical Conditioning in Young and Middle-aged Men," in Larson OA, Malmborg RO (Eds): *Coronary Heart Disease and Physical Fitness*, pp 21-26, Baltimore: University Park Press, 1971.
21. Haggendal J, Hartley LH, Saltin B: Arterial noradrenaline concentration during exercise in relation to the relative work level. *Scand J Clin Lab Invest* 26:348-353, 1970.
22. Clausen JP: Circulatory adjustments to dynamic exercise and effect of physical training in nor-

mal subjects and in patients with coronary artery disease. *Prog Cardiovasc Dis* 18:459-495, 1976.

23. Cooper KH, Pollock ML, Martin RP, et al: Physical fitness levels vs selected coronary risk factors. *JAMA* 236:166-169, 1976.

24. Skinner JS, Holloszy JO, Toro G, et al: "Effects of a Six-Month Program of Endurance Exercise on Work Tolerance, Serum Lipids and ULF-Ballistocardiograms of Fifteen Middle-aged Men," in Karvonen MJ, Barry AJ (Eds): *Physical Activity and the Heart*, pp 79-96, Springfield, Illinois: Charles C Thomas, 1967.

25. Carlson LA, Pernow B: Studies on blood lipids during exercise. I: Arterial and venous plasma concentrations of unesterified fatty acids. *J Lab Clin Med* 53:833-841, 1959.

26. Åstrand PO, Rodahl K: *Textbook of Work Physiology*, p 476, New York: McGraw-Hill, 1970.

27. Weinsier RL, Fuchs RJ, Kay TD, et al: Body fat: its relationship to coronary heart disease, blood pressure, lipids and other risk factors measured in a large male population. *Amer J Med* 61:815-824, 1976.

20

Control and Modification of Stress Emotions Through Chronic Exercise

Carlyle H. Folkins, PhD
Ezra A. Amsterdam, MD

Psychological stress, according to Lazarus,[1] plays a key role in many illnesses. When people perceive threat, either from internal or external sources, the body mobilizes as part of an effort to cope with the threat; when this mobilization is excessive or prolonged, disease may result. Lazarus suggested that most diseases could be stress-related, since the organ systems of the body tend to function poorly under stress-filled conditions. Thus, the stress emotions have been viewed as one factor of clinical importance contributing to the development of coronary heart disease.

This chapter deals with exercise and its role in controlling and modifying the stress emotions that affect the heart. The term "stress emotions" refers to a variety of unpleasant emotions, eg, fear, anxiety, tension, anger, depression, *etc*, all of which are accompanied by distressing visceral reactions. In this chapter, the "stress emotions" of greatest concern include those affective states labeled stress, tension and anxiety. These stress emotions are most often assumed to be potentially critical variables in the etiology and treatment of coronary heart disease.

Role of Stress Emotions in Coronary Heart Disease

Experimental and clinical studies have indicated an association between emotional stress and coronary heart disease (CHD). Reviews of the psychological and social precursors of CHD have highlighted a variety of environmental stresses, behavioral responses and physiological reactions that are more prevalent among people with CHD.[2-4] It has been generally assumed that the values and demands of western civilization create excess stress emotions which may promote clinical CHD,[2, 5, 6] while simpler life patterns are correlated with a lower incidence of CHD. The very low prevalence of CHD among Benedictine and Trappist monks is cited in support of this hypothesis.[7]

Stress may be considered to contribute to CHD in two basic ways. It has been implicated as an etiologic factor in the development of coronary artery athero-sclerosis and it can play a role in provoking the signs, symptoms and com-plications of established CHD, including angina pectoris, myocardial in-farction, cardiac failure, arrhythmias and sudden death. Furthermore, CHD it-self can create emotional stress which may exacerbate the clinical problem and hamper its management.

Stress Emotions and the Etiology of CHD—Although a relation between per-sonality and behavioral factors and increased risk of coronary heart disease has been suggested by a number of observers, Friedman, Rosenman and colleagues have provided the most systematic approach to this problem.[2, 8, 9] On the basis of laboratory, clinical and epidemiologic studies, they have described the coro-nary-prone personality, which is characterized by a specific type of behavior pat-tern—type A. Type A behavior consists of excesses of competitiveness, achieve-ment drive, aggressiveness, haste, impatience, and feelings of time urgency and the challenge of responsibility. The opposite behavior pattern, characterized by a relaxed, unhurried, satisfied style, is type B. Prospective studies by Friedman, Rosenman et al [8] in which behavior pattern was analyzed as an independent risk factor, have consistently revealed an incidence of clinical CHD more than twice as great in type A subjects as in type B.

Although the mechanisms by which behavior and central nervous system function might influence the development of CHD are obscure, experimental and clinical findings have suggested a basis for an etiological role of these fac-tors. An association between two of the major coronary risk factors, serum lip-ids and hypertension (see Chapter 1), and the stress emotions has been demon-strated, suggesting that one mechanism by which stress may be related to CHD is through an effect on these risk factors. Increases in serum cholesterol [10-14] and triglycerides [14] have been noted during heightened stress related to occupation-al demands and other situations. Elevations of blood pressure are a consistent finding during stress in experimental animals [15-17] and in man.[15, 16, 18] In laborato-ry studies, sustained increase in blood pressure has occurred after withdrawal of stress.[17] Alterations in hemostatic mechanisms which enhance intravascular thrombosis and may contribute to atherogenesis (see Chapter 8) are also asso-ciated with stress. Coagulation of blood is accelerated [19] and the elevated levels of plasma catecholamines provoked by emotional stress [20] can increase platelet aggregability.[21, 22]

Stress Emotions and Clinical Manifestations of CHD—The role of the stress emotions in provoking clinical manifestations of CHD in patients is readily understood in terms of the pathophysiology of the disease (see Chapter 2). In addition, important clinical cardiac episodes have been precipitated by stress in individuals with no demonstrable heart disease.

Myocardial ischemia, the pathophysiologic basis of the signs and symptoms of CHD, occurs when cardiac oxygen demand exceeds supply. Of the major factors determining myocardial oxygen demand, heart rate, blood pressure and contractility are readily elevated by increased sympathoadrenal activity through circulating catecholamines and the sympathetic nerves,[23] a characteristic accompaniment of emotional stress.[20] Augmented hemodynamic activity, reflecting increased sympathetic stimulation and raising myocardial oxygen demand, has been well demonstrated in man during mental stress associated with intellectual tasks or anxiety.[18, 24-27] In patients with CHD, stress has been associated with angina pectoris [18, 25] and electrocardiographic [18] and metabolic evidence [26] of myocardial ischemia. Indeed, emotional stress is a common provoking factor of angina pectoris,[28] as noted by Heberden [29] in his original description of the disorder over 200 years ago. In the sleeping state, angina may result from emotional stimulation by dreams.[30] In these settings, myocardial ischemia and angina are related to the augmented cardiovascular activity produced by sympathetic stimulation, resulting in excessive myocardial oxygen demand in the presence of coronary heart disease.

If cardiac ischemia due to the foregoing series of reactions is severe enough, myocardial infarction can result, and an association between emotional stress and infarction has been noted.[31, 32] The increased coagulability of blood related to emotional stress [19] may also play a role in coronary thrombosis and consequent infarction. Experimental studies have shown that excessive catecholamine stimulation can, itself, produce myocardial necrosis in the absence of coronary heart disease.[33]

Myocardial ischemia can also result in cardiac arrhythmias and sudden death. The myocardial stimulatory effects and altered cardiac electrophysiologic activity produced by catecholamine stimulation and provoked by emotional reactions can also produce serious arrhythmias and even sudden death in individuals without heart disease. In laboratory studies increases in heart rate have been induced by a variety of emotionally stressful situations.[18, 34, 35] Even more significant are the effects of the stress emotions of daily life on cardiac rate and rhythm. Portable electrocardiographic monitoring has demonstrated that tachycardia and cardiac arrhythmias are associated with such activities as routine tasks,[36] delivering a speech [18, 37] and driving in traffic.[38] Serious arrhythmias are more likely to occur in patients with CHD than in normal individuals.[39] The potentially deleterious effect of the emotions on cardiac rhythm is demonstrated by a CHD patient we evaluated in whom frequent ventricular ectopic beats consistently occurred during discussion of personal crises, whereas maximal treadmill exercise was performed without any arrhythmia.

Sudden cardiac death is usually due to a lethal ventricular arrhythmia [40] and the importance of psychologic stress in the genesis of these arrhythmias has been demonstrated in experimental animals [41] and in man.[42 43] The relation of emotionally stressful events to sudden death has long been noted [42] and it has been proposed that "in at least 50% of the patients with sudden death, psychological and social factors are associated with the time of sudden death."[44]

In patients with cardiac disease of varying etiologies, emotionally stressful situations may precipitate congestive heart failure.[45] Cardiac failure in this setting may be related to the hemodynamic stress produced by catecholamine stimulation accompanying the emotional reaction.[20, 23] In CHD, increased ischemia could place an added burden on a diseased myocardium and contribute to failure. In terms of Selye's "general adaptation syndrome,"[46] a chronic excessive workload on the heart resulting from continuing psychophysiologic stress could contribute to cardiac dysfunction and decompensation.

Stress Emotions and the Treatment of CHD—Emotional stress and tension are also a problem in the rehabilitation of the coronary patient. Some years ago a psychoanalyst suggested that the heart provides a rhythm which serves as a framework for experiencing body sensations during a person's development, and as such is fundamental in determining the self-concept.[47] A person's view of his heart may also be important for identity formation at a social-psychological level—people frequently identify themselves and others as goodhearted, hardhearted, softhearted or weakhearted, *etc*. It should not be surprising, therefore, that malfunction of this unique organ is often a severe blow to psychological stability. Indeed, a number of researchers have found that coronary patients are generally more anxious than healthy people or even presurgery patients.[47-51] "There seems little doubt that the sudden death-dealing implications of myocardial infarctions produce psychological disturbance in the coronary patient in the form of anxiety, hostility directed inward, or depression. . . ."[49] Coronary patients, especially the younger ones, may be more anxious because of the fear of physical decline and death. Thus, Rodda et al [50] studied anxiety and depression patterns in 31 coronary patients every 6 weeks for 15 months, and compared these patients with 46 healthy controls. The coronary patients had higher anxiety scores, but even more striking was the finding that the patients under age 50 were five times more anxious than the controls.

Not all coronary patients manifest high levels of emotional stress. A good number are successful in denying the threat to their physical integrity, and on the surface they appear secure and relatively unconcerned. Nevertheless, high levels of emotional stress in many coronary patients may aggravate their disease as well as interfere with their interpersonal relationships at home and at work. But, more important to the physician, the heightened anxiety experienced by a CHD patient may render that patient quite susceptible to further problems stemming from the actions, words or demeanor of the treating physician. Special treatment considerations may be necessary to avert further aggravating stress.[52]

Exercise and Stress Emotions

Somatopsychic Theory [53]—There is good reason to assume that the body affects the mind just as the mind affects the body. A vast amount of research has emerged from the psychosomatic perspective, but until recently little was done to demonstrate somatopsychic phenomena, *ie*, that body changes alter mental attitude. A somatopsychic theory is needed to develop testable hypotheses regarding the effects of exercise. Harris [53] suggested that physical activity may produce a positive psychological response in much the same way as altering a negative psychic state can improve a somatic condition. The somatopsychic concept provides a unifying theme for viewing the relationship of physical activity to the stress emotions.

Physical educators have long assumed that physical fitness is associated with emotional health, and most studies have confirmed this association.[54] Recently, a number of studies have focused more specifically on the effect of chronic exercise on stress variables.

The Effects of Exercise on Stress Emotions—The first systematic investigation of the psychological correlates of exercise was begun in 1953 by Cureton [55] at the Physical Fitness Research Laboratory, University of Illinois. Over a 10-year period his staff studied 2,500 adults who were followed individually through physical conditioning programs. From interview and check list data they found that "nervous tension disappears" with the help of a physical exercise program. Cureton was firmly convinced that inactivity has a negative effect on tension release while movement (exercise) relieves tension. However, controlled studies of this observation did not emerge until recently.

Cooper's [56] book, *Aerobics*, further promoted the notion that exercise can relieve stress emotions. He cited numerous cases where exercise was assumed to be the critical factor in controlling or eliminating stress emotions. The work of Cureton and Cooper inspired a number of researchers to investigate the relationship between exercise and the stress emotions.

In a correlational study, Murphy et al [57] conducted an exercise program as part of a multidimensional 12-week treatment for 93 alcoholics at the Veterans Hospital, Salem, Virginia. They found that fitness change scores correlated significantly with changes on the Psychasthenia scale of the MMPI, a measure of reported anxiety and obsessive worrying. While significant, this correlation was very low (.21) and provides little support for the stress release hypothesis.

DeVries [58] investigated the short-term and long-term effects of exercise on the neuromuscular system, using surface electromyography to evaluate activity of the neuromuscular system before and after exercise. In one experiment, 29 college students were tested before and one hour after a 5-minute bench-stepping exercise; the same procedure was used on a control day when a rest period was substituted for the exercise. Results showed that electrical activity in the muscles was reduced 58% after exercise, as compared to no change on a control day. DeVries concluded that neuromuscular activity (tension) does indeed drop after an exercise session. In a second experiment to assess the long-term effects of exercise, 11 middle-aged men were tested before and after 17 one-hour exercise sessions which included weight training and running. The subjects exercised between two and three times a week until 17 sessions were recorded.

Seven moderately active control subjects agreed to maintain a constant level of physical activity during the experimental period. The experimental group showed a decrease of 25% in electrical activity, while the control group increased 24%. Much of the decreased activity for the experimental group, however, was contributed by six out of the 11 subjects who originally reported extreme nervousness (neuromuscular hyperactivity), while none of the controls initially reported such high distress. These six subjects accounted for 80% of the total mean decrease in electrical activity for the experimental group. Could it be that "normals" have little to gain in the way of stress and tension release from exercise?

There have been several studies that have focused on exercise as a natural means of dealing with stress emotions among "normal" adults and children. In a recent review, Layman [59] presented several studies which supported the proposition that exercise reduces anxiety levels. Karbe [60] found anxiety measures were substantially reduced for 92 female college students after a 16-week swimming class, consisting of 40 minutes twice a week. Hanson [61] found that anxiety levels of 4-year-old children who were assigned to a 10-week movement behavior program were reduced in comparison to a control group that participated in the regular school program.

In addition to Cureton's pioneering work, several studies have been carried out at the University of Illinois on the effects of physical fitness training on manifest anxiety. Popejoy [62] found improvement in psychological and physiological measures of anxiety for 22 previously sedentary women who participated in a 20-week physical fitness program. Jette [63] studied 75 men, who at one time had participated in one of Cureton's fitness programs, and who had continued an exercise program regularly, or continued irregularly or had discontinued altogether. He gave each group Catell's 16 Personality Factor Questionnaire and concluded that the regular exercisers were more tough-minded, prudent and relaxed, compared to the nonexercisers. In this study, however, it is not known if the differences found were related to regular exercise or simply to group differences which were previously present. Obviously, one group was more motivated to continue exercising and this motivational difference may have been linked to a more "tough-minded" character structure.

Ismail and Young [64] studied 56 middle-aged male faculty members at Purdue University who participated in a physical fitness program 3 days a week over a 4-month period. Using Catell's 16 Personality Factor Questionnaire, they compared personality factor scores of 14 low-fitness subjects with the 14 high-fitness subjects, both before and after the training program. In the pre-test, the high-fitness subjects demonstrated significantly more emotional stability and imagination. In the post-test, the high-fitness group still was more imaginative and unconventional and now was also more confident and unshakable. But the low-fitness group appeared significantly more self-sufficient and resourceful as compared to the high-fitness group and, furthermore, they no longer demonstrated low emotional stability. Hence, lack of physical fitness was related to emotional instability before fitness training, and this relationship disappeared after the fitness training. The authors concluded: "This may have been due to the treatment effect, namely, the physical fitness program."[64] The meaning of the changes in Catell's factor scores is not easily understood in this study, although the data do suggest that exercise and fitness enable a person to better cope with emotional stress.

We have studied normal junior college students in a semester-long jogging course.[65] Forty-two junior college students who took the course and 42 students enrolled in archery and golf courses were compared on psychological measures of anxiety, depression, self-confidence, adjustment, work efficiency and sleep behavior. In each group, half of the subjects were men and half were women. Improved physical fitness among the joggers was noted from time trials and resting heart rate. Subjects were timed over a one and three-quarter–mile course before and after the training period. At the beginning, the average jogging time for all subjects was almost 18 minutes, and after 25 jogging sessions the average time for all subjects was 14 minutes and 43 seconds. Men improved from 14 minutes and 54 seconds to 12 minutes and 51 seconds, but women dropped dramatically from 20 minutes and 43 seconds on the first time trial to 16 minutes and 35 seconds at the end of the course. Using Cooper's point system, the group as a whole moved from a poor fitness rating to a fair-to-good level of fitness. Furthermore, resting heart rate decreased an average of 8.76 beats/min for all subjects. Again, the women showed greater improvement. A direct comparison of the experimental and control subjects on psychological variables was not feasible because the students who elected the jogging course, especially the women, were more distressed than the controls at the outset. Nevertheless, significant differences between the pre-test and post-test scores were found on anxiety, depression, self-confidence, adjustment and sleep behavior measures, while no significant changes were found on these variables for the control group. The women in the exercise group contributed the major source of variance for the observed changes. Men alone showed no significant changes. The men initially rated better psychologically and physically, than the women. As in the DeVries study, those subjects that were in the poorest shape initially showed the greatest improvement.

We suspected that college students who are relatively active and physically fit would have less to gain psychologically from an exercise program than an older group of relatively unfit individuals. Hence, we arranged a study of middle-aged men who participated in a 19-session exercise program, consisting primarily of jogging.[66] Thirty-six men (mean age, 46.5) completed an exercise program and were tested before and after the program; 34 men (mean age, 43.5) did not participate in an exercise program but completed pre- and post-measures. The Multiple Affect Adjective Check List instrument, which was also used in the previous study, was used to measure the stress emotions—anxiety, depression and hostility. The joggers showed significantly greater reductions in all three stress emotions as compared to the no-exercise control group.

Results of this study indicate that exercise by middle-aged men can provide considerable relief from their stress emotions. Since men of this age group are at increased risk for CHD, the stress-relief benefits of exercise may have extra significance in favorably altering risk for this group.

Exercise and Sleep Behavior—An examination of the effects of exercise on sleep behavior may be an indirect but meaningful approach to the study of the effects of exercise on the stress emotions, since restless sleep is so often associated with stress emotions, especially depression. Baekeland and Lasky [67] studied the sleep EEG's of ten college athletes and found that subjects had more deep sleep (delta sleep) on days when they exercised as compared to no-exercise days. Subjects never went more than two days without exercise, however, so the effect of exercise on sleep could not be determined. In a follow-up study, Baekeland [68] examined the effects of exercise deprivation on sleep patterns and other psychological reactions. The sleep patterns of 14 normal college students who were accustomed to regular exercise, and who were also free from psychiatric or medical problems, were studied over a one-month period on 2 days when they exercised as usual and then on 4 days when they did not exercise at all. Deep sleep tended to be greater on the second night of exercise as compared to the first night of no exercise, but more significant was the obvious psychological stress experienced by the subjects when they were deprived of their usual exercise. Wakefulness, first REM latencies, and REM sleep increased during the deprivation period. These changes were viewed as indices of anxiety or increased arousal. The subjects themselves reported that they experienced impaired sleep, increased sexual tension and an increased need to be with others. Baekeland [68] suggested that physical activity allows greater benefit from sleep, and this effect may help explain the frequent report, by those who habitually exercise, that they feel better and more alert during the day.

These studies on sleep behavior are of special relevance to understanding stress factors in CHD patients, since the rehabilitation of a CHD patient always begins at a point when he has been deprived of normal activity routines, no matter how minimal those routines may have been. Apparently, any form of physical confinement may generate stressful experience and some attempt to return to a normal exercise level is, perhaps, critical in managing stress emotion levels.

Exercise in Coronary Heart Disease—In a carefully controlled study, McPherson et al [69] examined the effects of an exercise program on postinfarct patients. They divided 18 men with previous acute myocardial infarctions into an exercise and a control group and compared them with nine exercising normals and nine sedentary normals. The exercise groups engaged in a graduated exercise program two evenings a week for 24 weeks. The cardiac controls also met weekly to assess the possible social-psychological benefits of socializing. Cattell's 16 PF Questionnaire and a semantic differential inventory were used to evaluate psychological changes. After the program cardiac and normal exercisers, as well as cardiac controls, showed reduced manifest anxiety scores while nonexercising normal subjects experienced increased anxiety. On the semantic differential inventory cardiac exercisers experienced more favorable changes in mood states than the other groups.

McPherson [69] noted that the cardiac subjects showed greater maladjustment than the normals at the beginning of the program and, therefore, had a greater potential for improvement. Most of these men were "tense, aloof, taciturn, fickle, emotional, hurried, and aggressive" compared to the normal subjects, perhaps partly because of the enforced sedentary existence since their myocardial infarctions. The exercise helped them gain self-confidence and optimism, which "led to a reduction of anxiety and tension. . . ."[69]

Another study [70] evaluated psychological changes experienced by 36 men employed in county police and fire departments who had recently been identified as having a high prevalence of coronary risk factors. Subjects were matched by age, occupation and risk factors and assigned to an exercise or control group. The exercise group participated in three exercise sessions a week for a 3-month period. They experienced a significant drop in anxiety, as measured by the Multiple Affect Adjective Check List, as compared to no change for the controls. Interestingly, these recently identified high risk subjects did not differ from the normal population on personality variables or pretraining anxiety. Possibly, in contrast to McPherson's subjects who were recovering from myocardial infarctions, these subjects were able to successfully deny the threat value of their high risk status.

Theories of Exercise Effect

The psychological and physiological processes by which exercise may afford control and modification of stress emotions have been the subject of recent speculation. Ismail and Trachtman [71] presented a general psychological theory to explain this relationship. They suggested that changes occur when an individual confronts a challenge (eg, a strenuous exercise program) and overcomes it. The positive outcome, or mastery of the challenge, provides a sense of accomplishment or self-control. Presumably, this psychological state allows for more adaptive responses to distressing situations.

Others have assumed that the experience of exercising in a group could provide social-psychological benefits that would assist in stress management. Also, improved self-image, especially body image, might be seen to bolster the resources needed to deal with stress and tension.

Ismail and Trachtman [71] also presented the general viewpoint that psychological changes are the direct effect of physiological and biochemical changes resulting from exercise. They suggested that increased circulation to the brain increases availability of glucose, which is essential to cerebral metabolism. Thus, improvement in oxygen transport may enhance mental function.

Elsewhere we have speculated that a number of physiological changes, when received at the cognitive level, would lead to an appraisal of lower stress emotion level.[65] For example, the reduced electrical activity to the muscles, as noted by DeVries,[58] could provide an important cue for an appraisal of "less tension." Also, the response of the heart to psychological stress changes with improved fitness. The fit jogger's heart responds to stress with greater stroke volume, rather than increased rate [72] (see Chapter 4). This type of response is, presumably, more efficient, because it is associated with the release of smaller amounts of adrenalin than would occur with increased heart rate; it also does not lead to a stress associated cue, a racing heart.

Several studies [65, 67, 68] have demonstrated that exercise may be critical to restful sleep patterns. Improved sleep could produce the "sense of well-being" reported by many chronic exercisers who also report less disturbing encounters with everyday stresses.

Finally, a physiological cause theory has been built around Selye's theory of stress. Selye promoted the concept that exercise can serve as a therapy for stress because it interrupts the stereotyped response pattern which often contributes to physical and mental illness. In a review of the literature concerning the effects of exercise on the adrenal glands and the autonomic nervous system, Michael [73] offered strong support for this idea: "The evidence reported here supports the theory that repeated exercise 'conditions' the stress adaptation mechanism. The studies point out that the adrenocortical activity along with the autonomic nervous system are involved in adjusting to stress. This ability to adjust is helped with exercise if we assume that the more sensitive response to stress reduces the time necessary to elicit a response and therefore lessens the duration of the adjusting phase. The evidence indicates that adaptation to exercise produces a degree of protection against emotional stress. The increased adrenal activity resulting from repeated exercise seems to cause an increased reserve of steroids available to counter a stress. A lack of activity was reported to reduce the ability to withstand stress, as if the reaction to a shock is a 'learned' process."[73]

A commonsense explanation of how exercise leads to the control and modification of stress emotions would include all of the above processes. That is, a variety of psychological and physiological shifts most likely follow from improvements in physical fitness and each provides input, in varying degrees, for different individuals, which allows greater control of the stress emotions.

Perspective on Exercise in Attenuation of Stress

Most of the research on exercise and its effects on stress emotions supports the conclusion that chronic exercise, which results in improved physical fitness, does indeed reduce stress emotion levels. Evidence supporting this conclusion has emerged from studies on children, male and female college students, normal adult men, and men with coronary heart disease. Those studies that evaluated exercise effects in some detail also demonstrated that those individuals who were most unfit physically and/or psychologically initially experienced the most improvement from an exercise program.

Since CHD patients are generally more anxious than normal subjects, they are good candidates for some type of stress reduction treatment. And, since exercise is also beneficial to circulatory function (See Chapter 4, 9, 24, 25, 26), its indirect effects on the stress emotions would naturally lead one to assume it was the "best" prescription for controlling the stress emotions. Such an assumption may not be warranted, however.

There are numerous popular approaches besides exercise to the regulation of stress emotions. Lazarus [1] provided a conceptual framework for viewing the variety of coping maneuvers available for dealing with stress. In direct action approaches, the person tries to alter or master the perceived threat by attack, avoidance, flight or preparation (eg, studying for an examination). When direct action is ineffective, *palliation* occurs. Palliative modes for coping with stress emotions involve attempts to control the emotion itself or its somatic correlates. Examples of such modes of control are ego defenses (denial, intellectualization, *etc.*), tranquilizers, alcohol, relaxation training, meditation, hypnosis, biofeedback therapy and exercise. All of these palliative modes may lower stress emotion levels and allow an individual to function at a higher level.

What should be of concern to the individual who might be treating a person, such as a CHD patient, with high levels of stress emotion, is that there are clearly numerous approaches to this problem. More important, a strategy that is appropriate for one person might not be effective for another. Unfortunately, little research has attempted to evaluate coping dispositions.[1] Generally however, one might be able to determine whether a particular prescription for stress release would fit with a person's usual coping style. As an illustration, patients with CHD show a great range of change in their activity level following the onset of the disease. Some become more active in response to this threat; others reduce their activity levels dramatically. According to Mordkoff and Rand,[74] adaptation to CHD is generally consistent with personality makeup. "To the extent that the patient's mode of adjustment is consistent with his general adaptational structure, it will minimize the propensity for the kind of psychological trauma which might precipitate a recurrence of an infarction or death."[74] Therefore, if one were concerned about reducing stress in the person who tends to show increased activity when threatened, that person would probably not respond to a relatively passive approach like relaxation training or meditation, nor would he be agreeable to suggestions that he slow down or avoid excessive challenge and stress. He might, however, be quite willing to fit an exercise session into a busy daily schedule. In contrast, a person who decreases his activity level might respond better to a more supportive approach such as family or group therapy, tranquilizers or relaxation training.

Regular exercise is a difficult habit to promote, even in individuals who are activity-oriented. But, increasingly, the public is learning that the long-term effects of exercise can lead to a gratifying sense of well-being and, for some, a kind of high or "flow" experience.[75] Yet it would appear that efforts at prevention and rehabilitation with the coronary patient must incorporate individual counseling sessions which allow some degree of exploration of an individual's preferred coping style, so that an agreeable approach to stress-emotion relief can be offered. To some extent, the patient may be considered as an expert in determining the best approach for himself.

Summary

There is abundant evidence supporting a role for the stress emotions in coronary heart disease. Through its stimulatory effect on sympathetic neurohumoral transmission and thereby on hemodynamic function, emotional stress can provoke the clinical manifestations of underlying coronary heart disease. Stress also influences certain coronary risk factors unfavorably, and in this manner may contribute to the etiology of the disease. Emotional stress may also hamper management of the coronary patient. Physical activity can attenuate the stress emotions and improve psychological function. Exercise has been associated with improved sense of well-being and has been correlated with objective demonstration of reduced psychological and physiological indices of factors such as anxiety, depression and hostility. Favorable effects of exercise on sleep have been documented and the converse has been shown with lack of physical activity, suggesting one means by which exercise may contribute to improved subjective and objective function during daily activities. Improvement in psychological parameters in relation to exercise is greatest in those individuals who are initially most unfit physically and psychologically. Although the mechanisms by which exercise may confer a beneficial effect on the stress emotions are not clear, it is likely that a variety of psychological and physiological processes are involved. Exercise is one potential means of reducing stress emotions, and its application should be considered in terms of an individual's overall characteristics and needs.

References

1. Lazarus RS: Psychological stress and coping in adaptation and illness. *Int J Psychiat Med* 5:321-333, 1974.
2. Jenkins CD: Recent evidence supporting psychologic social risk factors for coronary disease. *New Eng J Med* 294:987-994, 1033-1038, 1976.
3. Johns MW: Stress and coronary heart disease. *Ergonomics* 16:683-690, 1973.
4. Wheeler EO: "Emotional Stress: Cardiovascular Disease and Cardiovascular Symptoms," in Hurst JW, Logue RB, Schlant RC, et al (Eds): *The Heart*, pp 1548-1562, New York: McGraw-Hill, 1974.
5. Minc S: Psychological factors in coronary heart disease. *Geriatrics* 20:747-755, 1965.
6. Eliot RS, Forker AD: Emotional stress and cardiac disease. *JAMA* 236:2325-2326, 1976.
7. Russek HI: Role of emotional stress in the aetiology of clinical coronary heart disease. *Dis Chest* 52:1-9, 1967.
8. Rosenman RH, Brand RJ, Jenkins D, et al: Coronary heart disease in the western collaborative group study. Final follow-up experience of 8½ years. *JAMA* 233:872-877, 1975.
9. Jenkins CD, Zyzanski SJ, Rosenman RH: Risk of new myocardial infarction in middle-aged

men with manifest coronary heart disease. *Circulation* 53:342-347, 1976.

10. Dreyfus F, Czaczkes JW: Blood cholesterol and uric acid of healthy medical students under stress of an examination. *Arch Intern Med* 103:708-711, 1959.

11. Wolf S, McCabe WR, Yamamoto J, et al: Changes in serum lipids in relation to emotional stress during rigid control of diet and exercise. *Circulation* 26:379-387, 1962.

12. Rahe RH, Rubin RT, Gunderson EKE, et al: Psychologic correlates of serum cholesterol in man. A longitudinal study. *Psychosom Med* 33:339-410, 1971.

13. Friedman M, Rosenman RH, Carroll V: Changes in serum cholesterol and blood clotting time in men subjected to cyclic variation of occupational stress. *Circulation* 17:852-861, 1958.

14. Wolf S, McCabe WR, Yamamoto J, et al: Changes in serum lipids in relation to emotional stress during rigid control of diet and exercise. *Circulation* 26:379-387, 1962.

15. Henry JP, Cassel JC: Psychosocial factors in essential hypertension. Recent epidemiologic and animal experimental evidence. *Amer J Epidemiol* 90:171-200, 1969.

16. Gutman MC, Benson H: Interaction of environmental factors and systemic arterial blood pressure: a review. *Medicine* 50:543-553, 1971.

17. Forsyth RP, Harris RE: Circulatory changes during stressful stimuli in rhesus monkeys. *Circ Res* 27 (suppl 1):13-20, 1970.

18. Schiffer F, Hartley LH, Schulman CL, et al: The quiz electrocardiogram: a new diagnostic and research technique for evaluating the relation between emotional stress and ischemic heart disease. *Amer J Cardiol* 37:41-47, 1976.

19. Dreyfus F: Coagulation time of the blood, level of blood eosinophile and thrombocytes under emotional stress. *J Psychosom Res* 1:252-257, 1956.

20. Theorell T, Lind E, Froberg J, et al: A longitudinal study of 21 subjects with coronary heart disease: life changes, catecholamine excretion and related biochemical reaction. *Psychosom Med* 34:505-516, 1972.

21. Ardlie NG, Glew G, Schwartz CJ: Influence of catecholamines on nucleotide-induced platelet aggregation. *Nature* 212:415-417, 1966.

22. Haft JI, Kranz PD, Albert FJ, et al: Intravascular platelet aggregation in the heart induced by norepinephrine. *Circulation* 46:698-708, 1972.

23. Marshall RJ, Shepard JT: "Catecholamines," in Marshall RJ, Shepard JT (Eds): *Cardiac Function in Health and Disease*, pp 141-167, 1968.

24. Hickam JB, Cargill WH, Golden A: Cardiovascular reactions to emotional stimuli. Effect on the cardiac output, arteriovenous oxygen difference, arterial pressure and peripheral resistance. *J Clin Invest* 27:290-298, 1948.

25. Brod J, Fencl V, Hejl Z, et al: Circulatory changes underlying blood pressure elevation during acute emotional stress (mental arithmetic) in normotensive and hypertensive subjects. *Clin Sci* 18:269-279, 1959.

26. Amsterdam EA, Manchester JH, Kemp HG, et al: Spontaneous angina pectoris (SAP): hemodynamic and metabolic changes (abstract). *Clin Res* 17:225, 1969.

27. Moss AJ, Wynar B: Tachycardia in house officers presenting cases at grand rounds. *Ann Intern Med* 72:255-256, 1970.

28. Lane FM: Mental mechanisms and the pain of angina pectoris. *Amer Heart J* 85:563-568, 1973.

29. Heberden W: Some account of a disorder of the breast. *Med Trans Coll Physicians (London)* 2:59-67, 1772.

30. Nowlin JB, Troyer WG, Collins WJ, et al: The association of nocturnal angina pectoris with dreaming. *Ann Intern Med* 63:1040-1046, 1965.

31. Dreyfuss F: Role of emotional stress preceding coronary occlusion. *Amer J Cardiol* 3:590-596, 1959.

32. Levene DL: Correspondence: psychological factors in the genesis of myocardial infarction. *Canad Med Ass J* III:499-501, 1974.

33. Raab W: The sympathogenic biochemical trigger mechanism of angina pectoris. Its therapeutic suppression and long-range prevention *Amer J Cardiol* 9:576-590, 1962.

34. Folkins CH, Lawson CD, Opton EM, et al: Desensitization and the experimental reduction of threat. *J Abnorm Psychol* 73:100-113, 1968.

35. Folkins CH: Temporal factors and the cognitive mediators of stress reaction. *J Personality Soc Psychol* 14:173-184, 1970.

36. Hinkle LE Jr. Carver ST, Stevens M: The frequency of asymptomatic disturbances of cardiac rhythm and conduction in middle-aged men. *Amer J Cardiol* 24:629-650, 1969.

37. Taggart P, Carruthers M, Somerville W: Electrocardiogram, plasma catecholamines and lipids, and their modification by oxprenolol when speaking before an audience. *Lancet* II:341-346, 1973.
38. Bellet S, Roman L, Kostis J, et al: Continuous electrocardiographic monitoring during automobile driving: studies in normal subjects and patients with coronary disease. *Amer J Cardiol* 22:856-862, 1968.
39. Amsterdam EA, Vismara L, Brocchini R, et al: Relation of ventricular arrhythmias to coronary artery disease (abstract). *Circulation* 48 (suppl IV):138, 1973.
40. Lown B, Wolf MA: Approaches to sudden death from coronary heart disease. *Circulation* 44:130-142, 1971.
41. Corbalan R, Verrier R, Lown B: Psychologic stress and ventricular arrhythmias during myocardial infarction in the conscious dog. *Amer J Cardiol* 34:692-696, 1974.
42. Engel GL: Sudden and rapid death during psychological stress. Folklore or folk wisdom? *Ann Intern Med* 74:771-782, 1971.
43. Lown B, Temte JV, Reich P, et al: Basis for recurring ventricular fibrillation in the absence of coronary heart disease and its management. *New Eng J Med* 294:623-629, 1976.
44. Greene WA, Goldstein S, Moss AJ: Psychosocial aspects of sudden death. *Arch Intern Med* 129:725-731, 1972.
45. Perlman LV, Ferguson S, Bergum K, et al: Precipitation of congestive heart failure: social and emotional factors. *Ann Intern Med* 75:1-7, 1971.
46. Selye H: *The Stress of Life*, New York: McGraw-Hill, 1956.
47. Schneider DE: The image of the heart and the synergic principle in psychoanalysis (psychosynergy). *Psychoanal Rev* 41:197-215, 1954.
48. Cleveland SE, Johnson CJ: Personality patterns in young males with coronary disease. *Psychosom Med* 24:600-610, 1962.
49. Miller CK: Psychological correlates of coronary artery disease. *Psychosom Med* 27:257-265, 1965.
50. Rodda BE, Miller MC, Bruhn JG: Prediction of anxiety and depression patterns among coronary patients using a Markov process analysis. *Behav Sci* 16:482-489, 1971.
51. Jenkins CD: Psychologic and social precursors of coronary disease (first of two parts). *New Eng J Med* 284:244-255, 1971.
52. Hurst JW: "Iatrogenic Problems and Heart Disease," in Hurst JW, Logue RB, Schlant RC, et al (Eds): *The Heart*, pp 1558-1562, New York: McGraw-Hill, 1974.
53. Harris DV: *Involvement in Sport: A Somatopsychic Rationale for Physical Activity*, Philadelphia: Lea and Febiger, 1973.
54. Kane JE: *Psychological Aspects of Physical Education and Sport*, Boston: Routledge and Kegan Paul, 1972.
55. Cureton TK: Improvement of psychological states by means of exercise-fitness programs. *Assoc Phys Mental Rehab* 17:14-17, 1963.
56. Cooper KH: *Aerobics*, New York: Bantam Books, 1968.
57. Murphy JB, Bennett RN, Hagen JM, et al: Some suggestive data regarding the relationship of physical fitness to emotional difficulties. *Newsletter for Research in Psychology* 14:15-17, 1972.
58. DeVries HA: Immediate and long-term effects of exercise upon resting muscle action potential level. *J Sports Med* 8:1-11, 1968.
59. Layman EM: "Psychological Effects of Physical Activity," in Wilmore JH (Ed): *Exercise and Sports Sciences Reviews*, New York: Academic Press, 1974.
60. Karbe WW: The relationship of general anxiety and specific anxiety concerning the learning of swimming. PhD Thesis, New York University, 1966.
61. Hanson DS: The effect of a concentrated program of movement behavior on the affective behavior of four-year-old children at University Elementary School. Edd Thesis, University of California, Los Angeles, 1970.
62. Popejoy DI: The effects of a physical fitness program on selected psychological and physiological measures of anxiety. PhD Thesis, University of Illinois, Urbana, 1967.
63. Jette M: Habitual exercisers: a blood serum and personality profile. *J Sports Med* 3:12-17, 1975.
64. Ismail AH, Young RJ: The effect of chronic exercise on the personality of middle-aged men by univariate and multivariate approaches. *J Human Ergol* 2:47-57, 1973.
65. Folkins CH, Lynch S, Gardner MM: Psychological fitness as a function of physical fitness. *Arch*

Phys Med Rehab 53:503-508, 1972.

66. Lynch S, Folkins CH, Wilmore JH: Relationships between three mood variables and physical exercise. Unpublished data, February 1973.
67. Baekeland F, Lasky R: Exercise and sleep patterns in college athletes. *Perceptual and Motor Skills* 23:1203-1207, 1966.
68. Baekeland F: Exercise deprivation. *Arch Gen Psychiat* 22:365-369, 1970.
69. McPherson BD, Paivio A, Yuhasz MS, et al: Psychological effects of an exercise program for post-infarct and normal adult men. *J Sports Med Phys Fitness* 7:61-66, 1967.
70. Folkins CH: Effects of physical training on mood. *J Clin Psychol* 32:385-388, 1976.
71. Ismail AH, Trachtman LE: Jogging the imagination. *Psychology Today* 6:79-82, 1973.
72. Chapman CB, Mitchell JH: Physiology of exercise. *Sci Amer* 212:88-96, 1965.
73. Michael ED: Stress adaptation through exercise. *Res Quart* 28:50-54, 1957.
74. Mordkoff AA, Rand MA: Personality and adaptation to coronary artery disease. *J Consult Clin Psychol* 32:648-653, 1968.
75. Furlong WB: The fun in fun. *Psychology Today* 10:35-38, 80, 1976.

21

Physical Fitness Programs for Adults

Karl G. Stoedefalke, PhD

In a recent national physical fitness survey conducted for the President's Council on Physical Fitness and Sports,[1] 3,875 men and women over the age of 22 years were interviewed. The results indicated that 55% of adult Americans, 60 million persons, engage in some form of exercise. Of these 60 million it is estimated that 44 million walk, 18 million bicycle, 14 million swim, 14 million do some type of calisthenics and 6.5 million jog. Many active adults participate in more than one form of exercise.

Although more than half of adult Americans engage in some physical activity, many are not physically educated. They must be helped to make intelligent decisions on the selection of physical activities. And they must be informed about the importance of the frequency of participation, the duration of activity sessions, as well as the intensity of the energy expenditure during exercise. Frequency, duration and intensity and type of exercise are the key words in fitness programs for adults.

Research has provided the scientific basis for exercise decisions: frequency, duration and intensity. It is a matter of time before this information is translated and written in meaningful terms for the general public. In the meantime the American adult relies on the guidance of physicians and physical educators. All too often he does not seek counsel. He relies on past experience and initiates an exercise program on his own. The activity he selects and the intensity of his effort may result in unnecessary pain and discomfort. Sometimes sudden death occurs. This is a high price to pay for an honest attempt to achieve physical fitness.

Programs of physical fitness are available to the public through government publications and the popular press. The books and pamphlets are attractively presented and read by millions of Americans. Each publication has its own special way of convincing adults to do something about the "middle-age troika": weak musculature (especially of the abdomen), lack of flexibility and low endur-

TABLE I

$\dot{V}O_2$ max Relative to Age for Moderately Active Men

Age	$\dot{V}O_2$ max (ml/kg per min)	Age	$\dot{V}O_2$ max (ml/kg per min)	Age	$\dot{V}O_2$ max (ml/kg per min)	Age	$\dot{V}O_2$ max (ml/kg per min)
20	52.8	30	48.4	40	44.0	50	39.6
21	52.4	31	48.0	41	43.6	51	39.2
22	51.9	32	47.5	42	43.1	52	38.7
23	51.5	33	47.1	43	42.7	53	38.3
24	51.0	34	46.6	44	42.2	54	37.8
25	50.6	35	46.2	45	41.8	55	37.4
26	50.2	36	45.8	46	41.4	56	37.0
27	49.7	37	45.3	47	40.9	57	36.5
28	49.3	38	44.9	48	40.5	58	36.1
29	48.8	39	44.4	49	40.0	59	35.6

Reproduced with permission from Hodgson JL: Age and Aerobic Capacity of Urban Midwestern Males, PhD dissertation, University of Minnesota, 1971.

ance capability. The reader has his choice among programs whose requirements range from a few minutes of daily activity to 60 minutes of exercise a day, 6 days a week. Fortunately, each publication also recommends that the reader consult his personal physician before beginning an exercise program. Accordingly, the intent of this chapter is to provide the physician with an understanding of the principles of exercise programs that will enable him to provide intelligent counsel to his patient.

Motivation

Adults decide to exercise for a variety of reasons—health, recreation or relaxation, opportunities for social contact or factors related to personal image and self-esteem. Many Americans believe that exercise is "good for you" and, if performed regularly, will confer health benefits. Some believe that exercise controls body weight. Others maintain that exercise strikes the balance between work and play or serves as a vehicle to ameliorate tensions and frustrations. Man is a social being. Exercise programs, sport and games present an opportunity to meet others with similar interests. A reason for exercise may be to achieve a feeling of euphoria, a feeling that is difficult to quantify or explain. All of these reasons are valid and have one thing in common: they are endogenous. The final and conclusive reason for exercise is the physician's recommendation that if the patient doesn't begin to change his life style and become physically active he may soon have serious medical problems. A previously sedentary adult will benefit from an exercise program if he is motivated. Exercise leaders and physicians must allow for differences in attitude toward exercise and prescribe programs that meet individual needs. A man's adherence to an exercise program depends almost entirely on his motivation.

Scientific Evaluations

Table I, developed by Hodgson,[10] presents data on maximal oxygen uptake ($\dot{V}O_2$ max) for moderately active men aged 20 to 59 years. The equation ($\dot{V}O_2$ max, ml/kg per min $= 61.6 - 0.44$ age) used to construct Table I was developed from mean values reported in nine studies with a total of 302 men plus data from lumberjacks referred to by Andersen.[11] Like these moderately active men, sedentary men, after a period of conditioning, showed a similar reduction in $\dot{V}O_2$ max with age, but their data were not included. In these studies, moderately active was defined to include men who were former athletes or were active by occupation or recreation. Table I provides the physician with objective data against which he can measure his patient's capabilities. A reliable assessment of performance capability is a critical aspect of an exercise prescription. A laboratory assessment of aerobic capacity provides the physician with the objective criteria needed for diagnosis and recommendation.

Types of Programs

It has been well established that there is a high degree of specificity in physical fitness programs. Fitness programs can be designed for specific goals. If the desired goal of the exercise program is muscular strength, strength-producing types of activities (dynamic weight training, static isometric exercise) will result in higher levels of strength during performance. If increased range of motion of the joints is the desired goal, exercise programs can be designed to increase a subject's flexibility. If cardiorespiratory endurance is the goal, programs of aerobic training that include a wide variety of human movements will result in increased endurance capability. Many agency-sponsored programs (Jewish Community Centers, Young Men's Christian Associations) attempt to incorporate all three goals in an exercise session: strength, flexibility and endurance. Published programs for the general public may emphasize the importance of only one factor. All three factors are important, but priority and emphasis should be placed on the cardiorespiratory organs. Aging man needs a frequent training stimulus to the heart and circulatory system.

Ideally a physical fitness training session should consist of a warm-up period, an endurance phase, a game (optional) and a cooling down period.

Warm-up (3 to 5 minutes)—The warm-up period is recommended to prepare the body for sustained activity. A warm-up period increases blood flow and stretches postural muscles. It is a period of adaptation. Rhythmic movements of the segments and trunk are precautions against the occurrence of skeletal muscle strain.

Endurance (15 to 30 minutes)—The training of the oxygen transport system is

---

TABLE II

Activities That Improve Endurance of Performance

---

1. Walking
2. Jogging
   a. In place
   b. Moving
3. Running
4. Cycling
5. Swimming
6. Rope skipping

7. Skiing
   a. Alpine
   b. Nordic
8. Ice skating
9. Roller skating
10. Rowing
11. Bench or stair climbing

---

essential. The cardiopulmonary system should be stressed by activities of graduated intensity. The intensity of work loads is changed when adaptation occurs. Table II lists some typical activities that improve endurance of performance.

Games, Fun (10 to 15 minutes)—A game is defined as any competition in which the object is to gain a temporary advantage over one's opponent. In prophylactic exercise programs the games portion has a single goal—fun. Participation in games should be physical self-expression for its own sake. Winning or losing should be secondary to play. Men who are symptomatic or at risk of coronary disease need creative outlets for their energy expenditure. The need to win or to be first is often the reason why a man becomes an early candidate for myocardial infarction. Games with few rules and many participants are ideally suited for a structured or group exercise program.

Cooling down (3 to 5 minutes)—At the completion of an exercise session some time should be devoted to the cooling down process. Exercise raises core temperature and increases heart rate and arterial pressures. The last few minutes of exercise should include gross body movements. The intensity of these movements should be gradually decreased. Activities that maintain or improve range of motion of the joints are desirable.

Exercise Studies of Middle-aged Men

Since 1964, nineteen studies have been published on the effect of physical training on maximal aerobic power.[12-27] These studies ranged from 5 weeks to 2 years in duration; the subjects, all male, ranged in age from 20 to 60 years and exercised 2 to 6 days a week. All 19 studies reported increases in maximal oxygen uptake between the initial and final testing sessions. A 6% increase was reported by Wilmore et al;[23] Cureton and Phillips [27] reported an increase of 38%. Thirteen of the 19 studies reported increases in aerobic power in excess of 15% of the baseline measures.

The subjects of these studies participated in a variety of aerobic training activities including calisthenics, jogging, running, walking, bench-stepping, bicycling and swimming. Some programs included games of handball, paddleball or volleyball. The results indicate that aerobic power increases with training and that this training effect occurs at all age levels. The degree of improvement depends upon the type of activity, the frequency of training and the intensity of the exercise sessions.

Frequency—Research has not determined how frequently exercise should be performed for optimal cardiorespiratory improvement. An acceptable recommendation is three times weekly. This schedule permits an adequate period of recovery between activity sessions.

Intensity—The intensity of training is critical to improvement in aerobic capacity. The best estimate at this time is that an intensity of 70% of a person's maximal aerobic power is sufficient to afford cardiorespiratory gains. Activity performed at a greater intensity produces change, but of a much smaller magnitude. Determining the appropriate intensity of the activity for each individual depends upon the baseline measures obtained during a progressive exercise test. Training regimens can be based on the concept of METS (1 MET = 3.5 ml oxygen/kg per min) or target heart rates. The monitoring of heart rates during activity sessions is important. In an asymptomatic adult, activity heart rates during the endurance phase of training are maintained at levels of 120 to 160 beats/min.

Duration—Cardiorespiratory benefits occur when an exercise session is more than 10 minutes in duration. In programs of prevention, intervention and rehabilitation, sessions are usually 20 to 45 minutes long.

Research indicates that adults reach an optimal training level some time after 20 to 30 weeks of regular physical activity. At approximately 6 months, maximal aerobic power gains tend to plateau. The degree of improvement is related to the state of deconditioning; that is, the lower the level of initial performance capability, the greater the expected improvement.

Adherence—Improvement in endurance, strength and range of joint motion requires adherence to an exercise regimen. Problems of muscle or joint soreness occur frequently. Foot, ankle, knee and back pains are not only irritants but seriously impair attendance and participation. These problems can be minimized if the introduction to an exercise program is gradual. Moderation is important. Occasionally a man reports that his interest has waned because of the monotony of the exercise regimen. Other dropouts from physical activity programs report that the time required for exercise deprived them of time spent on the job or with their family. Complaints of orthopedic problems or monotony can be avoided by skillful exercise leaders and informed physicians who counsel their patients in the proper selection of activity. The time spent away from one's job or family cannot be avoided, but it is not a large price to pay for improvement in health status.

No one is ever too old to have a good time. Exercise should be a pleasant experience. A preoccupation with distance, number of repetitions or a stop watch may provide incentives but is of secondary importance in adult fitness programs. The primary emphasis should be on participating in activities that are safe and enjoyable. When this goal is achieved, people will sustain and adhere to their exercise commitment.

Conclusions

There is a national awareness of the need to improve the physical fitness of adults. Physical activity of a progressive nature produces functional changes. Through exercise, people can increase their endurance capabilities, muscular strength and range of motion of the joints. A progressive exercise test that includes monitoring of the subject's electrocardiogram and arterial blood pressures is the objective assessment necessary to the exercise prescription. Programs should be designed or recommended to meet individual needs. Special attention should be paid to gradual orientation to the exercise regimen. Initially low levels of energy expenditure are desirable. The concepts of intensity, frequency and duration are important. Adaptation to the stress of exercise requires time. Every effort should be made to support the adult in his participation. Successful patient management rests with the cooperative effort and communication of a patient, his physician and the leader of physical activity.

Before a physician recommends an individual exercise regimen or group program, he should carefully evaluate it. Answers to the following questions are important to his evaluation: Does the program allow for individual differences? Is the subject gradually eased into the exercise program? Are the exercise leaders competent? Is adequate supervision available in programs where participants are at high risk? What factors determine the intensity of the exercise session? Are allowances made for participants who have special medical problems (arthritis, emphysema, diabetes, asthma)? What are the avenues for communication and feedback on the patient's progress?

The assessment of human performance is a science. Individually prescribing activity is an art.

Summary

The sedentary habits, occupational stresses and high caloric intake of adults have spurred an interest in physical exercise. Participation in some form of physical activity is necessary to maintain acceptable levels of muscular strength, range of motion of the joints and endurance. Ideally, each person over the age of 35 years should have a progressive exercise test administered by a physician before undertaking an exercise program. An exercise prescription must take into account the type of activity, intensity of training, frequency of participation and duration of each exercise session. Both an understanding of exercise physiology and a knowledge of exercise programs are essential to sound patient counseling and management.

Acknowledgment—James Hodgson, Mitchell McKirnan and Gale Miller provided assistance. Cal Shearburn computed the table of aerobic power estimations.

References

1. Newsletter. President's Council on Physical Fitness and Sports, May 1973.
2. Åstrand PO: Health and Fitness. Skandia Insurance Company Ltd. and The Swedish Information Service, Stockholm, Sweden, 1972.
3. Adult Physical Fitness. President's Council on Physical Fitness and Sports. Washington, DC, US Government Printing Office.
4. Royal Canadian Air Force Exercise Plans for Physical Fitness. Canada, Pocket Books, 1962.
5. Bowerman WJ, Harris WE: *Jogging*, New York: Grosset & Dunlap, 1967.
6. Cooper KH: *The New Aerobics*, New York: M Evans, 1970.
7. Roby FB, Davis RP: *Jogging for Fitness and Weight Control*, Philadelphia: WB Saunders, 1970.
8. Kasch FW, Boyer JL: *Adult Fitness: Principles and Practice*, Palo Alto, California: Mayfield, 1968.
9. Cureton TK: *Physical Fitness and Dynamic Health*, New York: Dial Press, 1965.
10. Hodgson JL: *Age and Aerobic Capacity of Urban Midwestern Males*, unpublished PhD dissertation, University of Minnesota, 1971.
11. Andersen KL: "Fitness for Work of Convalescence Improved by Various Types of Conditioning Exercise," in Evang K, Andersen KL (Eds): *Physical Activity in Health and Disease*, Baltimore: Williams & Wilkins, 1966.
12. Pollock ML, Cureton TK, Greninger L: Effects of frequency of training on working capacity, cardiovascular function, and body composition of adult men. *Med Sci Sports* 1:70-74, 1969.
13. Pollock ML, Broida J, Kendrick Z, et al: Effects of training two days per week at different intensities on middle-aged men. *Med Sci Sports* 4:192-197, 1972.
14. Saltin B: Physiological effects of physical conditioning. *Med Sci Sports* 1:50-56, 1969.
15. Hanson JS, Tabakin BS, Levy AM, et al: Long-term physical training and cardiovascular dynamics in middle-aged men. *Circulation* 38:783-800, 1968.
16. Kasch FW, Phillips WH, Carter JEL, et al: Cardiovascular changes in middle-aged men during two years of training. *J Appl Physiol* 34:53-57, 1973.
17. Maksud MG, Contts KD, Tristani FE, et al: The effects of physical conditioning and propranolol on physical work capacity. *Med Sci Sports* 4:225-229, 1972.
18. Naughton J, Nagle F: Peak oxygen intake during physical fitness program for middle-aged men. *JAMA* 191:899-901, 1965.
19. Pyörälä K, Kärävä R, Punsar S, et al: "A Controlled Study of the Effects of 18 Months' Physical Training in Sedentary Middle-aged Men with High Indexes of Risk Relative to Coronary Heart Disease," in Larsen OA, Malmborg RO (Eds): *Coronary Heart Disease and Physical Fitness*, Copenhagen: Munksgaard, 1971.
20. Ribisl PM: Effects of training upon the maximal oxygen uptake of middle-aged men. *Int Z Angew Physiol* 27:454-460, 1969.
21. Siegel W, Blomqvist GB, Mitchell JH: Effects of a quantitated physical training program on middle-aged sedentary men. *Circulation* 41:19-29, 1970.
22. Tzankoff SP, Robinson S, Pyke FS, et al: Physiological adjustments to work in older men as affected by physical training. *J Appl Physiol* 33:346-350, 1972.
23. Wilmore JH, Royce J, Girandola RN, et al: Physiological alterations resulting from a 10-week program of jogging. *Med Sci Sports* 2:7-14, 1970.
24. Pollock ML, Miller HS Jr, Janeway R, et al: Effects of walking on body composition and cardiovascular function of middle-aged men. *J Appl Physiol* 30:126-130, 1971.
25. Brynteson P, Sinning WE: The effects of training frequencies on the retention of cardiovascular fitness. *Med Sci Sports* 5:29-33, 1973.
26. Mann GV, Garrett HL, Farlin A, et al: Exercise to prevent coronary heart disease: an experimental study of the effects of training on risk factors for coronary disease in man. *Amer J Med* 46:12-27, 1969.
27. Cureton TK, Phillips EE: Physical fitness changes in middle-aged men attributable to equal eight-week periods of training, nontraining, and re-training. *J Sports Med* 4:87-93, 1964.

22

Physical Fitness Programs for Children

John L. Boyer, MD
Jack H. Wilmore, PhD

Cardiovascular diseases are presently the leading cause of death in the adult American population, constituting 54% of all deaths at all ages.[1] Coronary heart disease secondary to atherosclerosis had an estimated prevalence of 3.99 million individuals in the United States during 1973.[1] It is becoming increasingly clear that primary prevention is the preferred approach to controlling the atherosclerotic disease process. This appears to be the only approach that will substantially alter the risk of the American population as a whole.[2]

Kannel and Dawber [3] recently stated that atherosclerosis is not only a disease of the aged but is primarily a pediatric problem, since the pathologic changes which lead to atherosclerosis begin in infancy and progress during childhood. This is exemplified in the work of Enos, Holmes and Beyer,[4] who demonstrated that 70% of autopsied Korean war casualties, with an average age of 22.1 years, already had at least moderately advanced coronary atherosclerosis. In a more recent study, McNamara et al [5] found evidence of atherosclerosis in 45% of Vietnam war casualties, with 5% demonstrating severe coronary atherosclerosis. Mason [6] and Rigal et al [7] reported similar results. Fatty streaks or lipid deposits, which are considered to be the probable precursors to fibrous plaques and atheromatous ulcerations, are common in children by the age of 3 to 5 years.[3]

The natural history of atherosclerosis can be divided into three stages: (1) An incubation period which starts early in life and continues through adolescence [8]; (2) A latent period which is asymptomatic but in which definite pathological changes can be demonstrated at an early age [9, 10]; and (3) A clinical period during which signs and symptoms first appear. The incubation period is manifested by a fatty streak in the arterial wall. This is the earliest gross pathological alteration that can be seen. By three years of age, fatty streaks are present in the aorta of almost all children regardless of their geographic location or diet or both. During the latent period, beginning in the second decade, the fatty streaks increase in number, size and distribution and first become evident in the coronary arteries. The fatty streak is considered a reversible lesion. If there is no intervention with the progress of the fatty streak, the most commonly accepted hypothesis suggests that the fatty streak progresses to the fibrous plaque during the third decade (between 20 and 30 years).[11] This lesion appears early in the vessels of individuals in Western, industrialized societies, and less frequently in population areas of the world where there is a low incidence of coronary heart disease. This stage of the fibrous plaque is considered irreversible. The clinical period of the disease is that period of time in which the fibrous plaque has progressed to produce hemodynamically significant narrowing of the coronary artery lumen with consequent diminution of coronary flow reserve, at which stage the lesion is often calcified. This occurs most often after the end of the fourth decade and is responsible for the clinical manifestations of angina pectoris, myocardial infarction, sudden death, cerebral infarction and peripheral vascular disease.

Risk Factor Identification

Over the past twenty years, epidemiologists have attempted through both prospective and retrospective studies to determine the basic etiology of the atherosclerotic process. As a result, certain factors have been identified which, when present, place the individual at an increased risk for the premature development of coronary heart disease. These factors include hypertension, elevated blood lipids, cigarette smoking, diabetes mellitus, obesity, anxiety and tension, electrocardiographic abnormalities, family history and inadequate physical activity.[12-18] Evidence is now available which suggests these risk factors can be identified early in life.[19-22] Furthermore, studies of college students indicate that coronary and stroke mortality rate can be predicted at this early age.[23-25]

Friedman,[20] in a study of 2,260 children, found 26% to have serum cholesterol levels in excess of 160 mg/100 ml. Wein and Wilcox [26] reported 33 and 35% of their sample in excess of 200 mg/100 ml in two groups of 7 to 9 and 9 to 12-year-old children. The mean cholesterol concentration in children has been found to be between 165 and 180 mg/100 ml.[19, 27-29] Lee [30] studied serum cholesterol levels in a group of 35 boys and 28 girls over a ten-year period. The values ranged between 100 and 250 mg/100 ml. Wilmore and McNamara [21] reported 19.8% of their sample to have cholesterol values in excess of 200 mg/100 ml and 5.2% to have triglyceride values in excess of 120 mg/100 ml. Lauer et al [22] found a mean serum cholesterol level of 182 mg/100 ml in 4,829 school children, 6 to 18 years of age, with 24% of this sample in excess of 200 mg/100 ml. Serum triglyceride levels in excess of 140 mg/100 ml were identified in 15% of these children. Drash [19] suggested 200 mg/100 ml as the upper limit for normal cholesterol values in children. Mitchell et al [31] suggested that cholesterol levels in excess of 230 mg/100 ml and/or triglycerides above 140 mg/100 ml warrant further evaluation of the hyperlipidemia.

Zinner et al [32] demonstrated that the process of hypertension begins at a very early age. Elevated blood pressures were found in children between the ages of 2 and 14 years. Their results suggest that adult hypertension can be predicted in childhood. By contrast, Haggerty et al [33] found only nine children under 14 years of age who exhibited essential hypertension over a 14-year period in a large Boston hospital. Masland et al [34] identified 1.4% of 1,795 adolescents to have a blood pressure of at least 140 systolic and 90 diastolic. Wilmore and McNamara [21] were unable to detect hypertension in a large group of 8 to 12-year-old boys, and Lauer et al [22] found no hypertension in their 6 to 9-year-old group, but found 8.9% systolic and 12.2% diastolic hypertension in their 14 to 18-year-old group. The varied findings in these studies may be at least partially attributable to the problem of defining hypertension in children.

The incidence of abnormal resting and exercise electrocardiograms is rare in youth. Wilmore and McNamara [21] found no evidence of ST-segment depression during exercise testing in a group of 95 eight to 12-year-old boys whom they studied. Although Goldberg [35] reported that 5% of normal children demonstrated 1 or 2 mm ST-segment depression during exercise, it is unclear whether he was referring to displacement of the J point alone or to horizontal ST-segment depression. He found arrythmias to be infrequent but of great significance.

Obesity has been identified as one of the most prevalent health problems in the United States today.[36] It is not only an established risk factor for coronary heart disease, but is also associated with an increased risk for hypertension, diabetes mellitus, and abnormal cardiopulmonary and metabolic function.[36] The prevalence is difficult to assess because of the inadequacies of the traditional height-frame size method of selecting ideal weight, but there is evidence that the adult male and female population will be over 20% above their "best weight" in 12 to 46% of the population between 20 and 59 years of age.[36]

Obesity has also been identified at an early age. Exact standards are difficult to establish, however, as the body composition of the child is rapidly changing. Due to the differences in total body water and the density of bone, the whole body density of children cannot be evaluated by adult standards. In addition, the ratio of total body fat to subcutaneous fat is higher in children.[37] Stunkard et al [38] identified obesity in 29 and 40% of lower class girls and boys at the age of 6 years. They found a definite relationship between obesity and social class. Wilmore and McNamara [21] found 37.5% of 96 boys between the ages of 8 and 12 years to have body densities lower than 1.053, which represents a relative fat in excess of 20.0%. Hampton et al [39] found 11 to 14% of their male and 11 to 17% of their female populations to be obese when followed longitudinally between the ninth and twelfth grades.

The Role of Physical Activity

A number of research studies have identified inadequate physical activity as a risk factor in coronary artery disease. These studies have been recently summarized by Fox and Haskell,[40] Fox, Naughton and Haskell,[41] Clarke,[42] and Fox, Naughton and Gorman.[43] Naughton and Bruhn [44] reported the incidence of myocardial infarction in sedentary populations to be approximately twice that found in men who are physically active either in their jobs or in their recreational pursuits. They suggested that the clinical manifestations of coronary heart disease should be preventable, providing suitable activity programs are instituted early in life. Fox, Naughton and Haskell [41] concluded that the existing evidence suggests, but falls short of proving, that an increase in habitual physical activity is beneficial in the prevention of coronary heart disease. These studies point to the critical need for a longitudinal study of sufficient magnitude and scope which will begin in childhood and continue through at least middle age, when clinical manifestations of coronary heart disease begin to appear.

In addition to being a significant risk factor in itself, physical activity has been shown to have a favorable influence on most of the other risk factors. Physical training has been shown to reduce elevated blood pressure,[45-52] overweight and obesity,[53-61] blood cholesterol and triglyceride levels,[62-72] and depression, anxiety and tension.[73-75] The data regarding the role of exercise in significantly reducing blood pressure and cholesterol levels is somewhat equivocal at the present time as several well-controlled studies have failed to demonstrate changes with physical conditioning.[64, 66, 68, 76-78]

New Approaches to Exercise Programs

Much of the organized, competitive, emotionally stressful life of the adult has been transmitted to our children through the various physical activities in which children engage today. Many children's games are adult organized, adult supervised and attended by adult spectators. There are the adult organized team sports with emphasis on winning at almost any cost. The joy and self-expression of vigorous play has been replaced by competition, pressure and stress placed upon children often at an early age. The solution, of course, is to teach our children early in life how to play and to engage in activities which they can continue throughout their entire life span. The emphasis on physical activity for children should stress those activities which develop cardiovascular endurance, neuromuscular coordination, muscular strength and flexibility. Skill games with the major emphasis on the endowed youngster with good hand-eye coordination should be de-emphasized. All children, regardless of natural athletic skill, can engage in proper lifelong physical activity. Adult attitudes toward physical activity and fitness are formed in childhood. If a child is to lead an active life in later years, he must learn to enjoy activity while he is young. Like eating habits, physical habits are formed early. The best way to teach children lifelong physical habit patterns is for families to engage in activities together. Family physical activity togetherness occurs in father-son bicycle clubs, hiking clubs, canoeing clubs and family hiking, cycling, skiing and swimming. We need opportunities for family backpacking, family surfing and family cross-country skiing. If the weather is inclement, there are many indoor activities which have excellent cardiovascular, endurance, flexibility and strength components, such as square dancing and folk dancing. Aerobic dancing is also a fine family activity that is vigorous, rhythmic and fun. Note that the emphasis is on individual activities that are done with others. Individual fitness does not depend upon natural skill or athletic endowment. Anyone can become physically fit regardless of his or her athletic ability.

There is an overemphasis on sports and competitive athletics beginning at an early age. But let's look at physical development. At the elementary school level, a child's large arm and leg muscles are more fully developed than his fine hand and finger muscles. Hand-eye coordination is incomplete. His heart grows less rapidly than his body. Attention span is short. Competitive athletics and skill programs are of no value at this time. During this period the physical program should concentrate on basic total body activities such as running, jumping, throwing and activities to develop whole body control, body strength and endurance. In this age group, tumbling, relays, swimming, cycling, hiking and whole body rhythms are most desirable. There should be a de-emphasis of competitive athletics with its pressure on the child to win just to please the parents. Neuromuscular and motor skill developments are such that he is not ready for intense competition.

At the junior high school age, a child's bones are not fully calcified. His arms and legs are growing rapidly and body framework and muscular development do not coincide. Awkwardness is prevalent at this time. During this period, the child should engage in a wide variety of physical activities rather than specialize in one or two skill sports. Soccer, basketball, volleyball, gymnastics and aquatics help his total body development. He needs to ride his bicycle, walk and hike a great deal. Contact sports such as tackle football, ice hockey, wrestling and boxing should be avoided.

At the high school age, a wide variety of individual and team performance sports can be tried. Competition can be at a greater intensity but not so great as in college. Muscular strength, flexibility and cardiovascular endurance activities should still be emphasized at this time. The concepts of running, hiking, cycling and swimming should remain important but they can be channeled into more competitive team activities during the high school period. Soccer, basketball, volleyball, the racquet games and track and field are excellent ways to maintain endurance and muscular and flexibility fitness but still allow the fun of competition.

Physical activity appears to be beneficial only when it operates above a certain threshold level, ie, a level at least 70 to 75% of a person's work capacity.[79] We need new games that are continual and rhythmic and enjoyable and also require enough work to increase cardiovascular endurance. These activities should begin early in the school years, certainly by the first grade. Most elementary schoolyard games are largely passive, with short bursts of activity. Activity that is vigorous and imaginative with running, jumping and climbing would be more constructive. Rhythmic, continual group exercises to music and group gymnastics can also be utilized. Schoolyards need jumping pits, horizontal ladders, obstacle courses, balance beams, large ropes to swing on and large areas for running. Changes are required in the usual sterile playground consisting of some swings, a softball area and a jungle gym. These should be replaced with innovative, interesting and challenging types of programs and equipment that can contribute to the development of the cardiovascular system in a protective way. Competitive sports should be de-emphasized and lifelong physical activity emphasized. The physical education plants in our schools (the playgrounds, swimming pools, athletic fields and gymnasiums) represent millions of taxpayers' dollars. They are for the use of the entire student body and the surrounding community, not just for a limited number of varsity lettermen.

Treatment of coronary heart disease must be prevention-oriented rather than crisis-oriented as it is now, with coronary care units and mobile resuscitation units. We need planned human maintenance beginning early in life with special attention to the period of growth and development. These early years represent the period in which lifelong habits and behavior patterns are established. It is during these "pivotal" years (birth through adolescence) that the caliber of an individual's total life is often determined. The potential benefits of a comprehensive program directed toward improving cardiovascular health are indeed monumental. The lack of significant, associated disadvantages further emphasize its rationale and virtue.

References

1. American Heart Association: *Heart Facts 1976*, New York, 1976.
2. Blumenthal S: Prevention of atherosclerosis. *Amer J Cardiol* 31:591-594, 1973.
3. Kannel WB, Dawber TR: Atherosclerosis as a pediatric problem. *J Pediat* 80:544-554, 1972.
4. Enos WF, Holmes RH, Beyer J: Coronary disease among United States soldiers killed in action in Korea. *JAMA* 152:1090-1093, 1953.
5. McNamara JJ, Molot MA, Stremple JF, et al: Coronary artery disease in combat casualties in Vietnam. *JAMA* 216:1185-1187, 1971.
6. Mason JK: Asymptomatic disease of coronary arteries in young men. *Brit Med J* 2:1234-1237, 1963.
7. Rigal RD, Lovell FW, Townsend FM: Pathologic findings in the cardiovascular systems of military flying personnel. *Amer J Cardiol* 6:19-25, 1960.
8. Neufeld HN, Vlodaver Z: Structural changes in the coronary arteries of infants. *Proc Ass Europ Pediat Cardiol* 4:35-39, 1968.
9. Neufeld HN, Vlodaver Z: "Structural Changes of Coronary Arteries in Young Age Groups," in Brest AN, White PD (Eds): *International Cardiology, Cardiovascular Clinics Series*, vol 2, pp 55-78, Philadelphia: F.A. Davis, 1971.
10. Strong WB, Rao PS, Steinbaugh M: Primary prevention of atherosclerosis: a challenge to the physician caring for children. *Southern Med J* 68:319-328, 1975.
11. Strong WB: Is atherosclerosis a pediatric problem? *Med Times* 104:65-75, 1975.
12. Chapman JM, Massey FJ: The interrelationship of serum cholesterol, hypertension, body weight, and risk of coronary disease: results of the first ten years follow-up in the Los Angeles Heart Study. *J Chronic Dis* 17:933-949, 1964.
13. Dawber TR, Kannel WB, McNamara PM: The prediction of coronary heart disease. *Trans Ass*

Life Insur Med Dir Amer 47:70-101, 1964.

14. Doyle JT: Risk factors in coronary heart disease. *New York J Med* 63:1317-1320, 1963.

15. Doyle JT, Kannel WB: Coronary risk factors: 10 year findings in 7,446 Americans. Pooling Project, Council on Epidemiology, American Heart Association. Read before the VI World Congress of Cardiology, London, September 1970.

16. Inter-Society Commission for Heart Disease Resources Report: Primary prevention of the atherosclerotic diseases (abstract). *Circulation* 42:55-95, 1970.

17. Kannel WB: Physical exercise and lethal atherosclerotic disease. *New Eng J Med* 282:1153-1154, 1970.

18. Paul O, Lepper MH, Phelan WH, et al: A longitudinal study of coronary heart disease. *Circulation* 28:20-31, 1963.

19. Drash A: Atherosclerosis, cholesterol, and the pediatrician. *J Pediat* 80:693-695, 1972.

20. Friedman G: A pediatrician looks at risk factors in atherosclerotic heart disease (abstract). *Clin Res* 20:250, 1972.

21. Wilmore JH, McNamara JJ: Prevalence of coronary heart disease risk factors in boys, 8 to 12 years of age. *J Pediat* 84:527-533, 1974.

22. Lauer RM, Connor WE, Leaverton PE, et al: Coronary heart disease risk factors in school children: the Muscatine study. *J Pediat* 86:697-706, 1975.

23. Paffenbarger RS, Notkin J, Krueger DE, et al: Chronic diseases in former college students. II: Methods of study and observations on mortality from coronary heart disease. *Amer J Public Health* 56:962-971, 1966.

24. Paffenbarger RS, Wing AL: Characteristics in youth predisposing to fatal stroke in later years. *Lancet* I:753-754, 1967.

25. Thomas CB: Familial and epidemiologic aspects of coronary disease and hypertension. *J Chronic Dis* 7:198-208, 1958.

26. Wein EE, Wilcox EB: Serum cholesterol from pre-adolescence through young adulthood. *J Amer Diet Ass* 61:155-158, 1972.

27. Aldersberg D, Schaefer LE, Steinberg AG, et al: Age, sex, serum lipids, and coronary atherosclerosis. *JAMA* 162:619-622, 1956.

28. Clarke RP, Merrow SB, Morse EH, et al: Interrelationships between plasma lipids, physical measurements, and body fatness of adolescents in Burlington, Vermont. *Amer J Clin Nutr* 23:754-763, 1970.

29. Owen GM, Lubin AH: Nutritional status of preschool children. Program of the Midwest Society for Pediatric Research, November 1971.

30. Lee VA: Individual trends in the total serum cholesterol of children and adolescents over a ten-year period. *Amer J Clin Nutr* 20:5-12, 1967.

31. Mitchell S, Blount SG Jr, Blumenthal S, et al: The pediatrician and atherosclerosis. *Pediatrics* 49:165-168, 1972.

32. Zinner SH, Levy PS, Kass EH: Familial aggregation of blood pressure in children. *New Eng J Med* 284:401-404, 1971.

33. Haggerty RJ, Maroney MW, Nadas AS: Essential hypertension in infancy and childhood. *J Dis Child* 92:535-549, 1956.

34. Masland RP, Heald FP, Goodale WT, et al: Hypertensive vascular disease in children. *New Eng J Med* 255:894-897, 1956.

35. Goldberg SJ: "Exercise in Cardiac Patients," in Moss AJ, Adams FH (Eds): *Heart Disease in Infants, Children, and Adolescents*, Baltimore: Williams and Wilkins, 1968.

36. *Obesity and Health*, U.S. Department of Health, Education, and Welfare. U.S. Public Health Service. U.S. Government Printing Office, 1966.

37. Parízková J: Total body fat and skinfold thickness in children. *Metabolism* 10:794-807, 1961.

38. Stunkard A, d'Aquili E, Fox S, et al: Influence of social class on obesity and thinness in children. *JAMA* 221:579-584, 1972.

39. Hampton MC, Huenemann RL, Shapiro LR, et al: A longitudinal study of gross body composition and body conformation and their association with food and activity in a teen-age population. *Amer J Clin Nutr* 19:422-435, 1966.

40. Fox SM III, Haskell WL: Physical activity and the prevention of coronary heart disease. *Bull NY Acad Med* 44:950-967, 1968.

41. Fox SM III, Naughton JP, Haskell WL: Physical activity and the prevention of coronary heart disease. *Ann Clin Res* 3:404-432, 1971.

42. Clarke HH (Ed): Physical activity and coronary heart disease. *Physical Fitness Research Digest* 2:1-13, 1972.
43. Fox SM III, Naughton JP, Gorman PA: Physical activity and cardiovascular disease. *Mod Conc Cardiovasc Dis* 41:17-30, 1972.
44. Naughton J, Bruhn J: Emotional stress, physical activity and ischemic heart disease. *Disease-a-Month*, pp 1-34, July 1970.
45. Boyer JL, Kasch FW: Exercise therapy in hypertensive men. *JAMA* 211:1668-1671, 1970.
46. Mann GV, Garrett HL, Billings FT, et al: Exercise and coronary risk factors. *Circulation* 36 (suppl 2):181-182, 1967.
47. Naughton J, Nagle FJ: Peak oxygen intake during physical fitness programs for middle-aged men. *JAMA* 191:899-1005, 1965.
48. Naughton J, Shanbour K, Armstrong R, et al: Cardiovascular responses to exercise following myocardial infarction. *Arch Intern Med* 117:541-545, 1966.
49. Pederson-Bjergaard O: "The Effect of Physical Training in Myocardial Infarction," in Larsen OA, Malmborg RO (Eds): *Coronary Heart Disease and Physical Fitness*, p 114, Baltimore: University Park Press, 1971.
50. Rudd JL, Day WC: A physical fitness program for patients with hypertension. *J Amer Geriat Soc* 15:373-379, 1967.
51. Stone WJ: The effects of physical training on post-coronary patients (abstract). 1972 Convention of the American Association for Health, Physical Education and Recreation, p 63.
52. Wilmore JH, Royce J, Girandola RN, et al: Physiological alterations with a 10-week program of jogging. *Med Sci Sports* 2:7-14, 1970.
53. Boileaú RA, Buskirk ER, Horstman DH, et al: Body composition changes in obese and lean men during physical conditioning. *Med Sci Sports* 3:183-189, 1971.
54. Dempsey JA: Anthropometrical observations on obese and non-obese young men undergoing a program of vigorous physical exercise. *Res Quart* 35:275-287, 1964.
55. Moody DL, Kollias J, Buskirk ER: The effect of a moderate exercise program on body weight and skinfold thickness in overweight college women. *Med Sci Sports* 1:75-80, 1969.
56. Moody DL, Wilmore JH, Royce J, et al: The effects of a jogging program on the body composition of normal and obese high school girls. *Med Sci Sports* 4:210-213, 1972.
57. Parízková J: The development of subcutaneous fat in adolescents and the effects of physical training and sport. *Physiol Bohemoslov* 8:112-117, 1959.
58. Parízková J: Impact of age, diet and exercise on man's body composition. *New York Acad Sci Ann* 110:661-674, 1963.
59. Parízková J, Poupa O: Some metabolic consequences of adaptation to muscular work. *Brit J Nutr* 17:341-345, 1963.
60. Skinner JS, Holloszy JO, Cureton TK: Effects of a program of endurance exercises on physical work. *Amer J Cardiol* 14:747-752, 1964.
61. Wilmore JH, Royce J, Girandola RN, et al: Body composition changes with a 10-week program of jogging. *Med Sci Sports* 2:113-117, 1970.
62. Berkson DM, Whipple JT, Sime WE, et al: Experience with a long-term supervised ergometric exercise program for middle-aged sedentary American men (abstract). *Circulation* 36 (suppl 2): 67, 1967.
63. Daniel BJ: The effects of walking, jogging and running on the serum lipid concentration of the adult Caucasian male. Doctoral dissertation, University of Southern Mississippi, 1969.
64. Holloszy J, Skinner J, Toro G, et al: Effect of six-month training program of endurance exercise on serum lipids of middle-aged men. *Amer J Cardiol* 14:753-760, 1964.
65. Mann GV, Teel K, Hayes O, et al: Exercise in the disposition of dietary calories. *New Eng J Med* 253:349-355, 1955.
66. Montoye HJ, VanHuss WD, Brewer WD, et al: The effects of exercise on blood cholesterol in middle-aged men. *Amer J Clin Nutr* 7:139-145, 1959.
67. Naughton J, McCoy JF: Observation on the relationship of physical activity to the serum cholesterol concentration of healthy men and cardiac patients. *J Chronic Dis* 19:727-733, 1966.
68. Oscai LB, Patterson JA, Bogard DL, et al: Normalization of serum triglycerides and lipoprotein electrophoretic patterns by exercise. *Med Sci Sports* 4:63-64, 1972.
69. Phillips L: Physical fitness changes in adults attributable to equal periods of training, non-training, and re-training. Doctoral dissertation, University of Illinois, 1957.
70. Pollock MJ: "Effects of Frequency of Training on Serum Lipids, Cardiovascular Function and

Body Composition," in Franks BD (Ed): *Exercise and Fitness*, p 161, Chicago: Athletic Institute, 1969.

71. Tosshi A: Effects of three different durations of endurance exercises upon serum cholesterol (abstract). *Med Sci Sports* 3:i, 1971.

72. Wilmore JH, Haskell WL: Use of the heart rate-energy expenditure relationship in the individualized prescription of exercise. *Amer J Clin Nutr* 24:1186-1192, 1971.

73. deVries HA: Immediate and long-term effects of exercise upon resting muscle action potential level. *J Sports Med* 8:1-11, 1968.

74. deVries HA, Adams GM: Electromyographic comparison of single doses of exercise and mephrobamate as to effects on muscular relaxation. *Amer J Phys Med* 51:130-141, 1972.

75. Morgan WP, Pollock ML: Physical Activity and Cardiovascular Health: Psychological Aspects. Read before the International Congress of Physical Activity Sciences, Quebec City, Canada, July 12, 1976.

76. Brunner D, Lobel K, Altman S: Influence of manual labor on lipid values and their relation to the incidence of coronary artery disease (abstract). *Circulation* 26:693, 1962.

77. Johnson T, Wong H, Shim R, et al: The influence of exercise on serum cholesterol, phospholipids and electrophoretic serum protein patterns in college swimmers (abstract). *Fed Proc* 18:77, 1959.

78. Kilbom A, Hartley L, Saltin B, et al: Physical training in sedentary middle-aged and older men. *Scand J Clin Lab Invest* 24:315-322, 1969.

79. Pollock ML: "The Quantification of Exercise Programs," in Wilmore JH (Ed): *Exercise and Sport Sciences Reviews*, New York: Academic Press, 1973.

PART V

Exercise in
Coronary Heart Disease
Rehabilitation

23

Medical Screening of Patients with Coronary Artery Disease: Criteria for Entrance into Exercise Conditioning Programs

Malcolm M. McHenry, MD

The advent of coronary artery bypass surgery has not eliminated the need for continued medical treatment of patients with coronary artery disease. During the last decade, interest in exercise conditioning programs for such patients has increased because of clinical and experimental evidence of benefit.[1, 2] Carefully designed training protocols have been developed to observe, train and record results in such patients.[3] Unfortunately, the majority of exercise programs are unsupervised and frequently undertaken by the patient on his own. However, neither supervised nor unsupervised training has resulted in significant mortality.[3] The increasing awareness of exercise benefits both to the patient with coronary artery disease and to persons at risk of such disease suggests that the exercise fad itself may eventually become a risk factor.

The nonuniformity of training programs is paralleled by a similar inconsistency in preexercise medical screening. A "good history and physical examination" are not in themselves sufficient to protect the exercising subject.[4] Although these procedures are prerequisites for prevention of complications, they represent a somewhat crude assessment of participant risk. Yet, when they are combined with more subtle assessments, such as exercise stress testing, it is possible to eliminate most unsuitable subjects.

A review of published reports reveals few data on preliminary medical evaluation for stress testing and training. This chapter therefore presents guidelines for patient safety and rejection, emphasizing key aspects of the evaluation and the differences between a routine examination and medical screening for a conditioning program.

Who Should Be Screened?

All patients with known or suspected coronary artery disease deserve careful screening. In addition, all adults of 40 years or over contemplating exercise training should be evaluated, as should persons of any age with potentially complicating illnesses, coronary risk factors or a possible past history of heart disease.

Screening Aims

The screening analysis has three major aims: assessment of motivation, elimination of undue risk, and evaluation of potential benefit. These factors can be investigated by a specific history and physical examination in association with some laboratory procedures.

Motivation

Motivation, often neglected in preexercise evaluation, is a major factor in program adherence and patient safety. Cardiovascular conditioning may be necessary for months to years at levels of activity requiring a high heart rate and oxygen consumption at 65 to 85% of the maximal rate. Thus, poorly motivated subjects are frequently training failures. Overly motivated or overly competitive subjects may be dangerous to themselves or to the program. Such persons tend to follow rules and protocol poorly and may challenge the most fit members of the group or exceed their musculoskeletal and cardiorespiratory capacities.[7] The dropout rate of poorly or overly motivated subjects may be high. Motivation is assessed principally through a carefully taken history that stresses the patient's personal and social habits.[8] The five principal factors that influence adherence to an exercise program are: (1) Prior history of habitual exercise or participation in sports; (2) Competitive personality traits; (3) Fear of incapacitation; (4) Desire for good health and feeling of well being; and (5) Enjoyment of exercise without boredom.

People agreeing to train expect certain rewards. In general, these are positive feelings of health and well-being and the belief that exercise will favorably affect survival and functional capacity. Such feelings encourage program participants to continue even though training may be difficult and time-consuming. In addition, people who are likely to adhere to a program typically enjoy exercise. In many cases they have previously participated in exercise programs or sports and the return to training represents a combination of therapy and relaxation. Lastly, well motivated subjects, although questioning, may indicate that they have a competitive personality, have control of their aggressive drives, have a positive attitude toward exercise and are not bored by exercise, realizing that it is therapy,

---

TABLE I

Clinical Assessment of Undue Risk

History
1. Increasing angina
2. Duration since myocardial infarction
3. Congestive heart failure or low cardiac output
4. Symptomatic arrhythmias
5. Medication
6. Severe systemic diseases
7. Exertional hypotension or syncope

Physical Examination
1. Congestive heart failure
2. Abnormal precordial pulsation or thrill
3. Murmurs consistent with valvular disease
4. Diminished or abnormal arterial pulsations
5. Elevated diastolic blood pressure with retinopathy

Laboratory Evaluation
1. Specific abnormal electrocardiographic patterns
2. Chest X-ray abnormalities
3. Abnormal results of blood studies

---

not merely an enforced, meaningless obligation.

The screening physician must also obtain other information that may affect adherence to the program.[9] Does the subject understand the program? Does his working or professional schedule allow it? Can he agree to participation and supervision in a group program in which he will receive data about his performance and his physical safety will be assured? Has he performed well in past programs and adhered realistically to dietary or other measures designed to reduce risk factors? Finally, the reasons for referral of a patient to a training program must be scrutinized. Often a subject is referred only because medical treatment has failed him.

Undue Risk

The second major aim of screening is to identify and reject patients who could be harmed by an exercise conditioning program. For this purpose, a thorough and total medical evaluation must be made. The assessment must include an incisive review of the patient's history, a careful physical examination and specific laboratory procedures (Table I). Patient safety and program success require that this evaluation, although brief, reviews both the gross and subtle features of actual or potential disease.

History: From the history, the examiner can determine whether the subject is threatened by inordinate myocardial oxygen requirements, the hemodynamic consequences of medication during training, or other systemic diseases. Patients with coronary artery disease may remain well compensated when metabolic demand and vascular supply are matched. Because exercise may alter this relation, evidence of inadequate oxygen supply must be sought in the history.

Unstable Angina—Although unstable angina is the most common deterrent to training, it is often difficult to identify. Standard questioning may not reveal that the subject who now has pain on moderate effort also has spontaneous ischemic pain, nocturnal pain, an increasing need for nitrites, more prolonged periods of angina or has had to pace himself to a lower level of energy expenditure. This changing anginal pattern may assume many forms. There may be an obvious and severe intensification of ischemic symptoms (crescendo or preinfarction angina), or the signs may be insidious and more slowly progressive. Retrospective analysis of the patterns of pain leading to myocardial infarction frequently shows a slow and gradual intensification of complaints culminating in an acute coronary event. So-called anginal variants exist. In addition to the well-known Prinzmetal variant (angina typically occurring at rest and not associated with exertion), it is clear that myocardial ischemia can occur without pain. Exertional symptoms of dyspnea or fatigue due to elevated left heart filling pressure or transient decrease in cardiac output due to ischemia are now being retrospectively identified. The screening physician must appreciate these subtle changes if he is to ensure that patients with these symptoms do not enter the training program. In patients who are convalescing from a myocardial infarction, myocardial oxygen consumption should not be inordinately augmented until complete healing has occurred. A period of about 3 months is a standard interval for ensuring safety.

Reduced Ventricular Function and Myocardial Reserve—Patients with symptomatic congestive heart failure or low cardiac output (weakness on effort, dyspnea, fatigue and malaise) have reduced ventricular function and myocardial reserve. Increasing myocardial oxygen requirements in such patients can only be harmful.[10] The occurrence of symptomatic tachycardiac arrhythmias increases oxygen demand inappropriately. The arrhythmia must first be identified by type and then treated. For this reason, ambulatory electrocardiographic monitoring is recommended as part of the medical work-up to ensure that significant or dangerous ectopic activity does not occur occultly with effort. All of the aforementioned situations that inappropriately increase myocardial oxygen requirements can be identified by a carefully taken history, then treated and potentially controlled. Upon return to a stable condition, the patient may again be considered for training.

Medications—Certain medications are absolute or relative contraindications to training. Patients with systemic hypertension taking ganglionic blocking agents should be excluded. The hypotension on standing at rest associated with further peripheral vasodilatation on effort may reduce coronary perfusion to a significant degree. A relative contraindication exists with the use of beta adrenergic blocking agents. Although beta adrenergic blockade simulates some of the effects of training (reduced exercising heart rate and decreased myocardial oxygen requirements),[11] it also causes depression of myocardial function.[12] If in fact a significant benefit of training in patients with coronary artery disease is a redistribution of peripheral blood flow to active muscle[13] and a decrease in myocardial oxygen consumption through a reduction in ejection time, heart rate and peripheral resistance,[14] inhibition of myocardial function would not appear to have a salutary effect and might negate other benefits. The use of digitalis, quinidine and other agents that alter the repolarization characteristics of the electrocardiogram could be considered relative contraindications only if the intent of training is in part to observe electrocardiographic improvement or exercise-induced changes in ischemic electrocardiographic thresholds.[15]

Systemic Diseases—Several systemic diseases may significantly affect or contraindicate exercise. These include brittle insulin-dependent diabetes mellitus, cerebrovascular and peripheral vascular insufficiency, severe systemic hypertension and pulmonary emphysema when associated with hypoxia, hypercarbia and pulmonary hypertension. Exertional syncope or a history of hypotension also indicates undue risk.

Physical Examination: Careful examination of the cardiovascular system may disclose a patient at risk. Hyperthyroidism, congestive heart failure and abdominal aortic aneurysm are easily identified. A thorough preexercise cardiovascular screening attempts to identify more subtle lesions by particular attention to inspection, palpation of peripheral arteries, palpation and auscultation of the heart and close examination of the eye grounds.

A precordial thrill may indicate an acquired postinfarction ventricular septal defect or papillary muscle dysfunction. An apical impulse may indicate left ventricular hypertrophy or a ventricular aneurysm. A left parasternal impulse may indicate right ventricular hypertrophy of many causes or left atrial hypertension. All these conditions merit further clinical evaluation.

Cardiac auscultation is a critical part of the examination. Murmurs suggestive of acquired or congenital valvular disease must be identified. Patients with aortic stenosis of significant degree tolerate effort poorly, as manifested by exertional syncope and occasionally by sudden death. Similarly, the effects of chronic exercise training have not been explored in subjects with aortic or mitral insufficiency; such stress could excessively tax their marginal cardiac reserve. Training may theoretically benefit patients with mild to moderate mitral valve stenosis.[10] In this lesion, the expected training effect of slowing of the submaximal heart rate and prolongation of diastolic filling period might reduce the end-diastolic mitral gradient. But training is not generally recommended as profitable for subjects with congenital or acquired valvular lesions.

Patients with severe systemic hypertension (defined as a diastolic blood pressure greater than 120 mm Hg accompanied by advanced retinopathy) should be rejected for training. Although training can reduce diastolic pressure elevations of mild to moderate degree,[16] this reduction would not be expected in more severe hypertension.[17] The effects of exercise on fixed vascular resistance have not been defined clearly enough to exclude significant risk.

   Contrarily, patients with low resting blood pressure or mild hypotension must be critically evaluated since this finding may be a subtle indication of depressed myocardial function. Hypotension, especially when accompanying the onset of exertionally induced angina, has been associated with severe compromise of coronary blood flow due to multivessel obstruction.[18]

Laboratory Examinations: A limited number of laboratory procedures are essential to the careful preexercise screening. These consist basically of a resting electrocardiogram, a chest roentgenogram and blood chemistry determinations with special attention given to blood sugar, electrolytes and myocardial enzymes.

   Electrocardiogram—Analysis of the electrocardiogram is probably the most important laboratory procedure. Evidence of increasing ischemia, unsuspected or clinically undetected infarction and specific arrhythmias and conduction disturbances contraindicate entrance into training. Ventricular arrhythmias, particularly multifocal premature ventricular beats, require delay of training and prompt treatment. Conduction disturbances such as complete right bundle branch block and left bundle branch block produce only insignificant hemodynamic changes in subjects without major coronary artery disease.[18-20] However, the occurrence of bundle branch block in acute infarction increases mortality [21, 22] and is indicative of extensive myocardial damage. Therefore, the combination of bundle branch block and coronary artery disease indicates an added risk or contraindication to training.

   Two specific conduction disturbances merit discussion because of their potentially lethal consequences during exercise. They are type II (Mobitz) second degree atrioventricular block and bilateral bundle branch block. In both, destructive infranodal lesions are assumed.[23-25] With exercise, the normally expected shortening of atrioventricular refractoriness does not occur and the accelerated atrial rate finds ventricular unresponsiveness.[26] Complete heart block has been documented on occasion when such rate increases occur,[27] and bilateral bundle branch block appears to be the most common electrophysiologic mechanism of complete heart block.[28]

   Roentgenogram—X-ray examination of the chest for heart size is another simple technique for identifying a subject with reduced cardiac reserve. Cardiomegaly of any cause requires investigation and may indicate extensive myocardial damage. The identification on X-ray or fluoroscopic study of coronary arterial calcification has been correlated angiographically and pathologically with severe atherosclerotic obstruction [29] and may indicate undue training risk.

Patient Benefit

   The final screening analysis is concerned with the assurance of patient benefit. One can assume that benefit will occur if the subject has met the motivational, historical, clinical and laboratory standards described. However, training bene-

---

TABLE II

Major Causes for Rejecting Patients

---

1. Clinically unstable or inadequately treated disease
2. Clinically important complicating illnesses
3. Specific medications
4. Diseases mimicking coronary artery disease
5. Poor motivation

---

fit is restricted to subjects with coronary artery disease; exercise programs in other forms of heart disease are both untested and potentially harmful. Therefore, the precise nature of the disease process causing ischemic pain must be known.

Patients may have angina pectoris without having coronary artery disease. This is dramatically seen in severe valvular aortic stenosis, idiopathic hypertrophic subaortic stenosis, other forms of cardiomyopathy and severe pulmonary hypertension, especially that due to mitral stenosis or occurring with congenital heart disease. Training programs in these conditions are not beneficial and may be lethal.

Conclusions

When thoughtful and carefully performed screening procedures are applied, few patients in organized training protocols will suffer. When basic guidelines for patient rejection are followed (Table II), risk is minimized, the subject is protected and the yield of good results should be enhanced.

There can be no substitute for adequate medical control and management of patients with coronary artery disease. These measures include treatment of increasing angina, control of the symptoms of heart failure and low cardiac output and treatment of coexisting systemic diseases. Before a patient enters a training program, his medications must be reviewed to ensure that their effects will not be reversed by exercise, and diseases producing ischemic pain and mimicking arteriosclerotic heart disease must be excluded. Finally, the patient must be properly motivated.

Summary

Although considerable emphasis has been placed on stress testing and physical training of patients with coronary artery disease, data on safe and thorough preliminary medical evaluation are scarce. Because the routine history and physical examination are not sufficient to protect the exercising subject, medical screening attempts a thorough analysis of the patient's motivation, physical status, possible risk factors and the probability of benefit.

Motivation is a critical factor since training for prolonged periods of time at high levels of heart rate and oxygen consumption may be required. Patients who have unstable angina or who may be harmed by increased myocardial oxygen requirements must be excluded. Concomitant influencing diseases and certain medications may also be causes for rejecting a patient. Valvular heart disease and severe systemic hypertension are not associated with benefit from exercise conditioning. The screening physician must exclude patients with certain abnormal electrocardiographic patterns, such as bilateral bundle branch block and type II second degree atrioventricular block, and he must be assured that he is dealing with coronary artery disease, not a pathologic process that mimics it. When these principles are applied, few persons in organized programs of exercise conditioning should suffer, and the yield of good results should be enhanced.

References

1. Redwood DR, Rosing DR, Epstein SE: Circulatory and symptomatic effects of physical training in patients with coronary artery disease and angina pectoris. New Eng J Med 286:959-965, 1972.
2. Fox SM III, Haskell WL: Physical activity and the prevention of coronary heart disease. Bull NY Acad Med 44:905-967, 1968.
3. Haskell WL: Cardiovascular complications during medically supervised exercise training of cardiacs (abstract). Circulation 52(suppl 2):118, 1975.
4. Hellerstein HK: Exercise therapy in coronary artery disease. Bull NY Acad Med 44:1028-1047, 1968.
5. Fox SM III, Naughton JP, Gorman PA: Physical activity and cardiovascular health: the exercise prescription, intensity and duration. Mod Concepts Cardiovasc Dis 41:21-24, 1972.
6. Siegel W, Blomqvist G, Mitchell JH: Effects of a quantitated physical training program on middle-aged sedentary men. Circulation 41:19-29, 1970.
7. Fox SM III, Naughton JP, Gorman PA: Physical activity and cardiovascular health. Mod Concepts Cardiovasc Dis 41:25-30, 1972.
8. Mann GV, Garrett HL, Farhi A, et al: Exercise to prevent coronary heart disease: an experimental study of the effects of training on risk factors for coronary disease in man. Amer J Med 46:12-27, 1969.
9. Stiles MH: Motivation for sports participation in the community. Canad Med Ass J 96:889-892, 1967.
10. Durbeck DC, Heinzelmann F, Schacter J, et al: The National Aeronautics and Space Administration–U.S. Public Health Service health evaluation and enhancement program: summary of results. Amer J Cardiol 30:784-790, 1972.
11. Rapaport E: Exercise responses in patients with heart failure or valvular or congenital heart disease. J SC Med Assoc 65 (suppl 1):61-64, 1969.
12. Epstein SE, Robinson BF, Kahler RL, et al: Effects of beta-adrenergic blockade on the cardiac response to maximal and submaximal exercise in man. J Clin Invest 44:1745-1753, 1965.
13. Sonnenblick EH, Braunwald E, Williams JF Jr, et al: Effects of exercise on myocardial force-velocity relations in intact, unanesthetized man: relative roles of changes in heart rate, sympathetic activity and ventricular dimensions. J Clin Invest 44:2051-2062, 1965.
14. Varnauskas E, Bergman H, Houk P, et al: Haemodynamic effects of physical training in coronary patients. Lancet II:8-12, 1966.
15. Robinson BF: Relation of heart rate and systolic blood pressure to the onset of pain in angina pectoris. Circulation 35:1073-1083, 1967.
16. Detry J-M, Bruce RA: Effects of physical training on exertional S-T-segment depression in coronary heart disease. Circulation 44:390-396, 1971.
17. Boyer JL, Kash FW: Exercise therapy in hypertensive man. JAMA 211:1668-1671, 1970.
18. Thomson PD, Kelemen MH: Hypotension accompanying the onset of exertional angina: a sign of severe compromise of left ventricular blood supply. Circulation 52:28-32, 1975.
19. Finkielman S, Worcel M, Agrest A: Hemodynamic patterns in essential hypertension. Circulation 31:356-368, 1965.

20. Schecter E: Effect of intermittent left bundle branch block on left ventricular function (abstract). *Circulation* 40 (suppl III):111-178, 1969.

21. Schecter E, Eber L, Lancaster MC: Meaning of acquired left bundle branch block (abstract). *Circulation* 46: (suppl II):8, 1972.

22. Lancaster MC, Schecter E, Massing GK: Acquired complete right bundle branch block without overt heart disease: clinical and hemodynamic study of 37 patients. *Amer J Cardiol* 30:32-36, 1972.

23. Norris RM, Croxson MS: Bundle branch block in acute myocardial infarction. *Amer Heart J* 79:728-733, 1970.

24. Scheidt S, Killip T: Bundle-branch block complicating acute myocardial infarction. *JAMA* 222:919-924, 1972.

25. Langendorf R, Pick A: Atrioventricular block, type II (Mobitz)—its nature and clinical significance. *Circulation* 38:819-820, 1968.

26. Blondeau M, Rizzon P, Lenègre J: Les troubles de la conduction auriculoventriculaire dans l'infarctus myocardique recent. II. Etude anatomique. *Arch Mal Coeur* 54:1105-1117, 1961.

27. Rosen KM, Loeb HS, Chuquimia R, et al: Site of heart block in acute myocardial infarction. *Circulation* 42:925-933, 1970.

28. Watanabe Y, Dreifus LS: Second degree atrioventricular block. *Cardiovasc Res* 1:150-158, 1967.

29. Stock JPP: *Diagnosis and Treatment of Cardiac Arrhythmias*, pp 184-186, New York: Appleton-Century-Crofts, 1970.

30. Narula OS, Scherlag BJ, Javier RP, et al: Analysis of the A-V conduction defect in complete heart block utilizing His bundle electrograms. *Circulation* 41:437-448, 1970.

31. Frink RJ, Achor RWP, Brown AL Jr, et al: Significance of calcification of the coronary arteries. *Amer J Cardiol* 26:241-247, 1970.

24

Long-term Physiologic Adaptations to Exercise with Special Reference to Performance and Cardiorespiratory Function in Health and Disease

William C. Adams, PhD
Malcolm M. McHenry, MD
Edmund M. Bernauer, PhD

The long-term effects of systematic physical exercise have been subjected to scientific investigation for at least 60 years. The first comprehensive review was completed by Steinhaus in 1933[1]; more recent discussions are included in exercise physiology textbooks, the most complete being that by Åstrand and Rodahl.[2]

Participation in properly designed exercise training programs increases capacity for muscular work by effecting morphologic and functional changes. These include: (1) Increased muscular strength and endurance, primarily as a result of enlargement of existing muscle fibers and an increase in the number of capillaries; (2) Better neuromuscular coordination, which reduces the energy requirement; (3) Altered body composition, generally involving an increase in muscle mass and a decrease in adipose tissue; and (4) Increased maximal oxygen uptake, due primarily to increases in blood volume, total hemoglobin, heart size and stroke volume, and a widened arteriovenous oxygen difference. The effects of training on other body functions and their relative importance to increased physical performance are not as well known.

Until recently, the effects of physical training were frequently attributed to differences between athletes and nonathletes. This supposition is not entirely valid, since athletes are genetically endowed according to the particular requisites of their sport,[3] and the distinction between constitutional dissimilarities and the effects of physical training is not amenable to definitive analysis. Primarily for this reason it is preferable to use the longitudinal approach, in which subjects are followed over an appropriate period of time. Although this method is not without objections from a scientific viewpoint,[2] with proper attention to subject sampling procedures, insistence on stable habitual life patterns during the investigation, motivation, careful monitoring of the intensity of the training program, and appropriate control groups, it is preferred. It has been demonstrated, however, in numerous epidemiologic, cross-sectional investigations that physically active men are less likely to have myocardial infarcts, and when they do, are less apt to die.[4] Although these studies have inherent weaknesses in design, they have provided impetus for the longitudinal investigation of exercise programs on work performance and physiologic variables related to coronary artery disease risk factors in middle-aged normal subjects. Within this context, the effects of physical training on work performance and cardiorespiratory function are reviewed.

Principles of Physiologic Adaptation to Training

Specificity of Training—Exercise training programs can be biased to achieve particular physiologic effects. Obviously, the effects of a weight training regimen are quite different from those achieved by gradually intensified jogging. But even with a particular activity, there are specific effects. For example, Clausen and Trap-Jensen [5] trained two groups to perform dynamic work on a bicycle ergometer, one group using the arms only and one using leg work only. The reduction in heart rate obtained by training the arm muscles only could not be transferred to an ergometer leg work task, and vice versa. Thus, it was concluded that local changes in the trained muscles are of importance for the effect of training on heart rate. A recent study of female twins with a similar level of maximal oxygen uptake demonstrated that the twin who had continued to engage in competitive freestyle swimming training used a much greater percentage of her maximal oxygen uptake and sustained a significantly faster swimming pace than the twin who had remained active but had given up swimming training 3 years previously.[6] The difference in maximal oxygen uptake was less pronounced in arm ergometer work, and it was concluded that the continued swimming training had, by unknown mechanisms, enabled one twin to achieve close adaptation of central and peripheral functions to the specific work of swimming.

Proper training may increase the size and, some evidence suggests, the number of myofibrils within a muscle fiber. This appears to be primarily the result of a strength training stimulus that affects particularly the white fibers. Utilization of a high resistance, low repetition training program in lifting weights is the most effective method for increasing muscle size and strength. On the other hand, utilization of a low resistance, high repetition program produces an endurance training stimulus that increases the number of capillaries, muscle mitochondria, energy-liberating enzymes in the sarcoplasm and electron transport capacity.[7]

Improved efficiency in terms of reduced energy expenditure is another train-

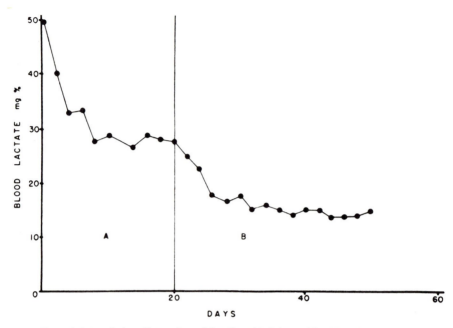

Figure 1. Interrelation of intensity and duration of training on blood lactate response to a standard work task. Training consisted of daily running on the treadmill for 20 minutes at 7 miles/hour for 20 days, followed by 15 minutes at 8.5 miles/hour for 30 days. Reproduced with permission from Brouha L: "Training," in Johnson WR, Buskirk E (Eds): *Science and Medicine of Exercise and Sports*, ed 2, p 280, New York: Harper, 1974.

ing effect specific to the particular activity engaged in. Brouha's studies [8] indicate that through training and practice in activities requiring mastery of skills (such as skiing and swimming), energy expenditure is reduced by elimination of unnecessary dynamic and static muscular contractions, more complete relaxation of muscular antagonists, and replacement of voluntary movement with reflex action. In activities that are uncomplicated technically, such as walking, there is no noticeable increase in efficiency as reflected by reduced oxygen consumption.

  Overload—Both intensity and duration are important factors influencing the degree of training effect. Depending on the particular requirements of their sport or event, athletes generally use maximal or near maximal efforts at appropriate rates and duration to enhance the rapid achievement of specific training effects.[7] However, when training middle-aged men, one is more concerned with the training threshold in achieving an optimal intensity. Karvonen [9] demonstrated a reduction in both work and resting heart rates when previously untrained medical students ran on a treadmill for 30 minutes 4 to 5 days per week with speed adjusted to attain a heart rate at 60% of the difference between the maximal and resting rates. At lower rates, the training effect was not seen and the speed of

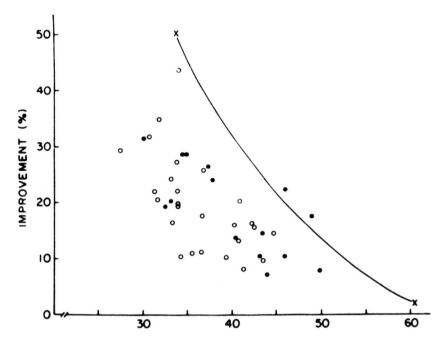

Figure 2. Individual values for percent improvement in relation to the pretraining level of maximal oxygen uptake in middle-aged men; the mean value for young men is included as a line. Reproduced with permission of the American College of Sports Medicine from Saltin B: Physiological effects of physical conditioning. *Med Sci Sports* 1:50-56, 1969.

running had to be increased for further improvement. The combined effect of intensity and duration is seen in Figure 1. Initially, a rather rapid decrease in blood lactate was effected, but was followed by a leveling off after 20 days until the training speed was increased to 8.5 miles/hour, and a further progressive decrease occurred for 10 days before again leveling off.[8]

In the training of middle-aged men, Siegel et al [10] postulated that the number of sessions a week, the total duration of training, the effective duration of each session and the intensity of exercise influence the degree of improvement. They found that training at an intensity necessitating a heart rate slightly in excess of 80% of predicted maximal rate, performed 2.6 times a week for an effective total of 30 minutes a week for 15 weeks, resulted in a significant increase in maximal oxygen uptake. The improvement was not maintained by continuing training for 10 effective minutes, 0.9 sessions a week.

Individual Differences—The response of a subject to a training stimulus is affected by his genetic potential, age and level of physical activity immediately before training. An inverse relation between the initial level of maximal oxygen uptake and percent improvement is shown in Figure 2.[11] Despite their relatively lower initial values, middle-aged men appear to be less trainable than younger

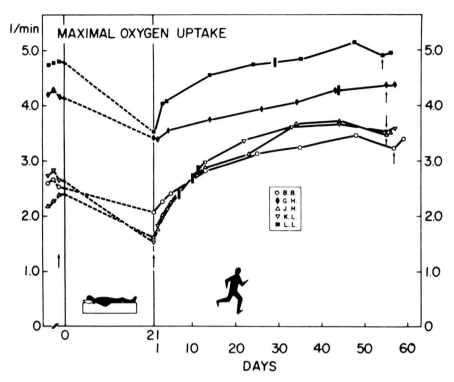

Figure 3. Changes in maximal oxygen uptake with bed rest and training. The heavy bars indicate the time during the training period at which the maximal oxygen uptake had returned to the control value before bed rest. Subjects G.H. and L.L. were in a trained state at the initiation of the experiment. Reproduced by permission of the American Heart Association, Inc. from Saltin B, Blomquist G, Mitchell JH, et al: Response to exercise after bed rest and training. *Circulation* 38 (suppl 7): 1-78, 1968.

subjects. However, this difference would be greatly attenuated if the improvement in percent of absolute $\dot{V}O_2$ max values was plotted against initial values expressed as a function of age adjusted mean values (eg, as percent of 47 ml/min per kg for the young men and 37 ml/min per kg for the middle-aged men).

The importance of the pretraining activity level is strikingly portrayed in Figure 3.[12] In three previously sedentary subjects, maximal oxygen uptake increased from an initial value of 2.52 to 3.41 liters/min (35%) with 55 days of hard aerobic training, whereas in the two previously active subjects it increased from 4.48 to 4.65 liters/min (4%). However, starting with the bed rest value after 21 days, the increases were from 1.74 to 3.41 liters/min (96%) and 3.48 to 4.65 liters/min (34%), respectively. If the bed rest were necessitated by disease processes in a vital organ, the deterioration in physical working capacity would be even greater. Furthermore, even if physical working capacity were known before the onset of disease, it would be difficult to ascertain the diminution due to disease

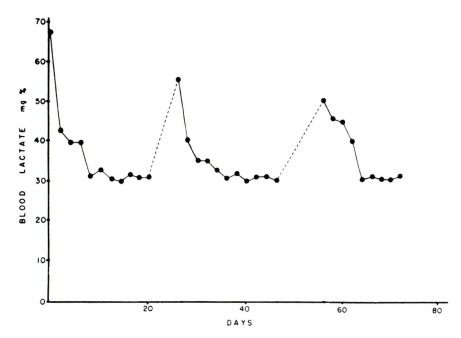

Figure 4. Effect of stopping exercise for a few days during a training period on blood lactate response to running on a treadmill for 10 minutes at 7.5 miles/hour. The dotted lines indicate two periods during which no exercise was performed. Reproduced with permission from Brouha L: "Training," in Johnson WR, Buskirk E (Eds): *Science and Medicine of Exercise and Sports*, ed 2, p 281, New York: Harper, 1974.

compared to that caused by inactivity.[2]

Transiency of Training—Most training studies have not been carried beyond several months duration. A notable exception is that of Katila and Frick,[13] who noted increased performance and lower submaximal heart rate in six subjects after 2 months of programmed training. Three subjects continued to train for 2 years and exhibited further training effects, whereas those who ceased training demonstrated exercise tolerance and heart rate characteristic of their pretrained state. Return to original pretraining values after cessation of training for 14 weeks has been observed.[10] In fact, significant training reversal may be a matter of several days, as is suggested in Figure 4.[8]

The longitudinal study of nine college cross-country runners provided an opportunity to assess the interrelated effects of increased maturity, work load (in terms of intensity and distance run), duration and transiency of training. After 3 months of training and competition, their maximal oxygen uptake increased from 62.1 to 66.6 ml/min per kg.[14] Six runners continued training and, when tested at peak training form 1 to 4 years later, demonstrated a further increase of 6.5 ml/min per kg to 72.0. They had no significant change in body weight during this period. Two of the three who ceased active training and were available for subsequent study had an initial maximal oxygen uptake of 61 ml/min per kg, which increased to 64.6 during training, but then regressed to 58.7 when measured 2 to 3 ½ years later. These subjects gained approximately 10% of body weight during the period of nontraining.

Selected Effects of Endurance-Oriented Training on Normal Middle-Aged Men

Body Composition—Physical training has a potentially profound influence on man's body composition, both increasing muscle mass and decreasing fat. However, since K^{40} has been found to be relatively constant in adults over a long period of time, some researchers maintain that change in body composition in the adult population is due to reduction in fat alone, and rarely to increased muscle mass.[15] Moreover, it is unlikely that substantially increased muscle mass is effected by rhythmic, relatively low resistance exercise characteristic of most middle-aged adult physical training programs. Conversely, the energy expenditure of walking, jogging or running over a speed range from 4.6 to 16 km/hour necessitates between 1.4 to 1.7 kcal/kg of body weight per mile traversed,[16] and could result in substantial fat loss.

Longitudinal studies on changes in body composition effected by physical training in middle-aged men have been summarized by Pollock et al.[17] In programs primarily entailing jogging 2 to 4 times a week for periods up to 1 hour for 10 to 24 weeks, the average loss in body weight was 1.4 kg and the mean decrease in percent of body weight as fat was 1.3. Apparently the amount of training is more important than intensity, in that training at 80 to 90% of maximal heart rate for 45 minutes 2 days a week for 20 weeks did not cause significant changes in body composition.[18] However, a saturation point apparently occurs, since subjects who trained 30 to 35 minutes for 2 to 3 days a week for 2 years revealed reductions of 3.8% of body weight after 6 months and 5.5% after 12 months, but had no additional change thereafter.[19]

Cardiorespiratory Effects—The primary measure of the quality of the cardiorespiratory system is $\dot{V}O_2$ max, which is the product of cardiac output and arteriovenous oxygen difference, and reflects both the performance of the heart as a pump and the efficiency of blood flow distribution and oxygen utilization.[20] For young untrained men, the mean value is approximately 50 ml/min per kg, which diminishes with age to about 30 ml/min per kg at age 70.[21] Values as high as 85 ml/min per kg have been noted in highly trained Olympic cross-country skiers and distance runners.[22]

Endurance-oriented physical training of middle-aged subjects for several months increases maximal oxygen uptake. The degree of increase appears to be an interrelation of age, activity level before training, and the intensity and duration of training (Table I, Figure 2 and 3), but accurate definition of the relative importance of each is presently lacking. Maximal heart rate is either unchanged or slightly lower, whereas oxygen pulse and pulmonary ventilation are in-

TABLE I

Comparison of Changes in Maximal Oxygen Uptake (V̇O₂ max) with Training in Middle-Aged Men

	Pollock et al [17]	Tzankoff et al [23]	Naughton & Nagle [24]	Mann et al [25]	Hanson et al [26]	Saltin et al [27]	Pollock et al [18]	Oscai et al [28]	Ribisl [29]	Wilmore et al [30]
# Subjects	16	15	18	62	7	50	22	14	15	7
Mean age (yr)	49	54	41	25-60	49	43	39	37	40	53
V̇O₂ max (ml/min per kg)										
Before training	29.9	30.2	31.3	34.0	35.1	36.0	37.1	38.5	40.1	40.3
After training	38.9	36.1	36.8	39.6	40.7	42.5	43.3	47.0	45.5	41.8
%Δ	30	20	18	16	16	18	17	22	14	10
Training duration (wk)	20	25	30	24	28	8-10	20	20	20	10
Frequency (sessions/wk)	4	2.3	3	5	3	2-3	2	3	3	3
Work time/session (excluding warm-up) (min)	40	55	30	40	60	20	45	30	35	12-24
Work intensity (% of maximal heart rate)	70	—	—	250-850 kcal/hour	—	90+	85	88	300-750 kcal/hour	600-700 kcal/hour
Type of activity	Walking	Games, walking, jogging	Running, calisthenics	Calisthenics, walking, running	Running, games, calisthenics	Running, walking, calisthenics	Running	Running	Running, calisthenics	Jogging

creased.[2] The increase in pulmonary ventilation is proportional to that in $\dot{V}O_2$ max, and since arterial blood gas studies indicate that ventilation and diffusion do not limit maximal performance under normal conditions, improvements secondary to training must primarily involve the circulation.[26] In young men this improvement may occur both by enlargement of cardiovascular dimensions (particularly heart volume, blood volume and total hemoglobin) and by improved function of the circulation itself, although the length of training appears critical to the former.[12]

At submaximal work loads in activities such as walking or riding a bicycle ergometer, there is no appreciable increase in skill with training and, thus, no reduction in oxygen consumption. There is, however, reduced physiologic strain as evidenced by a decreased percent of maximal oxygen uptake at submaximal work loads, and by absolute decreases in heart rate, pulmonary ventilation, blood lactate and ventilatory equivalent.[23, 26, 31] The reduction in submaximal heart rate is normally associated with an increased stroke volume and perhaps better vasomotor adjustments of blood flow to the working muscles, as is suggested by slightly reduced systemic blood pressures.[23] Because of this improved efficiency, work load capacity at a particular heart rate is augmented.[26] Since cardiac output and oxygen carrying capacity of the blood at submaximal work are the same, or nearly so, improved ventilatory efficiency appears to be due to peripheral factors. The lower level of blood lactate in submaximal work may be due to better distribution of the blood flow, or possibly to an increased activation of red muscle fibers with a more efficient energy yield from aerobic processes.[27] The biochemical mechanisms by which this could occur have been established by Holloszy,[32] but were derived from animal experiments. More recently, Kiessling et al [33] demonstrated that previously sedentary young men who ran 12 miles a week for 28 weeks increased the number of muscle mitochondria. More severe training, as evidenced by the study of elite endurance athletes, showed little difference in the number of mitochondria, but a pronounced size increase as compared to the trained normal young men. Further evidence of the peripheral cardiorespiratory changes effected by training is afforded by Varnauskas et al,[34] who observed a 44% increase in succinic dehydrogenase activity (an enzyme probably present only in the mitochondria).

Hemodynamic Response—After training, cardiac output is unchanged [35] or slightly reduced during submaximal work.[26, 36] Although there is a widened arteriovenous oxygen difference with training in young men,[11] both an increase at greater submaximal work loads [26] and no difference [35] have been noted after training in middle-aged men. Slightly reduced mean systemic arterial blood pressure at submaximal work loads in middle-aged men after training has been observed.[23, 35] Since cardiac output is little changed and heart rate and mean blood pressure are reduced at submaximal work, the reduced pressure must indicate that the contractile work of the left ventricle declines slightly.

There is a paucity of data on hemodynamic responses after physical training at maximal exercise levels in normal, middle-aged men. Hence, the hemodynamic

TABLE II

Summary of Findings During Maximal Work in Three
Longitudinal Studies on Hemodynamic Effects of Training in
Sedentary Young Men [11]

	Max V̇O$_2$ (liters/min)	a-v O$_2$ diff (vol %)	Q̇ (liters/min)	HR (beats/min)	SV (ml)
Minneapolis [37] (# = 6)					
Control	3.42	15.1	22.8	193	118
Training	3.87	16.3	23.8	186	128
Diff.(%)	+13.2	+8.0	+4.4	-3.6	+8.5
Stockholm [36] (# = 8)					
Control	3.10	13.8	22.4	200	112
Training	3.44	14.3	24.2	192	127
Diff.(%)	+11.1	+3.6	+8.0	-4.0	+13.4
Dallas [12] (# = 3)					
Control	2.52	14.6	17.2	192	90
Training	3.41	17.0	20.0	191	105
Diff.(%)	+35.3	+16.4	+16.4	-0.5	+16.7
Mean (# = 17)					
Control	3.11	14.4	21.5	196	110
Training	3.59	15.5	23.2	190	122
Diff.%	+15.4	+7.6	+7.9	-3.1	+10.9

a-v O$_2$ Diff = arteriovenous oxygen difference; HR = heart rate; Max V̇O$_2$ = maximal
oxygen consumption; Q̇ = cardiac output; SV = stroke volume

response at maximal performance in young men who have undergone endurance training is summarized in Table II. The 15.4% increase in maximal oxygen uptake is the result of a nearly equal increase in both arteriovenous oxygen difference and cardiac output. The increased cardiac output was entirely effected by a greater stroke volume, since maximal heart rate was reduced 3%. Hartley et al [35] studied the hemodynamic effects of training on middle-aged men during maximal work, and observed a 14% increase in maximal oxygen consumption which was almost entirely the result of increased cardiac output. There was no significant difference in arteriovenous oxygen difference and, since heart rate was slightly reduced, the increased cardiac output and maximal oxygen uptake were entirely a function of a 16% increase in stroke volume. There is a close relation between stroke volume and heart volume in young men, which has also been observed in active, middle-aged athletes.[38] Both stroke volume and heart volume increase with training in young men,[12] whereas in sedentary, middle-aged men the stroke volume was lower than would be expected from their heart volume, but increased with training concurrent with no change in heart volume,[35] thus suggesting possible improvement in myocardial contractility.

Mazzarella and Jordan [39] examined the possibility of reversing ischemic electrocardiographic exercise responses in seven middle-aged sedentary men who were asymptomatic at rest by subjecting them to 20 minutes of walking three times a week for 8 to 10 weeks. Six men showed less ST-segment depression in submaximal work after training, five showed improvement at maximal exercise, and only three exhibited ST-segment depression in their immediate postexercise electrocardiogram.

Adaptation to Endurance-Oriented Training in Coronary Artery Disease

With impetus provided by the early work of Hellerstein and Hornsten,[40] physical reconditioning has in the past decade become part of the armamentarium of treatment for patients with coronary artery disease. Several investigators [41-45] have shown that many patients with coronary artery disease can be retrained to perform better than sedentary normal subjects of similar age, although until recently the mechanisms effecting this improvement were not well elucidated.[46] The variability of response to physical training is greater in patients with coronary artery disease, presumably because the severity of the underlying disease limits some patients' ability to respond to the training stimulus.[41, 47]

Angina Pectoris—Although MacAlpin and Kattus [48] have demonstrated "walking through angina," most investigators have stopped such patients from exercising to the point of maximal effort because of pain; that is, they were symptom-limited.[49] Undoubtedly this procedure underestimates maximal work capacity, since an increase of 14.5% in maximal oxygen uptake has been observed in patients with angina after sublingual administration of 0.4 mg of nitroglycerin.[50] Detry and Bruce [51] observed increased maximal oxygen uptake (symptom-limited) after training, and others have noted a greater amount of work before onset of pain, which suggests decreased cardiac oxygen consumption or increased coronary blood supply, or both.[46, 52] In addition, Redwood et al [52] have made observations at the onset of angina which indicate that training might improve myocardial oxygen delivery. In submaximal work, heart rate, mean blood pressure, pressure-rate product, tension-time index and presumably myocardial oxygen requirements are reduced.[5, 52-54] In addition, reduced ST-segment depression has been noted.[40, 51] Hemodynamic studies have revealed little or no change in cardiac output, with a concurrent increase in stroke volume and nearly constant arteriovenous oxygen difference,[53, 54] whereas reduced muscle blood flow and a widened arteriovenous oxygen difference at low work loads [55] and

TABLE III

Basic Characteristics of Subjects

	Sedentary Normal (# = 45)	Trained After Infarction (# = 11)	Postoperative Bypass	
			Untrained (# = 17)	Trained (# = 4)
Age (yr)				
Mean ± 1 SD	50.0 ± 5.8	47.6 ± 8.0	50.6 ± 5.6	53.7 ± 8.2
Range	38.9-60.3	38.4-60.9	42.3-62.0	45.0-62.0
Height (cm)				
Mean ± 1 SD	178.9 ± 7.2	175.2 ± 4.8	174.7 ± 4.8	175.3 ± 3.5
Range	165.0-190.2	165.7-182.1	165.4-184.2	171.6-179.4
Weight (kg)				
Mean ± 1 SD	81.3 ± 11.4	74.9 ± 7.6	77.4 ± 9.5	71.4 ± 6.8
Range	63.9-103.4	62.8-85.5	64.0-94.6	64.0-78.4
BSA (m^2)				
Mean ± 1 SD	1.98 ± 0.2	1.89 ± 0.1	1.91 ± 0.1	1.85 ± 0.1
Range	1.70-2.28	1.67-2.03	1.75-2.18	1.75-1.94

increased muscle blood flow at heavier loads of submaximal work,[5] have been observed. The latter finding suggests that peripheral factors may also improve myocardial performance, as has recently been substantiated by Detry and Bruce,[51] who found no difference in the tension-time index, ST-segment depression relation at symptom-limited levels of maximal oxygen uptake after training.

Myocardial Infarction—Relatively few studies have been made of the effects of physical training on patients after myocardial infarction without significant concurrent angina. Early studies of such patients [40, 42-44, 47] demonstrated reduced heart rate, ST-segment depression and decreased indirect blood pressure and tension-time index at submaximal work loads. A variety of exercise programs, including walking, jogging, ergometer cycling and endurance calisthenics and games, involving sustained energy expenditures of up to 7 kcal/min (oxygen consumption 1.4 liters/min) for periods of 1 hour, 3 to 5 times a week, were utilized in these studies. Increased physical performance has also been demonstrated,[42, 43] as has increased maximal oxygen uptake.[41, 45]

Comparison of Submaximal and Maximal Cardiorespiratory Function of Patients After Myocardial Infarction and Coronary Bypass Grafting with that of Sedentary Normal Subjects—To safely test patients with various degrees of cardiac dysfunction, a slowly progressive multistage treadmill test that permits determination of maximal performance and attendant submaximal and maximal cardiorespiratory responses was developed. [56] The test is initiated at a speed of 50 meters/min, zero grade, and the work load increased every 3 minutes, first by increasing the speed 10 meters/min to a maximum of 80 meters/min, and then by increasing the inclination 2% to a maximum of 22% at 42 minutes. Exercise is continued to the point of maximal tolerable effort as defined by dyspnea, leg weakness or electrocardiographic contraindication. Heart rate is recorded periodically, whereas oxygen consumption and associated respiratory metabolism measures are derived by standard procedures from data collected by open circuit metabolism. [56]

A community search revealed 11 men who had trained for 6 months to 11 years after myocardial infarction. Ten were jogging 30 to 45 minutes, 3.5 times a week, and one patient swam 45 to 60 minutes, 5 times a week. Subsequently, 17 untrained men were studied 5 to 19 months after single or multiple aortocoronary bypass grafts. Thirteen had postoperative angiograms to confirm graft patency. One patient continued to have left ventricular failure with patent grafts, two patients had one of two grafts blocked, and one patient with residual angina had occlusion of his single anterior descending artery bypass. Forty-five sedentary normal men of similar ages (Table III) were used for comparative purposes. Student's t test was applied to determine if the mean differences between either of the two patient groups and the sedentary normal group were significant ($P = <0.05$). The comparisons of maximal performance and of submaximal and maximal cardiorespiratory function of the patient groups have inherent limitations and bias: (1) The subjects trained after infarction were not available for study before infarction or training; (2) Subjects trained after infarction and those who had undergone coronary artery bypass surgery are not strictly comparable because of differences in severity of disease and in training; and (3) Subjects trained after coronary artery bypass were not tested preoperatively since assessment of maximal tolerable effort did not seem justified before operation. Within these limitations, however, certain comparisons of the patient groups with the sedentary normal group are informative.

All subjects completed the first seven work loads (stages) encompassing 21 minutes, and only one subject who had undergone coronary artery bypass surgery failed to attempt stage 9 (80 m/min, 10% grade), which was accepted as the upper end of submaximal work. Graphic analysis of submaximal data in the three groups is shown in Figure 5 to 7. The close similarity in oxygen consumption values for all groups at submaximal work loads indicates that there was no significant difference in walking skill. Apparent differences between the patients trained after myocardial infarction and normal groups in heart rate, oxygen pulse, pulmonary ventilation and ventilatory equivalent were not statistically significant. On the other hand, differences in pulmonary ventilation and ventilatory equivalent between the normal group and patients who had undergone coronary artery bypass were significantly different over the whole range of submaximal work, while values for heart rate and oxygen pulse were significantly different after 15 minutes.

Mean values for walking time and selected cardiorespiratory responses at maximal tolerable effort for the three groups are summarized in Figure 8. The group values for patients trained after myocardial infarction were similar to those of normal subjects except for significantly lower heart rate and pulmonary

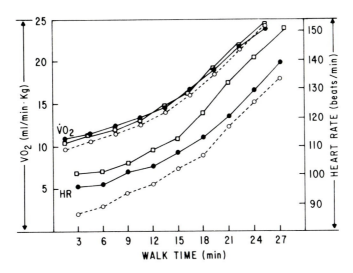

Figure 5. Heart rate (HR) and oxygen uptake ($\dot{V}O_2$) comparisons between a sedentary normal group and two groups with coronary artery disease at submaximal work loads. ● = sedentary normal; ○ = trained after infarction; □ = untrained after bypass surgery.

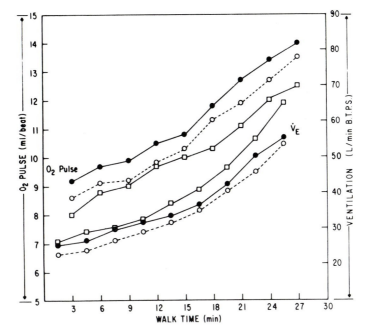

Figure 6. Oxygen pulse and pulmonary ventilation ($\dot{V}_E$) comparisons between a sedentary normal group and two groups with coronary artery disease at submaximal work loads. ● = sedentary normal; ○ = trained after infarction; □ = untrained after bypass surgery.

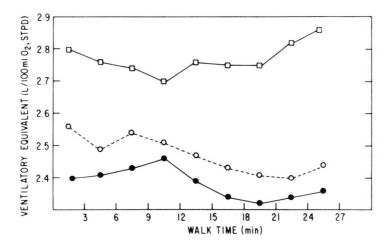

Figure 7. Ventilatory equivalent comparisons between a sedentary normal group and two groups with coronary artery disease at submaximal work loads. ● = sedentary normal; ○ = trained after infarction; □ = untrained after bypass surgery.

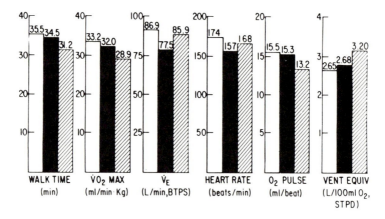

Figure 8. Comparisons of maximal performance data between a sedentary normal group and two groups with coronary artery disease. □ = sedentary normal; ■ = trained after infarction; ▨ = untrained after bypass surgery.

ventilation. In four subjects in the former group, maximal efforts should be considered symptom-limited; one patient had angina, one had leg cramps and two had marked ischemic ST-segment depressions and were stopped by the examiner before there was a clear tendency of the oxygen consumption to plateau. On the other hand, all of the coronary artery bypass patients walked to maximal effort, as evidenced by plateauing of oxygen consumption. Nevertheless, compared with the normal subjects, these patients had significantly

TABLE IV

Effect of Training 12 Weeks on Cardiorespiratory Function
in Four Coronary Artery Bypass Surgery Patients

Variable	Stage 1 (0-3:00) T_1	T_2	Stage 4 (9-12:00) T_1	T_2	Stage 7 (18-21:00) T_1	T_2	Stage 9 (24-27:00) T_1	T_2	Maximal Tolerable Effort T_1	T_2
Oxygen uptake (ml/min per kg)	8.0	8.9	13.7	13.8	19.2	19.5	24.1	25.2	28.6	31.7
Heart rate (beats/min)	88	87	97	101	122	126	144	150	160	170
Oxygen pulse (ml/beat)	6.5	6.9	10.4	9.2	11.5	10.3	12.1	11.2	12.7	12.5
Ventilation (liters/min, BTPS)	23.1	24.4	29.6	30.9	41.4	40.7	55.5	54.5	73.5	75.7
Ventilatory equivalent ($L\dot{V}_E/100$ ml $\dot{V}O_2$, STPD)	3.29	3.39	2.54	2.80	2.54	2.67	2.69	2.69	3.03	3.15

T_1 and T_2 indicate, respectively, test results before and after training

shorter walking time, lower maximal oxygen uptake, heart rate and oxygen pulse, and a higher ventilatory equivalent. Electrocardiographic evidence of myocardial ischemia increased with effort in five patients, four of whom had patent grafts as assessed by angiography. Seven had no change in resting ischemic electrocardiographic changes with effort; the remaining five exercised to maximal level with normal tracings.

Cardiorespiratory Adaptation to Training After Coronary Artery Bypass— Four of the subjects studied after coronary artery bypass surgery consented to enter a quantitative reconditioning protocol, training at least 3 days a week, 40 minutes a day for 12 weeks by walking and jogging at an intensity necessitating a heart rate of 75 to 85% of maximum. Data after training (Table IV) indicate no appreciable change in oxygen consumption in submaximal work, but heart rate in the later work stages increased 4 to 6 beats/min. As a result, the oxygen pulse after training was somewhat lower. Submaximal pulmonary ventilation was essentially the same after training, whereas the response to training of ventilatory equivalent was variable. Clearly, there were no classic training effects at submaximal work of the type seen in normal subjects [27] and patients after myocardial infarction.[44, 45, 54] Data at maximal work loads reveal higher heart rate and maximal oxygen uptake, but little change in oxygen pulse, pulmonary ventilation and ventilatory equivalent.

Significance of Cardiorespiratory Training Responses in Coronary Artery Disease— The group trained after myocardial infarction evidenced no atypical phys-

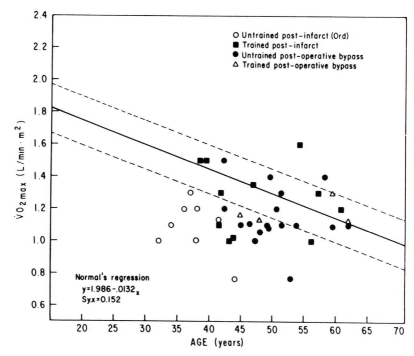

Figure 9. Individual values for untrained and trained subjects after myocardial infarction and coronary artery bypass. The solid line indicates the regression line for a sedentary normal group; the dashed lines represent 1 standard deviation above and below the regression line of the normal subjects.

iologic strain in providing submaximal energy requirements. Conversely, however, patients studied after coronary artery bypass did, as denoted by increased pulmonary ventilation, ventilatory equivalent and heart rate, and lower oxygen pulse. Furthermore, no significant changes in submaximal work responses occurred in the four subjects who underwent coronary artery bypass surgery and trained for 12 weeks. A substantially higher heart rate at submaximal work loads than that of sedentary normal subjects is characteristic of untrained patients after myocardial infarction,[49, 57, 58] whereas a reduced heart rate and decreased pulmonary ventilation at submaximal work loads have been observed in patients trained after myocardial infarction.[40, 45, 53-55] Hence, even though the submaximal heart rate of the subjects trained after infarction was not significantly lower than that of the normal group, it should not be assumed that there was no training effect in these patients. Further evidence supporting this contention is afforded in Figure 9. The bold line represents the regression line of maximal oxygen uptake (liters/min per m²) with age; the dashed lines represent ±1 standard deviation for 80 sedentary normal men aged 31 to 69 years [56]; the open circles indicate maximal oxygen uptake values from treadmill studies of untrained

TABLE V

Comparison of Maximal Oxygen Consumption in Untrained
and Trained Postmyocardial Infarction Patients

Study	# Subjects	Untrained	Trained	Training Duration	Training Time/ Week (min)
Ord [59]	8	27.4*	—	—	—
Kasch & Boyer [41]	11	19.9	30.6	6 months	210
Kasser & Bruce [49]	28	26.5†	—	—	—
Detry et al [45]	6	27.3	32.2	3 months	135
Present study					
Trained after infarction	11	—	32.0	6 months to 11 years	160
Untrained after CAB	17	28.6	—	—	—
Trained after CAB	4	28.6	31.7	12 weeks	120

CAB = coronary artery bypass surgery
*Assuming body surface area of 1.90 m^2 and body weight of 75 kg
†Calculated from formula for estimating maximal oxygen consumption from treadmill walking time,
assuming body weight of 75 kg

patients studied after myocardial infarction by Ord.[59] As can be seen, none of the values for these subjects fall within 1 standard deviation of the normal subjects' age-related regression line. On the other hand, the maximal oxygen uptake values of six of our subjects trained after myocardial infarction are above the line, and that of a seventh patient falls within 1 standard deviation. However, four values are significantly below the line (more than 1 standard deviation), thus emphasizing the individual variability of maximal exercise response in patients after myocardial infarction noted by others.[41, 47] The comparisons of group mean values for maximal oxygen consumption in Table V lend further credence to the assumption that a significant training effect had occurred in our subjects trained after myocardial infarction.

Of the 17 patients not trained after coronary artery bypass surgery, the values of nine were significantly below normal (more than 1 standard deviation) (Figure 9). Their heart rate and pulmonary ventilation were normal, but maximal oxygen pulse was significantly decreased, which is indicative of reduced stroke volume or arteriovenous oxygen difference, or both. Their ventilatory equivalent, which reflects the amount of ventilated air necessary for utilization of 100 ml of oxygen, was significantly greater. In view of the normal ventilatory capacity evidenced, increased ventilatory equivalent could be a reflection of decreased diffusing capacity in the lungs, but more likely is a secondary indication of reduced stroke volume or decreased capacity for oxygen utilization at the muscle cell level, or both. The maximal oxygen uptake of the subjects studied after coronary artery bypass was intermediate to that recorded in previous studies for untrained and trained patients after myocardial infarction (Table V). The four subjects who trained for 12 weeks sustained a 10.8% increase in maximal oxygen uptake to a value comparable with that of subjects trained after myocardial infarction. In addition, their walking time increased, as did their maximal heart rate (by 10 beats/min). Since oxygen pulse, pulmonary ventilation and ventilatory equivalent changed little, the primary mechanism for enhanced oxygen delivery at maximal effort appears to be an increased heart rate, which is uncharacteristic of trained normal subjects but has been noted previously in other subjects after myocardial infarction.[41, 45]

The primary distinction between the exercise response of our two patient groups is that the subjects trained after myocardial infarction evidenced no differences from normal subjects at submaximal work loads and had only slight evidence of reduced maximal energy production, whereas the untrained subjects who had undergone coronary artery bypass surgery demonstrated impaired performance at both submaximal and maximal work loads, as has also been noted in other untrained patients after myocardial infarction.[49] Although the four subjects trained after coronary artery bypass surgery had increased maximal energy production, they had no significant change in their atypical submaximal cardiorespiratory responses. The physiologic mechanisms for these findings are not readily discernible without appropriate hemodynamic measurements.

Conclusions

Our data indicate the following: (1) Most subjects trained after myocardial infarction can achieve the performance levels of normal, sedentary subjects, but some do not exhibit a classic training effect, probably because of residual myocardial dysfunction. (2) Successful coronary artery bypass surgery does not entirely normalize work performance, metabolic or hemodynamic function, although angina and electrocardiographic changes can be reduced. (3) Work performance and aerobic power of patients after coronary artery bypass can be further improved by physical training, although the physiologic mechanism for these changes is not readily apparent.

Physical training improves cardiorespiratory function, which may be indicative of improved myocardial function, and aids in reducing coronary artery disease risk factors.[4, 26] However, because of the relatively small number of patients studied longitudinally and the complex etiology of coronary artery disease, no conclusive evidence of less frequent recurrence rates or greater longevity has been demonstrated, although the recent report of Rechnitzer et al [60] indicates some encouraging initial findings.

Summary

Exercise training principles, including overload, individual differences and transiency, are discussed and examples of each presented. Disadvantages of the cross-sectional method, and values of the longitudinal method of ascertaining physical training effects are discussed. The effects of endurance-oriented exercise programs on middle-aged sedentary normal men and patients with coronary artery disease, emphasizing body composition and cardiorespiratory function and basic hemodynamic response to submaximal and maximal exercise, are reviewed. An original study of the effects of endurance-oriented training on patients after myocardial infarction and coronary artery bypass is presented. Emphasis is placed on cardiorespiratory function at submaximal and maximal exercise loads, and the patients' response is contrasted to that of a group of sedentary normal subjects of similar age.

It is concluded that most trained post-infarction patients can achieve the performance levels of sedentary normal subjects, but that their response to training is often restricted, presumably because residual disease effects myocardial dysfunction. Successful coronary artery bypass surgery seldom normalizes work performance and cardiorespiratory function, although it may ameliorate symptoms. However, physical training, in conjunction with bypass surgery, effects a further improvement in work performance and aerobic power.

This study was supported in part by the University of California Faculty Research Grant D-239, a grant from the Sacramento-Yolo-Sierra Heart Association, and U.S. Air Force Grants AFOSR-69-1659 and F 44620-72-C-0011.

References

1. Steinhaus AH: Chronic effects of exercise. *Physiol Rev* 13:103-147, 1933.
2. Åstrand P-O, Rodahl K: *Textbook of Work Physiology*, pp 373-430, New York: McGraw-Hill, 1970.
3. Tanner JM: *The Physique of the Olympic Athlete*, pp 111-113, London: Allen & Unwin, 1964.
4. Fox SM III, Haskell WL: Physical activity and the prevention of coronary heart disease. *Bull NY Acad Med* 44:950-967, 1968.
5. Clausen JP, Trap-Jensen J: Effects of training on the distribution of cardiac output in patients with coronary artery disease. *Circulation* 42:611-624, 1970.
6. Holmer I, Åstrand P-O: Swimming training and maximal oxygen uptake. *J Appl Physiol* 33:510-513, 1972.
7. Faulkner JA: New perspectives in training for maximum performance. *JAMA* 205:741-746, 1968.
8. Brouha L: "Training," in Johnson WR (Ed): *Science and Medicine of Exercise and Sports*, pp 403-416, New York: Harper, 1960.
9. Karvonen MJ: Problems of training of the cardiovascular system. *Ergonomics* 2:207-215, 1959.
10. Siegel W, Blomquist G, Mitchell JH: Effects of a quantitated physical training program on middle-aged sedentary man. *Circulation* 41:19-29, 1970.
11. Saltin B: Physiological effects of physical conditioning. *Med Sci Sports* 1:50-56, 1969.
12. Saltin B, Blomquist G, Mitchell JH, et al: Response to exercise after bed rest and training. *Circulation* 38 (suppl 7):1-78, 1968.
13. Katila M, Frick MH: A two-year circulatory follow-up of physical training after myocardial infarction. *Acta Med Scand* 187:95-100, 1970.
14. Adams WC: The effects of a season of training on selected anthropometric measures and maximum oxygen uptake of college cross-country runners. Unpublished data, April 1968.
15. Forbes GB: Nutritional implications of the whole body counter. *Nutr Rev* 21:321-324, 1963.
16. Margaria R, Cerretelli P, Aghemo P, et al: Energy cost of running. *J Appl Physiol* 18:367-370, 1963.
17. Pollock ML, Miller HS Jr, Janeway R, et al: Effects of walking on body composition and cardiovas-

cular function of middle-aged men. *J Appl Physiol* 30:126-130, 1971.

18. Pollock ML, Broida J, Kendrick Z, et al: Effects of training two days per week at different intensities on middle-aged men. *Med Sci Sports* 4:192-197, 1972.

19. Carter JEL, Phillips WH: Structural changes in exercising middle-aged males during a 2-year period. *J Appl Physiol* 27:787-794, 1969.

20. Mitchell JH, Sproule BJ, Chapman CB: The physiological meaning of the maximum oxygen intake test. *J Clin Invest* 37:538-547, 1958.

21. Robinson S: Experimental studies of physical fitness in relation to age. *Arbeitsphysiol* 10:251-323, 1938.

22. Saltin B, Åstrand P-O: Maximal oxygen uptake in athletes. *J Appl Physiol* 23:353-358, 1967.

23. Tzankoff SP, Robinson S, Pyke FS, et al: Physiological adjustments to work in older men as effected by physical training. *J Appl Physiol* 33:346-350, 1972.

24. Naughton J, Nagle F: Peak oxygen intake during physical fitness program for middle-aged men. *JAMA* 191:899-901, 1965.

25. Mann GV, Garrett HL, Farhi A, et al: Exercise to prevent coronary heart disease. An experimental study of the effects of training on risk factors for coronary disease in men. *Amer J Med* 46:12-27, 1969.

26. Hanson JS, Tabakin BS, Levy AM, et al: Long-term physical training and cardiovascular dynamics in middle-aged men. *Circulation* 38:783-799, 1968.

27. Saltin B, Hartley L, Kilbom A, et al: Physical training in sedentary middle-aged and older men. II: Oxygen uptake, heart rate, and blood lactate concentration at submaximal and maximal exercise. *Scand J Clin Lab Invest* 24:323-334, 1969.

28. Oscai LB, Williams BT, Hertig BA: Effects of exercise on blood volume. *J Appl Physiol* 24:622-624, 1968.

29. Ribisl PM: Effects of training upon the maximal oxygen uptake of middle-aged men. *Int Z Angew Physiol* 27:154-160, 1969.

30. Wilmore JH, Royce J, Girandola R, et al: Physiological alterations resulting from a 10-week program of jogging. *Med Sci Sports* 2:7-14, 1970.

31. Grimby G, Saltin B: Physiological effects of physical training. *Scand J Rehab Med* 3:6-14, 1971.

32. Holloszy JO: Biochemical adaptations in muscle. Effects of exercise on mitochondrial oxygen uptake and respiratory enzyme activity in skeletal muscle. *J Biol Chem* 242:2278-2282, 1967.

33. Kiessling K-H, Piehl K, Lundquist C-G: "Number and Size of Skeletal Muscle Mitochondria in Trained Sedentary Men," in Larsen OA, Malmborg RO (Eds): *Coronary Heart Disease and Physical Fitness*, pp 143-146, Baltimore: University Park Press, 1971.

34. Varnauskas E, Björntorp P, Fahlën M, et al: Effects of physical training on exercise blood flow and enzymatic activity in skeletal muscle. *Cardiovasc Res* 4:418-422, 1970.

35. Hartley LH, Grimby G, Kilbom A, et al: Physical training in sedentary middle-aged and older men. III: Cardiac output and gas exchange at submaximal and maximal exercise. *Scand J Clin Lab Invest* 24:335-344, 1969.

36. Ekblom B, Åstrand P-O, Saltin B, et al: Effect of training on circulatory response to exercise. *J Appl Physiol* 24:518-528, 1968.

37. Rowell LB: Factors Affecting the Prediction of the Maximal Oxygen Intake from Measurements Made During Submaximal Work. Doctoral dissertation, University of Minnesota, 1962.

38. Grimby G, Nilsson NJ, Saltin B: Cardiac output during submaximal and maximal exercise in active middle-aged athletes. *J Appl Physiol* 21:1150-1156, 1966.

39. Mazzarella JA, Jordan JW Jr: Effects of physical training on exertional myocardial ischemia in middle-aged men (abstract). *Circulation* 31 (suppl 2):147-148, 1965.

40. Hellerstein HK, Hornsten TR: "Reconditioning of the Coronary Patient: a Preliminary Report," in Likoff W, Moyer JH (Eds): *Coronary Heart Disease*, pp 448-454, New York: Grune & Stratton, 1963.

41. Kasch FW, Boyer JL: Changes in maximum work capacity resulting from six months training in patients with ischemic heart disease. *Med Sci Sports* 1:156-159, 1969.

42. Skinner JS, Holloszy JO, Cureton TK: Effects of a program of endurance exercises on physical work capacity and anthropometric measurements of fifteen middle-aged men. *Amer J Cardiol* 14:747-752, 1964.

43. Rechnitzer PA, Yuhasz MS, Pickard HA, et al: The effects of a graduated exercise program on patients with previous myocardial infarction. *Canad Med Ass J* 92:858-860, 1965.

44. Naughton J, Shanbour K, Armstrong R, et al: Cardiovascular responses to exercise following

myocardial infarction. *Arch Intern Med* 117:541-545, 1966.

45. Detry J-MR, Rousseau M, Vandenbroucke G, et al: Increased arteriovenous oxygen difference after physical training in coronary heart disease. *Circulation* 44:109-118, 1971.

46. Frick MH: The effect of physical training in manifest ischemic heart disease. *Circulation* 40:433-435, 1969.

47. Barry AJ, Daly JW, Pruett EDR, et al: Effects of physical training in patients who have had myocardial infarction. *Amer J Cardiol* 17:1-8, 1966.

48. MacAlpin RN, Kattus AA: Adaptation to exercise in angina pectoris. The electrocardiogram during treadmill walking and coronary angiographic findings. *Circulation* 33:183-201, 1966.

49. Kasser, IS, Bruce RA: Comparative effects of aging and coronary artery disease on submaximal and maximal exercise. *Circulation* 39:759-774, 1969.

50. Detry J-MR, Bruce RA: Effects of nitroglycerin on "maximal" oxygen intake and exercise electrocardiogram in coronary heart disease. *Circulation* 43:155-163, 1971.

51. Detry J-MR, Bruce RA: Effects of physical training on exertional S-T segment depression in coronary heart disease. *Circulation* 44:390-396, 1971.

52. Redwood DR, Rosing DR, Epstein SE: Circulatory and symptomatic effects of physical training in patients with coronary-artery disease and angina pectoris. *New Eng J Med* 286:959-965, 1972.

53. Frick MH, Katila M: Hemodynamic consequences of physical training after myocardial infarction. *Circulation* 37:192-202, 1968.

54. Clausen JP, Larsen OA, Trap-Jensen J: Physical training in the management of coronary artery disease. *Circulation* 40:143-154, 1969.

55. Varnauskas E, Bergman H, Houk P, et al: Haemodynamic effects of physical training in coronary patients. *Lancet* II:8-12, 1966.

56. Adams WC, McHenry MM, Bernauer EM: Multistage treadmill walking performance and associated cardiorespiratory responses of middle-aged men. *Clin Sci* 42:355-370, 1972.

57. Malmborg RO: A clinical and hemodynamic analysis of factors limiting the cardiac performance in patients with coronary heart disease. *Acta Med Scand* 177 (suppl 426):1-94, 1964.

58. Malmcrona R, Cramer G, Varnauskas E: Haemodynamic data during rest and exercise for patients who have or have not been able to retain their occupation after myocardial infarction. *Acta Med Scand* 174:557-572, 1963.

59. Ord JW: The evaluation of cardiac reserve in normal subjects and patients with heart disease by the maximal oxygen intake test. unpublished data, 1961.

60. Rechnitzer PA, Pickard HA, Palvio AU, et al: Long-term follow-up study of survival and recurrence rates following myocardial infarction in exercising and control subjects. *Circulation* 45:853-857, 1972.

25

Physical Activity Following Myocardial Infarction

William L. Haskell, PhD

Although definitive evidence is not yet available to determine if physical activity performed after myocardial infarction has a unique influence on subsequent cardiovascular morbidity or mortality, numerous studies have yielded favorable preliminary or short-term results. Selected patients after acute myocardial infarction have benefited from "appropriate increases in physical activity"; they have had fewer complications associated with bed rest,[1] made a more successful psychological adjustment to their disease,[2] shown improved cardiovascular function and physical working capacity,[3] returned to gainful employment earlier and more frequently,[4] and had fewer and less severe reinfarctions.[5]

Although additional research is required to more accurately determine the benefits derived by cardiac patients from increased activity and to define how these benefits can be achieved most economically, sufficient data and experience are available to provide useful guidelines for the organization and implementation of the physical activity aspect of a cardiac rehabilitation program.[6] Recommendations for integrating increased physical activity into a total program of cardiac rehabilitation have been described previously and should include, when necessary: medical therapy, health education, diet modification, reduction of mental stress or tension, abatement of cigarette smoking and psychological, social and vocational counseling.

The physical activity component of a comprehensive rehabilitation program should be implemented to meet the patient's specific needs during each stage of recovery. For the patient with uncomplicated myocardial infarction who has been admitted to the coronary care unit, a physical activity program can be organized into five rather arbitrary stages: coronary care unit, remainder of hospital stay, a 2 to 8-week period of posthospital convalescence, physical reconditioning and physical activity maintenance.

The activity at each stage of recovery should be systematically prescribed by a knowledgeable physician after a careful evaluation, and it should be supervised or monitored by a physician or other well-trained allied health personnel. The exact nature of the evaluation, supervision and monitoring will depend upon the patient's clinical and functional status. As recovery progresses, the specific activities performed and the immediate objectives of the exercise plan will change, but the general principles of clinical and functional evaluation, exercise prescription and reconditioning will remain the same.[7]

Coronary Care Unit Activity Program

The primary purposes of early performance of physical activity in the coronary care unit are to counter the potentially harmful deconditioning effects of prolonged bed rest and to minimize the psychological trauma of coping with the realities of surviving a myocardial infarction. In many cases the patient is unable to distinguish between a nonspecific consequence of extended inactivity and the debility directly produced by cardiovascular limitations resulting from the infarction. Conditions caused or aggravated by bed rest and alleviated to some extent by changes in posture and activity include decreased cardiovascular function manifested by orthostatic hypotension, venous thrombosis, reduced lung volume, atelectasis and reduced skeletal muscle tone and joint flexibility.[8]

Potential Hazards of Activity Early After Infarction—The major hazards of inappropriate exertion soon after acute myocardial infarction are considered to be the precipitation or aggravation of serious arrhythmias, congestive heart failure, aneurysm formation and cardiac rupture. However, only the hazard of an increase in premature ventricular beats during exercise by patients with coronary heart disease has been firmly documented.[9-11] There is conflicting evidence on the potential dangers of cardiac rupture or aneurysm formation with exertion immediately after infarction. The report of Jetter and White [12] that cardiac rupture occurred in 73% of severely psychotic patients who probably remained active during an acute myocardial infarction and died is not confirmed by recent studies of cardiac rupture occurring during sudden death in non-institutionalized adults.[13, 14] However, since in man most of the necrotic tissue resulting from the infarction is not replaced by connective tissue for about 2 weeks and complete healing requires 4 to 8 weeks,[15, 16] major increases in heart rate or blood pressure should probably be avoided for at least several weeks.

In animals, the effect of vigorous exercise soon after artificially induced myocardial infarction appears to be quite benign. Thomas and Harrison [17] found that after experimentally induced acute myocardial damage in rats, severe restriction of activity increased mortality, whereas enforced vigorous exercise had no detrimental effect. Kaplinsky et al [18] and Thompson et al [19] were not able to reproduce the earlier findings of Sutton and Davis [20] of an increase in aneurysm formation when dogs were exercised beginning 3 days after coronary artery ligation.

Kaplinsky et al [18] exercised dogs vigorously 1 hour daily for 5 weeks starting 3 days after acute myocardial infarction produced by coronary artery ligation; these animals had no increase in size of infarction, frequency or size of aneurysms, or instances of cardiac rupture or sudden death when compared to a nonexercised control group. Similar results were obtained by Thompson et al [19] when dogs were exercised vigorously (peak heart rates exceeding 220 beats/min) within 1 hour of total occlusion of the left anterior descending coronary artery. The results of such animal studies need to be considered with caution since they are not likely to be applicable to patients in a coronary care unit. Healthy dogs with a single artificially induced coronary occlusion without previous myocardial damage probably do not provide an acceptable model for the extrapolation of results to the diseased human heart with diffuse coronary atherosclerosis and previous myocardial necrosis.

The clinical rationale for early sitting and physical activity of patients after myocardial infarction was presented in 1940 by Levine [21] and in 1944 by Dock [22] and Harrison.[23] They cautioned against unnecessary bed rest and promoted the idea of frequent postural changes for the patient and early participation in self-care activities. Their primary concerns were the complications of phlebothrombosis, embolization and congestive heart failure associated with extended bed rest and the development of "cardiac neurotics" as a result of unnecessary and prolonged restriction. In the 1950's the concept of the "armchair" treatment was promoted by Levine.[24]

Levine and Lown [25] demonstrated that cardiac output was reduced by 23% when patients with a recent myocardial infarction changed from a supine position to sitting in a chair. Coe [26] found the mean cardiac work in such patients to be 23% less while sitting than while reclining. More recently, DeBusk et al [27] demonstrated that changes in posture or selected passive and active exercises can be performed by patients in the coronary care unit without significant increases in work of the heart (blood pressure–pulse rate product) or ventricular arrhythmias. Fareeduddin and Abelmann [28] concluded that the impaired orthostatic tolerance produced by complete bed rest in many patients after infarction is preventable or reversible by early ambulation or modified bed rest allowing passive movements and occasional sitting.

Activity Program in the Coronary Care Unit—For the patient with an uncomplicated myocardial infarction (no evidence of shock, heart failure, intractable angina or uncontrolled arrhythmia) low level passive and active isotonic or dynamic activities can normally be initiated in the coronary care unit. These activities should be carried out under the direction of the patient's physician or the medical director of the coronary care unit, or both. Acceptable activities and techniques for their instruction and supervision have been described in detail.[6, 27, 29, 30] Usually included at this time are self-care activities (self-feeding, washing of face and hands, shaving, use of bedside commode with assistance), active and passive movements of arms and legs while in bed and changes in posture to include sitting on the side of bed with feet supported or in a chair. All of these activities should be supervised by a well trained nurse or therapist with continuous electrocardiographic monitoring and periodic evaluations of blood pressure and symptoms.

Indications of an inappropriate increase in exertion during the coronary care unit activity phase include: unexpected fatigue; weakness or dyspnea; development of or increase in angina; significant rhythm or conduction disturbances; increased ischemic-type ST-segment displacement; increase in heart rate by more than 20 beats/min over the resting rate or a decrease by more than 10 beats; and a persistent decrease or substantial increase in systolic blood pressure (>40 mm Hg). If any of these responses occur during activity, bed rest should be resumed until the patient's status is evaluated and a revised activity plan developed.

Activity During Remainder of Hospital Stay

Upon transfer from the coronary care unit and in the absence of cardiovascular complications, the patient should continue a planned program of individually prescribed activity. The major objectives of physical activity during this stage are to continue to prevent the harmful physiologic and psychological effects of prolonged bed rest, reduce the duration of hospitalization and increase cardiovascular functional capacity to a level that will allow a reasonable degree of self-care after discharge and a more rapid return to work.

Mobilization of patients after discharge from the coronary care unit and the effects of a shortened hospital stay have been evaluated by several groups.[31-33] In general these studies have demonstrated that there are no adverse clinical effects from early mobilization in selected patients after myocardial infarction and that there may be some benefit by the reduction of physiologic and psychological complications and an earlier or more frequent return to work. Rose [34] has reviewed the rationale for and success rate of early mobilization and discharge after myocardial infarction.

Activity Program—Appropriate activities during this phase of recovery include longer periods of sitting in a chair; increased self-care activities; rhythmic exercises using arms, legs and trunk; and slow ambulation in the hospital room and later in the corridors. For patients who progress rapidly, limited stair climbing might be permitted during the latter portion of this phase.[35]

Increases in exertion should be performed by the patient at least several times a day unless contraindicated by signs or symptoms. Each activity session should have alternating periods of exercise and rest. These sessions should not be conducted immediately after meals and can be supplemented by calisthenics performed while in bed. Unnecessary isometric exercises, particularly in conjunction with a Valsalva maneuver, should be avoided. During and after each new activity the patient should be evaluated for changes in electrocardiogram, blood pressure and heart sounds.

During the latter stages of hospitalization, instructions should be provided to the patient and his family about particular activities to be performed or avoided after leaving the hospital. Topics that need to be covered include sexual activity, use of stairs, lifting and carrying of relatively heavy objects and activities in hot, cold or humid environments.

Testing of Functional Capacity—One means of improving the appropriateness of the recommendations on physical activity to the patient going home is to carefully evaluate his symptom-free functional capacity while he is still in the hospital. This can be achieved by monitoring the electrocardiogram, heart sounds, blood pressure and symptoms during ambulation in the corridor or during stair climbing. Low-level multistage exercise testing using either a stationary bicycle ergometer or treadmill as soon as 3 weeks after infarction has been demonstrated to be safe and can provide useful prognostic information as well as objective criteria for exercise prescription.[36]

Activity Program During Convalescence

After a patient has been discharged from the hospital following a myocardial infarction, one of his major concerns will be what he can or should do physically. He will have numerous questions regarding his job-related work and leisure time activities. He may want to know whether or not he should undertake an exercise program to help prevent new clinical manifestations, develop his cardiovascular capacity, lose weight or regain muscle strength. To tell him to just take it easy or to exercise moderately is no longer adequate advice. He needs specific information about activities he can perform relatively safely, instructions on how to perform these activities and advice about activities he should avoid. Each patient should be provided with a concise individualized exercise recommendation or prescription tailored to fit his functional capacity, needs and interests. His skill and experience at various physical activities need to be considered as well as accessibility of appropriate exercise equipment, facilities or programs. Within the limitations of current knowledge, an exercise recommendation for the cardiac patient should be developed with the same care and precision used in prescribing other therapies. An overdose of exercise can produce new clinical manifestations of coronary artery disease including cardiac arrest and sudden death while inappropriate restrictions can result in cardiovascular deconditioning, psychological trauma and economic disability.

The primary goals of an activity regimen during this phase of recovery are to gradually increase the frequency, duration and intensity of activity so that by the 8th to the 12th week after infarction the patient with an uncomplicated infarction has achieved a level of exertion commensurate with that required by the job to which he is scheduled to return, and to provide psychological support to the patient and family for the prospect of successful long-term recovery. If return to work is not a consideration or if the job requires a peak energy expenditure greater than 8 to 10 MET's (multiples of resting oxygen consumption), the activity level during this time should reach that necessary for complete self-care and the safe performance of selected leisure time activities, including sexual activity.

An objective evaluation of the effects of increased activity between the 4th and 12th weeks after infarction has been reported by Brock.[37] As a result of an 8-week exercise program (1 hour, three times a week) his patients had a small reduction in pulse rate at the same work load and a large (60 to 70%) increase in physical working capacity and peak oxygen consumption. The increases in working capacity and oxygen consumption are difficult to interpret because of a change in the criteria for terminating the exercise test from a pulse rate of 65% of the age-adjusted maximum before training to a pulse rate of 75 to 80% after training. How much of the improvement in physical working capacity during convalescence is due to the natural recovery from the infarction and bed rest and how much is due to the conditioning program has not been established.

Activity Program—Most usual light household and self-care activities can be permitted except floor scrubbing, hand washing and hanging of clothes, bed making and similar activities requiring prolonged or vigorous effort with the arms and shoulders. Again, isometric exercises using the arms, such as those required in carrying heavy objects like a suitcase, need to be avoided. Jackson et al [38] have demonstrated that this type of activity can create a disproportionate workload on the myocardium in relation to total body energy expenditure.

The patient who remains asymptomatic should gradually increase his level of activity at his own pace so that by the end of the 4th or 5th week after infarction he can walk a total of 1/2 to 1 mile a day comfortably. These walks should be divided into two or three periods of approximately equal duration. The program should remain within each patient's capabilities and he should remain symptom-free.

Before increasing the pace and distance of exercise further in the 6th through 8th weeks after infarction, the patient should be carefully re-evaluated by his physician. This assessment should include a medical history, with careful questioning about the level of daily activity the patient has reached and his symptomatic response to this activity, physical examination and appropriate laboratory tests including a resting electrocardiogram.

Functional Assessment—Cardiac function should be assessed by a multi-stage exercise test in which the highest workload performed is greater than that of the activities performed by the patient during the previous week, such as walking half a mile or stair climbing. The response to this effort test can serve as a valuable guide to the physician in regulating the patient's future activities. Adverse responses to the exercise test, which indicate a need to decrease rather than increase activities, include a disproportionately rapid and large rise in heart rate or blood pressure, a sustained reduction in systolic blood pressure of more than 10 mm Hg, significant changes in the electrocardiogram, increasing angina or a decrease in working capacity.

TABLE I

Peak Heart Rate and $\dot{V}O_2$ Responses to Exercise Testing
3 to 12 Weeks Following Myocardial Infarction (Mean Values)

Study	#	Age (yrs)	Duration* (weeks)	Heart Rate (beats/min)	$\dot{V}O_2$ or Work (ml/kg/min)	Test Protocol
Ericsson†[36]	100	< 65	3	118	100–600 kgm/min	TM
Atterhog [41]	12	58	3	124	370 kgm/min	Bicycle to HR 120–130
Styperek [42]	209	—	3	129	300–900 kgm/min	Clinical max
Hakkila [43]	74	< 65	3½	—	470 kgm/min	Max or HR 150
Brock [37]	64	54	4	102	13.0	TM to 65% max HR
Kentala [73]	144	53	6–8	128	484 kgm/min	Max or HR 150
Rousseau [44]	14	48	8	169	26.4	Max bicycle
Rousseau [45]	33	49	8	153	21.1	Max bicycle
Torkelson [46]	14	51	9	127		TM at 1.7 mph + 10%
Sanne [39, 40]	200	54	11–17	149	21.3	Max bicycle
Brock [37]	64	52	12	122	22.0	TM to 75–80% max HR
Benestad [47]	16	52	12	163	26.8	Max bicycle
Bergstrom [48]	52	54	12	—	625 kgm/min	Max bicycle

*Average duration since myocardial infarction
†Workload calculated in kgm/min = Sine $\alpha \times 60 \times$ a $\times$ b: when α = angle of inclination of treadmill in degrees; a = treadmill speed in m/sec; b = body weight in kg
HR = heart rate
TM = treadmill

Limited data are available regarding the objective assessment of functional capacity of patients prior to 12 to 16 weeks following infarction. In particular, there is limited serial data documenting the natural history of functional capacity during this period. Table I summarizes much of the literature available on exercise test response during early convalescence in postinfarction patients. From this data it appears that uncomplicated postinfarction patients have a functional capacity equivalent to 4 to 7 times resting energy requirement (MET's) during this time. The reasonably wide range of functional capacity is probably due to variations in patient age, preinfarction activity habits, severity of infarction and postinfarction activity status. Also, comparison of data from the various studies is difficult due to use of varying patient selection criteria, test protocols and criteria for terminating the tests. Of the reports listed in Table I, all but four utilized maximal or symptom-limited tests, while in the remaining studies effort was discontinued at an arbitrary heart rate or work load.

The patient with an improved exercise test response should be advised to increase the duration and speed of walking during the next several weeks in order to increase his endurance and strength in preparation for his return to work. In general, in the patient who has shown no adverse response to the preceding carefully monitored graduated activity program, a reasonable goal is to obtain a capacity for walking a mile in 20 to 25 minutes at least once a day, with a peak level of energy expenditure not exceeding 4 to 5 MET's. The principles of exercise prescription for coronary heart disease patients have been presented in detail by Hellerstein et al.[49]

Physical Reconditioning

Many patients without clinical complications 8 to 24 weeks after infarction become candidates for a program of higher intensity physical activity. The major objectives of such a physical conditioning program are to improve physical working capacity, decrease symptoms and signs of ischemic heart disease at rest and during exertion, increase speed and frequency of return to gainful employment, and reduce the chances of reinfarction or sudden death. Whether or not these changes take place appears to be dependent upon a combination of hemodynamic, metabolic and psychological alterations.

Hemodynamic and Metabolic Changes

In many respects the hemodynamic and metabolic changes that occur in cardiac patients with conditioning are quite similar to the changes seen in their age-matched asymptomatic, sedentary counterparts except that the magnitude of change is usually less and the interindividual variability is substantially greater for the former.[3] Some factors contributing to this variation in conditioning response include age, degree of myocardial necrosis and ischemia, interval after infarction, cardiovascular functional capacity at the start of training and the magnitude of the conditioning stimulus (intensity, duration and frequency). Also, the load (resting, submaximal or maximal) and body position (lying, sitting or standing) at which hemodynamic measurements are determined influence the nature and magnitude of measurable changes.

Improvement produced by physical conditioning in the working capacity and clinical manifestation of many patients after infarction results from a reduction in the discrepancy between myocardial oxygen supply and demand primarily due to a decrease in demand. A reduced myocardial oxygen demand at rest and submaximal exercise is reflected by a significant reduction in such indices of myocardial oxygen requirement as pressure-rate or double product,[50, 51] tension-time index [52, 53] and the triple product [54] (heart rate [beats/min] × systolic arterial pressure [mm Hg] × ejection time [seconds]) (Table II). The major change contributing to the lowering of these indices is bradycardia with a small decrease usually occurring in systemic arterial pressure.[55] The bradycardia is usually associated with a small increase in both stroke volume and arteriovenous oxygen (a-v O_2) difference [56] resulting from increases in skeletal muscle mitochondria size and number with augmented levels of activity by the mitochondrial respiratory enzymes.[57]

Increases in physical working capacity and aerobic capacity in patients not

TABLE II

Indices of Myocardial Oxygen Demand Before and After
Physical Conditioning by Male Coronary Heart Disease Patients

Study	#	Age (yrs)	Index	Rest Before	Rest After	Exercise Before	Exercise After	Exercise Intensity
Redwood et al [54]	7	48	Triple product	—	—	4300	3521	Same submaximal workload
						4300	4885	At onset of angina
Frick and Katila [52]	7	47	Tension-time index	2519	2941	5168	4382	Same submaximal workload
			Double product	103	107	262	242	Same submaximal workload
Clausen et al [53]	9	52	Tension-time index	2470	2380	3943	3393	Same submaximal workload
			Double product	—	—	204	166	Same submaximal workload
Hellerstein [51]	100	49	Double product	—	—	248	193	Same submaximal workload
Detry et al [50]	12	49	Double product	81	64	116	94	45% of pre-training $\dot{V}O_2$ max
						166	137	75% of pre-training $\dot{V}O_2$ max
Kasch and Boyer [58]	11	50	Double product	106	85	163	156	286 kgm* before—382 kgm after
						247	296	Maximal workload
Clausen and Trap-Jensen [55]	29	55	Double product	—	—	222	202	Same submaximal workload
						222	220	At onset of angina

Triple product = heart rate (beats/min) × systolic arterial pressure (mm Hg) × ejection time (seconds)
Tension-time index = area under systolic brachial artery pressure curve × heart rate (mm Hg sec/min)

$$\text{Double product} = \frac{\text{heart rate (beats/min)} \times \text{systolic arterial pressure (mm Hg)}}{100}$$

*kgm/min = kilogram meters of work per minute

limited by manifestation of ischemic heart disease before conditioning have been reported.[50, 54, 58, 59] Whether these changes result from an expanded a-v O_2 difference, a greater stroke volume or a combination of both as seen in healthy young adults has not been measured.[3] Extrapolations from hemodynamic measurements made during submaximal exercise indicate that increases in either a-v O_2 difference [50] or stroke volume [53] may be the major contributor to this enhanced capacity. Patients with substantial myocardial damage or ischemia resulting in poor left ventricular compliance are probably extremely limited in their ability to increase stroke volume with physical conditioning.

Changes in Coronary Circulation—Studies using coronary arteriography do not support the hypothesis that physical conditioning contributes significantly to coronary artery collateralization as observed in some animal studies.[60, 61] Ferguson et al [62] studied 14 patients with significant obstructions in one (6 patients) or two (8 patients) coronary arteries who exercised three times a week for 13 months. The average increase in maximal oxygen consumption was 25% (21.9 ± 4.8 to 27.4 ± 4.1 ml/kg per min) but only two patients with progressing obstructions manifested new collateral vessels. Similar results were observed by Connor et al [63] in patients who underwent 6 months of physical conditioning after myocardial infarction.

Redwood et al [54] found that as a result of physical conditioning the level of the triple product at which angina occurred was increased in some patients, possibly as a result of increased myocardial oxygen supply. Similar results using ST-segment displacement as a measure of ischemia have been reported by Kasch and Boyer,[58] but Detry and Bruce [59] found no significant decrease in ST-segment depression at the same double product. Such changes could result from a reduced myocardial oxygen requirement due to a more synchronous contraction and smaller heart volume during exertion or a slight increase in myocardial oxygen extraction without any increase in coronary blood flow.

Other alterations possibly resulting from physical conditioning activities but not well-defined in patients who have had a myocardial infarction include decreases in serum lipoproteins, especially triglycerides,[64] a reduction in plasma insulin,[65] enhancement of blood coagulation and fibrinolytic activity [66] and decreases in plasma catecholamine levels.[67] If some of these changes do occur they could reduce the patient's risk of reinfarction or sudden death.

Some of the improvements seen in the physical working capacity and physiologic responses to exercise by patients after myocardial infarction may be the result of psychological changes associated with their participation in a physical conditioning program. Both objective and subjective measures indicate that, for many such patients, physical conditioning results in a reduction in depression and hypochondriasis, an increase in self-confidence, particularly as it relates to the performance of physical tasks, and an improved sense of well-being.[51, 68] In general, the magnitude of psychological improvement appears to be related to the degree of neurosis or anxiety upon entrance into the program and may be due more to the attention received during supervised exercise programs than to the effects of the activity itself.[2]

Recurring Myocardial Infarction and Mortality

The influence of physical conditioning on the frequency and severity of recurring myocardial infarction has not been adequately defined using random allocation of a sufficiently large number of patients into exercise and control groups. Table III contains a comparison of the mortality rates reported for patients who participated in a program of active rehabilitation after infarction and patients with similar characteristics who did not participate in any structured program. A consistently more favorable mortality rate is shown for the rehabilitation program participants; however, there are serious questions as to the comparability of the active and nonactive groups in the first six studies regarding the severity of illness and the likelihood of reinfarction. Also, other coronary heart disease risk factors were not well controlled and sometimes intentionally altered as a part of the rehabilitation program.

Randomized Trials—Two studies have been reported in which post-infarction patients were randomly allocated into supervised exercise training

TABLE III

Deaths Due to Myocardial Infarction in Rehabilitation Program
Participants and Non-Participants

| Study | Death Rate Due to Recurrent Myocardial Infarction (# per 100 man years experience) | |
	Rehabilitation Program Participants	Comparison Group
Hellerstein [51]	1.95	4.5–6.0*
Gottheiner [69]	3.6	12.0
Brunner [70]	3.1	10.8
Kellerman [71]	0.8 (long-term group)	2.5
Bruce [72]	2.7 (men)	4.7 (program dropouts)
	0 (women)	3.8 (program dropouts)
Rechnitzer [5]	3.5	6.8 (matched control group)
Kentala [73]	6.3	5.2
Sanne [39, 40]	5.2†	8.4
	2.9**	8.3

*Usual mortality rate of comparable coronary subjects treated in traditional manner as stated by author
†Rate for total follow-up period (average = 1.85 years)
**Rate for 26 weeks postinfarction to end of follow-up period

and control groups and followed to determine reinfarction rate and mortality. In one study no difference in reinfarction or mortality was observed [73] while preliminary results from the other showed a significant reduction in total and coronary heart disease mortality for the training program participants.[39, 40]

Kentala [73] reported on a study of 298 consecutive male patients aged 65 or under who were treated in the University Central Hospital, Helsinki in 1969 with a diagnosis of acute myocardial infarction. Six to eight weeks after hospital admission, 158 met the criteria for a study of supervised physical activity. On the basis of their year of birth, the patients were randomly assigned during their hospital stay into control (odd year) and training (even year) groups. Control group participants received regular medical care; the training group members were requested to participate in a supervised exercise program approximately 1 hour three times a week during the first five months and then twice a week from the 5th to 12th months. During the first 20 months after initiation of the training program, of the 81 control patients, four had a nonfatal reinfarction and seven died from reinfarction; of the 77 training group patients, six had a nonfatal reinfarction and eight died from reinfarctions. These differences were not statistically significant. A major limitation of this study was the poor adherence by the training group patients to the supervised exercise program.

Using a study design similar to Kentala's, Sanne [39, 40] randomized 316 myo-

TABLE IV

Mortality in Exercise Training and Control Groups Postmyocardial Infarction
A Randomized Trial in 316 Patients [39]

	Randomized to Training	Randomized to Control
#	156	160
Surviving 3 months	151	153
Started training at 15 weeks	111	0
Mean follow-up time (yrs)	1.85	1.85
Mortality (since hospitalization)		
Total	18	26
Due to coronary heart disease	15	25
Mortality 25 weeks after myocardial infarction and later:		
Total	8 $p < 0.05$	19
Due to coronary heart disease	6 $p < 0.025$	18

cardial infarction patients at the time of hospitalization into training (n = 156) and control (n = 160) groups. The control group was provided "usual care" by their physician and the training group had "usual care" plus they participated in a supervised exercise program three sessions per week for 30 minutes each beginning 15 weeks postinfarction. When death rate was calculated from 6 months postinfarction until the end of the follow-up period (average = 1.85 years), the exercise training group had a lower total and coronary heart disease mortality rate than the control group (Table IV). Total mortality rate for the entire follow-up period was not significantly different even though there were 18 and 26 deaths, respectively, in the training and control groups.

As pointed out by the authors, a major problem encountered in this study was the high rate of drop out. After two years, only 25% of the patients randomly assigned to the training group were still participating in the supervised classes and 25% were in a home training program. Also, approximately 25% of those patients assigned to exercise training did not start training because of cardiac contraindications.

Return to Gainful Employment—Whether physical conditioning increases the speed and frequency at which patients who have had a myocardial infarction return to gainful employment has not been satisfactorily determined. Kentala [73] found no difference in his exercise and randomly allocated control groups, whereas Kellerman et al [74] observed an increase in frequency of return to work among rehabilitation program participants. For economic reasons, a definitive answer to this question needs to be determined but will be extremely difficult to obtain because the number of patients returning to work after a myocardial infarction depends, to a large extent, on factors other than their clinical status or physical working capacity.[75]

Supervised Conditioning Programs

Because patients who have had a myocardial infarction are at increased risk of exertion-induced cardiac arrest, it is generally recommended that their participation in physical conditioning programs be supervised by a knowledgeable exercise leader and physician or nurse trained and authorized to perform cardiopulmonary resuscitation.[72] How long patients should be under medical supervision while performing relatively high level exercise has not been established. Many cardiac rehabilitation programs in the United States graduate patients to nonsupervised conditioning exercise programs one year after infarction; others suggest supervision on an indefinite basis for safety reasons.[72]

A second reason for encouraging supervised programs is that patients who attend supervised exercise sessions after infarction tend to stop exercising if they are provided an exercise program to perform on their own.[71, 76] To determine which patients should have supervision and for what length of time, it is necessary to be able to accurately select those patients who are at very low risk of cardiac arrest or myocardial infarction produced or aggravated by exertion. Those patients at low risk can be encouraged to exercise on their own using an individualized exercise prescription based on and revised periodically according to the results of a medical re-evaluation. Because of advanced age, cardiovascular complications or other health problems, certain patients cannot increase their level of exertion above that achieved during the convalescent stage and should be discouraged from doing so.[77] The inability of patients with a low physical working capacity to increase their capacity after 6 months of regular participation in a conditioning program is considered an indication for re-evaluation and possibly alternative therapy.

Substantial experience gained from the operation of numerous cardiac exercise programs throughout the country has demonstrated the value of experienced medical supervision in providing exercise guidance, motivation and emergency care for major cardiovascular complications occurring during exercise, especially the resuscitation of sudden cardiac arrest. Thus, if the patient is to exercise on his own, the physician assumes more responsibility for providing the exercise prescription and in assuring that the patient knows exactly what is expected of him and what to expect.

Recently, 30 medically supervised outpatient cardiac exercise programs in the United States and Canada were asked to report any major cardiovascular complications that occurred at the time participants were at the exercise facility as well as the number of participant hours of supervised physical activity. All programs required exercise testing prior to participation and had on-site medical supervision. Major cardiovascular complications were defined as any cardiovascular complication requiring hospitalization. As of July 1976, these

30 programs reported 1,480,000 man hours of participation with the occurrence of 37 nonfatal cardiac arrests or myocardial infarctions and 14 fatal events. Of the nonfatal, 33 were listed as cardiac arrest and four as myocardial infarction. Of the fatal episodes, eight were listed as cardiac arrest, two as myocardial infarction, two as pulmonary embolism, one as pulmonary edema and one as shock. The event rate (number of man hours of participation divided by total of number of nonfatal and fatal events) for this survey was one major cardiovascular complication (nonfatal or fatal event) every 29,020 man hours of participation. The range within the various programs surveyed was from a high of one event per 4,600 man hours to a low of none in more than 200,000 man hours of exposure. It is impressive that of 41 cardiac arrests, 33 (80%) were successfully resuscitated, a much higher percentage than would be expected even with expert cardiopulmonary resuscitation capability immediately available.

Conditioning program activities usually include walking, jogging, running, stationary bicycling, swimming, calisthenics and selected games. The intensity, duration and frequency of activity should be prescribed on an individualized basis. Intensity for these types of activities can be at 60 to 80% of the patient's physical working capacity as measured by a multilevel exercise test.[48] Recommended duration is 30 to 60 minutes at a frequency of three to five times a week.

During the early phases of physical conditioning, exercise bradycardia occurs only when trained skeletal muscles are used. For example, Clausen et al [78] trained two groups of men using a bicycle ergometer; one group used their arms while the other used their legs. When tested with arm and leg cycling after training, the men had a lower heart rate only when using the trained limbs. Thus, if one of the objectives of the conditioning program is to improve physical working capacity for a task that requires arm work, then activities using the arms should be included. If arm exercises are used it is important to remember that the double product is higher for arm work than for leg work having the same total body oxygen requirement. Also, because of the low arm strength of many adults it is important to keep the resistance level in arm exercises low in order to avoid the rapid increase in myocardial oxygen demand resulting from a pressure response produced by isometric or heavy resistance activity.[38]

Maintenance Activity Program

Once a desirable cardiovascular functional capacity has been achieved, a long-term program of exercise maintenance should be considered. The goal of this program should be to provide the patient with a level of activity that will maintain his cardiovascular functional capacity and efficiency, assist in maintaining optimal body weight and help him to retain a physical working capacity commensurate with his occupational needs and leisure time interests.

A critical factor in the design of a maintenance program is the decision as to whether it should be performed only with medical supervision. Sufficient follow-up data are not available to determine the susceptibility of a particular patient to cardiac arrest or reinfarction precipitated by an increase in physical activity. In an attempt to make such a decision, all pertinent clinical and laboratory data on the patient should be considered with emphasis placed upon a recent near-maximal or maximal multilevel exercise test. Performance at a level of 10 to 12 MET's without symptoms or adverse effects would indicate that at least for the present time activity such as jogging, moderate intensity running, hiking, swimming, doubles tennis, badminton and most gardening are within the patient's capacity.

The maintenance plan should include a variety of activities that can be performed well within the patient's functional capacity, are of interest to him, and are primarily aerobic but still of sufficient duration and intensity to maintain an "appropriate functional capacity."

Participation in Sports and Games

Cardiac patients will frequently request advice from their physician regarding participation in various active sports, games or leisure time activities. For most patients this is a difficult question to objectively answer because of the substantial intraindividual as well as interindividual variation in both total body energy requirement and myocardial oxygen demand for many such activities. These variations are due to the intermittent nature of the intensity of many of the activities; differences in the skill or efficiency of the participant, his teammate(s) or opponent(s); variations in the competitiveness or aggressiveness of the participant; changes in the ambient environment (temperature, humidity, wind velocity and altitude); variations in the amount of upper body and isometric exercise performed and differences in the amount of excitement, thrill or danger associated with the activity. Activities which present these problems include competitive sports or games like handball, squash, tennis, badminton, volleyball or basketball; activities requiring isometric contractions or isotonic contractions against a very heavy resistance such as water skiing, weight lifting or weight training and activities with a component of speed, excitement and danger including snowmobiling, motorcycling or downhill skiing.

Before participating in sports or games, patients should be encouraged to first participate in a systematic program of reconditioning. Postinfarction patients should not participate in any high level games or recreational activities until 24 to 26 weeks postinfarction and then only after clearance by their physician.

Because of the difficulty in estimating the total body energy requirement or myocardial oxygen demand for a specific patient performing many of these activities, advice regarding participation should be given conservatively. Activities requiring sustained isometrics (more than 10 to 15 seconds) or heavy resistance should not be recommended for any patient. Clearance for participation in vigorous sports or games should include the performance of a maximal or symptom-limited multistage exercise test during which a workload is achieved that has an estimated energy requirement substantially higher than those listed for the planned activity without the patient developing signs or symptoms contraindicating unmonitored exercise of that intensity.

If the activity under consideration has a major component of arm or upper body activity, an exercise test using arm cranking might be appropriate. Also, monitoring of the patient during simulation of the activity in the clinic or office or the use of a Holter type ECG recorder to monitor the patient during actual performance of the activity can provide objective information on the appropriateness of many activities.

Patients who are cleared for participation in active games or sports should be cautioned to avoid the extremes of environmental conditions such as not playing tennis or hiking midday or on hot sunny or humid days or not to go skiing on the coldest days or at resorts located at the higher altitudes. Extremes in water temperature should be avoided when participating in water sports. Ideas on how to reduce the cardiovascular demand of an activity should be provided to the patient. Suggestions should include: play doubles instead of singles tennis, badminton or paddle ball; avoid highly competitive opponents or situations; plan to take frequent rest periods and carry loads in a backpack and not with the arms when hiking.

Whenever exercise is being recommended for a cardiac patient, regardless of whether it is to be medically supervised or not, guidelines should be followed to help insure that a relatively safe and effective plan is carried out by the patient. Adherence to these guidelines by the medical team and patient results in an increased likelihood that the exercise plan will be performed without major medical complications and with an enhancement in cardiovascular functional capacity. However, as with all other cardiovascular therapies, no absolute assurance regarding safety and benefit can be ascribed to exercise training for a specific patient.

Conclusions

Experimental and clinical research has provided substantial knowledge of the potential benefits and risks associated with the performance of physical activity by patients with uncomplicated myocardial infarction. This knowledge has resulted in earlier mobilization, a reduction in length of hospitalization, an increase in physical working capacity and a more successful return to work of many patients. These improvements have been associated with a variety of physiologic and psychological changes produced by increased activity during each stage of the patient's recovery. During hospitalization, changes in posture and low intensity activity minimize the cardiovascular and psychological complications caused by prolonged bed rest. After hospitalization, the most valuable benefit of regularly performed exercise appears to be a reduction in myocardial oxygen demand at rest and during submaximal exertion. In order to obtain definitive evidence as to the benefit of increased physical activity on future cardiovascular morbidity or mortality of patients with coronary artery disease a multi-center, cooperative secondary prevention trial is required. Concurrently with such a major research project, present knowledge of the benefits derived from effectively operated cardiac exercise programs justifies the expansion of these services and increased third-party payment for medically based programs. The unique contribution of increased physical activity to reducing the frequency and severity of reinfarction has not been adequately established but, when combined with other behavior designed to reduce risk factors, the preliminary results are favorable. For these benefits to be obtained without undue risk, exercise for the postmyocardial infarction patient needs to be individually prescribed and periodically re-evaluated.

This study was supported by a grant from the Educational Foundation of America to the Division of Cardiology, Stanford University School of Medicine.

References

1. Wenger NK: The use of exercise in the rehabilitation of patients after myocardial infarction. *J S Carolina Med Ass* 65 (suppl 1): 66-68, 1969.
2. McPherson BD, Paivio A, Yuhasz MS, et al: Psychological effects of an exercise program on post-infarct and normal adult men. *J Sports Med* 7:95-102, 1967.
3. Detry JM: *Exercise Testing and Training in Coronary Heart Disease*, p 56, Baltimore: Williams and Wilkins, 1973.
4. Acker JE: The Cardiac Rehabilitation Unit: Experiences with a program of early activation (abstract). *Circulation* 44 (suppl 2): 119, 1971.
5. Rechnitzer PA, Pickard HA, Paivio AU, et al: Long-term follow-up study of survival and recurrence rates following myocardial infarction in exercising and control subjects. *Circulation* 45:853-857, 1972.
6. Council on Rehabilitation, International Society of Cardiology: *Myocardial Infarction. How to Prevent, How to Rehabilitate*, 1973.
7. Hirsch EZ, Hellerstein HK, Macleod CA: "Physical Training and Coronary Heart Disease," in Morse RL (Ed): *Exercise and the Heart*, Springfield, Illinois: Charles C Thomas, 1972.
8. Irvin CW, Burgess AM: The abuse of bedrest in the treatment of myocardial infarction. *New Eng J Med* 243:486-489, 1950.
9. Bourne G: An attempt at the clinical classification of premature ventricular beats. *Quart J Med* 20:219-243, 1927.
10. Mann RH, Burchell HB: Premature ventricular contractions and exercise. *Proc Staff Meetings Mayo Clinic* 27:383-389, 1952.
11. Goldschlager N, Cake D, Cohn K: Exercise-induced ventricular arrhythmias in patients with coronary artery disease. *Amer J Cardiol* 31:434-440, 1973.
12. Jetter WW, White PD: Rupture of the heart in patients in mental institutions. *Ann Intern Med* 21:783-802, 1944.
13. London RE, London SB: Rupture of the heart: a critical review of 47 consecutive autopsy cases. *Circulation* 31:202-208, 1965.
14. Titus JL, Oxman HA, Norbega FT, et al: Sudden unexpected death as the initial manifestation of ischemic heart disease. Clinical and pathologic observations (abstract). *Amer J Cardiol* 26:662, 1970.
15. Mallory GK, White PD, Salcedo-Salgar J: The speed of healing of myocardial infarction. *Amer Heart J* 18:647-671, 1939.
16. Lodge-Patch I: The ageing of cardiac infarcts, and its influence on cardiac rupture. *Brit Heart J* 13:37-42, 1951.
17. Thomas WC, Harrison TR: The effect of artificial restriction of activity on the recovery of rats from experimental myocardial injury. *Amer J Med Sci* 208:436-450, 1944.
18. Kaplinsky E, Hood WB, McCarthy B, et al: Effects of physical training in dogs with coronary

artery ligation. *Circulation* 37:556-565, 1968.

19. Thompson PL, Jenzer HR, Lown B, et al: Exercise during acute myocardial infarction: an experimental study. *Cardiovasc Res* 7:642-648, 1973.

20. Sutton DC, Davis MD: Effects of exercise on experimental cardiac infarction. *Arch Intern Med* 48:1118-1125, 1931.

21. Levine SA: Management of patients with heart failure. *JAMA* 115:1715-1719, 1940.

22. Dock W: The evil sequelae of complete bed rest. *JAMA* 125:1083-1085, 1944.

23. Harrison TR: Abuse of rest as a therapeutic measure for patients with cardiovascular disease. *JAMA* 125:1075-1077, 1944.

24. Levine SA: The myth of strict bed rest in the treatment of heart disease. *Amer Heart J* 42:406-413, 1951.

25. Levine SA, Lown B: Armchair treatment of acute coronary thrombosis. *JAMA* 148:1365-1369, 1952.

26. Coe WS: Cardiac work and the chair treatment of acute coronary thrombosis. *Ann Intern Med* 40:42-48, 1954.

27. DeBusk RF, Spivack AP, VanKessel A, et al: The coronary care unit activities program: its role in post-infarction rehabilitation. *J Chronic Dis* 24:373-381, 1971.

28. Fareeduddin K, Abelmann WH: Impaired orthostatic tolerance after bed rest in patients with myocardial infarction. *New Eng J Med* 280:345-350, 1969.

29. Wenger NK: Cardiac inpatient conditioning program (Appendix 4). *J S Carolina Med Ass* 65 (suppl 1):102-104, 1969.

30. Cardiac Rehabilitation 1975. Report of a joint working party of the Royal College of Physicians of London and the British Cardiac Society on Rehabilitation After Cardiac Illness. *J Roy Coll Physicians* 9:281-346, 1975.

31. Harpur JE, Conner WT, Hamilton M, et al: Controlled trial of early mobilization and discharge from hospital in uncomplicated myocardial infarction. *Lancet* II:1331-1334, 1971.

32. Groden BM: The management of myocardial infarction: a controlled study of the effects of early mobilization. *Cardiac Rehabilitation* 1:13-16, 1971.

33. McThockcoth R, Ho SC, Wright H, et al: Is cardiac rehabilitation really necessary? *Med J Aust* 2:669-674, 1973.

34. Rose GA: Early mobilization and discharge after myocardial infarction. *Mod Conc Cardiovasc Dis* 41:59-64, 1972.

35. Acker J: "Early Ambulation of Post-Myocardial Infarction Patients. A. Early Activity After Myocardial Infarction," in Naughton JP, Hellerstein HK (Eds): *Exercise Testing and Exercise Training in Coronary Heart Disease*, New York: Academic Press, 1973.

36. Ericsson M, Granath A, Ohlsen P, et al: Arrhythmias and symptoms during treadmill testing three weeks after myocardial infarction in 100 patients. *Brit Heart J* 35:787-790, 1973.

37. Brock L: "Early Ambulation of the Post-Myocardial Infarction Patients. B. Early Reconditioning for Post-myocardial Infarction Patients: Spalding Rehabilitation Center," in Naughton JP, Hellerstein HK (Eds): *Exercise Testing and Exercise Training in Coronary Heart Disease*, pp 315-323, New York: Academic Press, 1973.

38. Jackson DH, Reeves TJ, Sheffield LT, et al: Isometric effects on treadmill exercise response in healthy young men. *Amer J Cardiol* 31:344-350, 1973.

39. Sanne H: Exercise tolerance and physical training of nonselected patients after myocardial infarction. *Acta Med Scand* (suppl 551):1-124, 1973.

40. Sanne H, Elmfeldt D, Wilhelmsen L: "Preventive Effect of Physical Training after a Myocardial Infarction," in Tibblin G, Keys A, Werko L (Eds): *Preventive Cardiology*, pp 154-160, Stockholm: Almqvist and Wiksell, 1972.

41. Atterhog JH, Ekelung LG, Kaijer L: Electrocardiographic abnormalities during exercise 3 weeks to 18 months after anterior myocardial infarction. *Brit Heart J* 33:871-877, 1971.

42. Styperek J, Ibsen H, Kjoller E, et al: Exercise-ECG in patients with acute myocardial infarction before discharge from the CCU (abstract). *Amer J Cardiol* 35:178, 1975.

43. Hakkila J, Kentala ES, Valtonen ES, et al: Control study of effects or early activation in acute myocardial infarction (abstract). *Circulation* 44 (suppl II):120, 1971.

44. Rousseau MF, Brasseur LA, Detry J-MR: Hemodynamic determinants of maximal oxygen intake on patients with healed myocardial infarction: influence of physical training. *Circulation* 48:943-949, 1973.

45. Rousseau MF, Degré S, Messin R, et al: Hemodynamic effects of early physical training after

acute myocardial infarction: comparison with a control untrained group. *Europ J Cardiol* 2:39-45, 1974.

46. Torkelson LO: Rehabilitation of the patient with acute myocardial infarction. *J Chronic Dis* 17:685-704, 1964.

47. Benestad AM: The deteriorative effect of myocardial infarction upon physiological indices of work capacity. *Acta Med Scand* 191:67-75, 1972.

48. Bergström K, Bjernulf A, Erickson U: Work capacity and heart and blood volume before and after physical training in male patients after myocardial infarction. *Scand J Rehab Med* 5:51-64, 1974.

49. Hellerstein HK, Hirsch EZ, Ader R, et al: "Principles of Exercise Prescription for Normal and Cardiac Subjects," in Naughton JP, Hellerstein HK (Eds): *Exercise Testing and Exercise Training in Coronary Heart Disease*, pp 129-168, New York: Academic Press, 1973.

50. Detry J-MR, Rousseau M, Vandenbroucke G, et al: Increased arteriovenous oxygen difference after physical training in coronary heart disease. *Circulation* 44:109-118, 1971.

51. Hellerstein HK: Exercise therapy in coronary disease. *Bull NY Acad Med* 44:1028-1047, 1968.

52. Frick MH, Katila M: Hemodynamic consequences of physical training after myocardial infarction. *Circulation* 37:192-202, 1968.

53. Clausen JP, Larson OA, Trap-Jensen J: Physical training in the management of coronary artery disease. *Circulation* 40:143-154, 1969.

54. Redwood DR, Rosing DR, Epstein SE: Circulatory and symptomatic effects of physical training in patients with coronary-artery disease and angina pectoris. *New Eng J Med* 286:959-965, 1972.

55. Clausen JP, Trap-Jensen J: Heart rate and arterial blood pressure during exercise in patients with angina pectoris. *Circulation* 53:436-442, 1976.

56. Clausen JP: Circulatory adjustment to dynamic exercise and effect of physical training in normal subjects and in patients with coronary artery disease. *Prog Cardiovasc Dis* 18:459-494, 1976.

57. Holloszy JO: Adaptations of muscular tissue to training. *Prog Cardiovasc Dis* 18:445-458, 1976.

58. Kasch FW, Boyer JL: Changes in maximum work capacity resulting from six months training in patients with ischemic heart disease. *Med Sci Sports* 1:156-159, 1969.

59. Detry J-MR, Bruce RA: Effects of physical training on exertional ST segment depression in coronary heart disease. *Circulation* 44:390-396, 1971.

60. Eckstein RW: Effect of exercise and coronary artery narrowing on coronary collateral circulation. *Circ Res* 5:230-235, 1957.

61. Stevenson J, Felek V, Rechnitzer P, et al: Effect of exercise on coronary tree size in rats. *Circ Res* 15:265-269. 1964.

62. Ferguson RJ, Petitclerc R, Choquette G, et al: Effect of physical training on treadmill exercise capacity, collateral circulation and progression of coronary disease. *Amer J Cardiol* 34:764-769, 1974.

63. Connor JE, La Camera F, Swanick EJ, et al: Effects of exercise on coronary artery collateralization—angiographic studies in six patients in a supervised exercise program. *Med Sci Sports* 8:145-151, 1976.

64. Oscai LB, Patterson JA, Bogard DL, et al: Normalization of serum triglycerides and lipoprotein electrophoretic patterns by exercise. *Amer J Cardiol* 30:775-780, 1972.

65. Bjorntorp P, Berchtold P, Grimby G, et al: Effects of physical training on glucose tolerance, plasma insulin and lipids and on body composition in men after myocardial infarction. *Acta Med Scand* 192:439-443, 1972.

66. Astrup T: "The Effects of Physical Activity on Blood Coagulation and Fibrinolysis," in Naughton JP, Hellerstein HK (Eds): *Exercise Testing and Exercise Training in Coronary Heart Disease*, pp 169-192, New York: Academic Press, 1973.

67. Banister EW, Licorish KA, Griffiths J, et al: Plasma catecholamine changes in response to rehabilitation therapy in postmyocardial infarction patients (abstract). *Med Sci Sports* 5:70, 1973.

68. Naughton J, Bruhn JG, Lategola MT: Effects of physical training on physiologic and behavioral characteristics of cardiac patients. *Arch Phys Med* 49:131-138, 1968.

69. Gottheiner V: Long-range strenuous sports training for cardiac reconditioning and rehabilitation. *Amer J Cardiol* 22:426-435, 1968.

70. Brunner D: Active exercise for coronary patients. *Rehab Rec* 9:29-31, 1968.

71. Kellerman JJ: Physical conditioning in patients after myocardial infarction. *Schweiz Med Wschr* 103:79-86, 1973.

72. Bruce EH, Frederick MS, Bruce RA, et al: Comparison of active participants and dropouts in CAPRI Cardiopulmonary Rehabilitation Programs. *Amer J Cardiol* 37:53-60, 1976.
73. Kentala E: Physical fitness and feasibility of physical rehabilitation after myocardial infarction in men of working age. *Ann Clin Res* 4 (suppl 9):1-84, 1972.
74. Kellerman JJ, Modan B, Levy J, et al: Return to work after myocardial infarction. *Geriatrics* 23:151-156, 1968.
75. Miller MG, Brewer J: Factors influencing the rehabilitation of the patient with ischemic heart disease. *Med J Aust* 1:410-416, 1969.
76. Barry AJ, Daly JW, Pruett EDR, et al: Effects of physical training in patients who have had myocardial infarction. *Amer J Cardiol* 17:1-8, 1968.
77. Kavanagh T, Shephard RJ, Doney H, et al: Intensive exercise in coronary rehabilitation. *Med Sci Sports* 5:34-39, 1973.
78. Clausen JP, Trap-Jensen J, Lassen NA: The effects of training on the heart rate during arm and leg exercise. *Scand J Clin Lab Invest* 26:295-301, 1970.

26

Cardiac Rehabilitation:
Principles, Techniques, Applications

John Naughton, MD

Cardiac rehabilitation is a form of longitudinal, comprehensive care through which selected patients are restored to and maintained at their optimal medical, physiological, psychological, social, vocational and recreational status. Secondary prevention of the underlying disease process is implicit in the concept, as is acceleration of the subject's return to either his pre-illness level of activity or a new and appropriate level of adjustment.

At its present state of development, cardiac rehabilitation is usually equated with the long-term care of survivors of myocardial infarctions. This appreciation stems from the fact that the techniques and principles which characterize the process have evolved from investigators whose interests have concentrated on the problems of coronary heart disease and myocardial infarction. However, the principles and techniques are available to and can be utilized in the care of patients with other cardiac disorders as well, including corrected congenital lesions, angina pectoris and aortocoronary bypass surgery.

Cardiac rehabilitation appears justified for a number of reasons. Myocardial infarction is the leading cause of physical impairment and disability in the United States. Among its sequelae are loss of physical working capacity as a result of reduced myocardial reserve and overall physical deconditioning, and an increase of psychological symptoms which are directly related to a loss of performance capacity and overall integrity. Although 80% of the survivors of a myocardial infarction should be able to return to work and/or near normal levels of activity,[1] many do not because of the presence of symptoms directly related to their physical deconditioning. The disease carries a high direct and indirect economic cost which has been estimated as ranging from as low as $17 billion to as high as $30 billion annually.

The components of cardiac rehabilitation include: optimal medical care; periodic measurements of adaptation to submaximal stress and of symptom-limited work capacity; participation in lifelong, graduated and prescribed physical activity; adequate psychological support; and patient and spouse education.

Onset of Rehabilitation

Rehabilitation begins with the onset of injury or illness. For survivors of myocardial infarction the process is initiated when the clinical status has stabilized and the imminent threat of death is removed. This is usually the second to fourth day on the coronary care unit. Several approaches to early ambulation and the hospital phase of cardiac rehabilitation have been reported and are reviewed in Chapter 25.

In the strictest sense, most of the efforts that are carried out from the onset of myocardial infarction until a patient is ready to return to work are designed to prevent physical deconditioning, enhance emotional outlook, and prepare the patient for participation in a long-term program of rehabilitation. The formal rehabilitation program is initiated when the patient is prepared to return to his pre-infarct life style. The time period can range from as little as 6 weeks after infarction for the uncomplicated, stabilized patient with a clerical or executive job, to as long as 16 to 20 weeks for patients with symptoms or those covered by special disability insurance programs. The rate and degree of return to usual levels of activity are apparently not directly related to the severity of myocardial infarction. Rather, the presence or absence of symptoms, and other social and vocational considerations affect this situation.

A comprehensive cardiac rehabilitation evaluation includes an appropriate cardiovascular history and physical examination, standard chest X ray, and a 12-lead electrocardiogram (ECG) recorded at supine rest. If the patient's condition is stabilized, and no contraindications are detected, the patient is permitted to perform a multistage exercise test to determine the quality and quantity of his cardiovascular adaptation to submaximal stress, the performance capacity, the abnormalities associated with physical effort, and the basis for developing the exercise prescription. The exercise stress test can be administered in the physician's office, a hospital-based laboratory, or a specialized referral center.

Exercise Stress Tests

An exercise stress test has become one of the keystone procedures associated with cardiac rehabilitation. For the known cardiac patient, it is not a diagnostic procedure. It is an evaluative procedure which defines a patient's limitations and potentials for physical activity. In this context, it is a procedure analogous to the BUN, blood pressure and the 12-lead ECG in that it is administered to define the patient's baseline status following recovery, and to define whether future interventions are associated with improvement, stability or deterioration of the patient's health status.

It is now well recognized that many reactions which might not be observed at rest can be precipitated during mild forms of physical stress. The application of the techniques and principles has aided in selecting patients for different forms of therapy including physical reconditioning programs.

Techniques—An exercise stress test can be administered with many types of devices. Those most often utilized in clinical practice are steps, a motor-driven treadmill or bicycle ergometer. The advantage of these instruments is that they lend themselves to quantitation of the external workloads; therefore, if a procedure is used in a standardized manner from one study to the next, the results are comparable either for individuals or for varying population groups.

An exercise stress test is standardized by determining the external oxygen requirement for various workloads, and by converting that workload to the per unit body weight. Thus total oxygen consumption for a given task may vary from individual to individual depending on total body weight, but the unit value should be similar. It is generally accepted, for example, that the oxygen requirement for supine, relaxed rest requires approximately 3.5 ml O_2/kg/min. This value has been described as a MET. Patients who walk on a level grade at 2.0 mph have an external oxygen requirement per kilogram, which is approximately 7.0 ml or 2 MET's. Patients who become limited at a workload approximating 35.0 ml/kg/min are said to have a working capacity of 10 MET's, and patients who can attain thresholds of 70 ml/kg/min possess a performance capacity of 20 MET's. In terms of man, the capacity for physical effort ranges from the extreme low of one MET to a peak of 20 to 21 MET's. Multistage exercise stress tests make it possible to define each patient's limitations or potentials rather critically.

The design of an exercise stress test protocol for use in cardiac rehabilitation is critical. The procedure should be sufficiently flexible to permit patients to be studied at a low workload in terms of the anticipated threshold capacity. Since the vast majority of nonrehabilitated cardiac patients will be limited at thresholds below 8 MET's, I have advocated a procedure in which treadmill belt speed is held constant at 2.0 mph and the slope of the treadmill bed is elevated gradually in 3.5% increments. This approach permits patients an opportunity to be evaluated at workloads of 2, 3, 4, 5, 6 and 7 MET's. If the patient is symptom-free and has a greater capacity than 7 MET's the treadmill slope can be decreased slightly and the belt speed increased. For example, at 2.0 mph on a 17.5% grade, a 7.0 MET threshold is reached; a reduction of slope to 12.5% with an increase of speed to 3.0 mph results in an increased O_2 requirement to 8 MET's; 2.5% increments thereafter can maintain the one MET increase programmed at the slower speeds.

Many physicians and investigators do not favor the above approach because of its time requirements. However, for the unconditioned cardiac patient, actual testing time should be 14 minutes or less, depending on the time used for each stage. In the clinical situation it is recommended that the slope can be increased every 2 minutes, because these small increments are not as challenging to the metabolic adjustments of the body as are other protocols. Most patients will reach their steady-state blood pressure and heart rate values within 60 to 90 seconds with the above approach, and therefore the values recorded during the last 30 seconds of each workload reflect the individual patient's adaptation to that external workload. This approach, therefore, is one which can assure an aerobic procedure.

The technique referred to here has the added advantage that the work tolerance can be correlated with the Functional Class schemata of the New York Heart Association (NYHA). A patient who becomes limited at 2.0 MET's or less should be Class IV; 3 or 4 MET's, Class III; 5 or 6 MET's, Class II; and a patient who attains 7.0 MET's or greater is considered Class I (see Table I, Chapter 16).

Measurements—Presence or absence of symptoms, development of abnormal physical signs, onset of abnormal ECG findings not detected at rest, and the adaptation of blood pressure and heart rate to each external workload should be measured and recorded. These should be performed routinely at rest, during each workload and for at least the first 5 minutes of recovery.

The symptoms most commonly precipitated by physical stress are chest discomfort, dyspnea, fatigue and claudication, all of which should be evaluated in order to determine whether they are cardiovascular in origin. If in the observer's judgment they are, the procedure should be terminated. Many patients will not be specific about a symptom, but will simply indicate a desire or need to terminate the procedure. It should be stopped. If the observer feels the reason for stopping was ambiguous or has a clinical indication for pursuing the issue further, the procedure can be rescheduled for another time.

Electrocardiographic abnormality, usually manifested as ischemic manifestations or in the form of ventricular arrhythmia is another common reason for terminating an exercise stress test. In the case of asymptomatic cardiac patients, it is recommended that the procedure be stopped if the ST segment is displaced upward or downward 3 mm (0.3mV) from that measured in the resting tracing. Multifocal ventricular extrasystoles and ventricular tachycardia are indications for stopping a procedure.

The presence of abnormal physical signs, reduction of systolic blood pressure, and increase of diastolic blood pressure are also reasons for stopping an exercise stress test. They apparently occur less frequently in the absence of symptoms, and therefore should be considered secondary end points.

From the foregoing, it is possible to construct those items that should be monitored and measured routinely during an exercise stress test. They are: (1) Symptoms. (2) ECG—If only one lead can be measured, it should be the one with the greatest QRS voltage. This will usually be precordial V_5 or for an exercise stress test, the simulated lead, CM_5. Preferably, multiple leads should be recorded, and in the ideal setting they should be II, aV_F, V_3, V_4, V_5 and V_6. (3) Blood Pressure—Systolic and diastolic blood pressure can be recorded adequately by auscultation provided an anesthetist's stethoscope is used and the tubing is restrained so as to minimize adventitious noise. (4) Heart Rate—This can be measured from the ECG, with a cardiotachometer, or by auscultation. (5) Abnormal Physical Signs—Onset of cyanosis or ataxia during the procedure is sufficient reason for stopping. As a matter of fact most abnormal physical findings will be found during recovery, especially S_3 and S_4 sounds, paradoxical movements, and diminished pulsations.

Normal and Abnormal Responses—SYMPTOMS—A sense of fatigue or exhaustion at high workloads might not be considered abnormal. However, if it occurs at extremely low effort it is indicative of reduced myocardial reserve. The onset of other symptoms is abnormal.

ECG—The PR and QT intervals shorten in response to increased cardiac rate. A physiologic J-point depression is considered a normal response. Any major changes not recorded at rest such as a significant degree of ST-T depression, multifocal ventricular extrasystoles, and onset of intraventricular block is considered abnormal.

SYSTOLIC BLOOD PRESSURE—The systolic blood pressure should increase in relation to the intensity of effort. A failure to increase or a decrease in value as work intensity increases is abnormal.

DIASTOLIC BLOOD PRESSURE—The diastolic blood pressure changes little in healthy, sedentary subjects. In athletes it decreases significantly as stress is increased. An increase above the resting measurement of 10 mm Hg or more is considered an abnormal response.

HEART RATE—Much has been made of the age-adjusted peak heart rate level. The uninitiated reader must be aware that these values hold for presumably healthy subjects, but not for cardiac patients. Approximately 15% of the cardiac population can achieve their peak adjusted heart rate levels without other abnormality. The remaining 85% will be limited with some abnormality at a heart rate level 85% or less than the age predicted peak heart rate estimate. Thus, the character of the heart rate response is probably more important. A steep heart rate increase will occur in the severely compromised patients, and a more gradual increase of slope in the less compromised patients. There are a few patients whose heart rate response will be lower than predicted at each workload. Ellestad[2] has used the term "chronotropic incompetence" to characterize this response. In his experience, he found this to have a bad prognostic implication.

SIGNS—The normal adaptation to physical stress is to develop a sweat, become slightly flushed and pleasantly tired. Ataxia and cyanosis or other visible signs of distress are clearly abnormal.

Recovery—The recovery phase of an exercise stress test is sometimes ignored. This is a mistake! Gooch[3] reported that the highest incidence of arrhythmia occurs within the first minute postexercise. Other investigators have reported additional findings during recovery. Examples include symptoms, ischemic changes on the ECG, and either postexercise hypertension or hypotension. A patient should be observed critically for at least 5 minutes after exercise (see Chapter 14). The observations should include auscultation for abnormal heart sounds not present in the pre-test situation and changes evidenced in the ECG, and measurement of blood pressure and heart rate during the first and fifth minutes. If the patient is comfortable and the clinical situation stable, he is permitted to prepare to leave the laboratory.

Many patients desire the opportunity to shower before departing the premises. This is permissible provided they are recovered, symptom-free and the shower is tepid.

Informed Consent—Most physicians recommend that the patient sign an Informed Consent prior to the exercise test. This form need not be complicated. It should detail the indications for an exercise stress test, list the measurements to be done, explain the benefits of the evaluation, describe the potential risks and hazards, and clarify what will be done in the event an emergency arises. It should be signed by the patient and the examining physician.

Some investigators still prefer to perform exercise stress tests without the requirement for a signed Informed Consent. The rationale for their attitude is related to the fact that such a procedure cannot be performed involuntarily. I have utilized a written consent form for almost 15 years, and to date no patient has refused to sign it. In this day and age of medico-legal concern, it seems a prudent adjunct to clinical practice.

Other Considerations—Although a stress testing facility need not be elaborate it should be well lighted, and maintained with a temperature between 68 and 72° F and humidity from 40 to 60%. The room should be large enough to contain the equipment, a patient and at least two staff members, and to permit cardiopulmonary resuscitation to be administered comfortably.

The staff should be certified in the principles of cardiopulmonary resuscitation. A properly equipped and stocked emergency cart should be on the premises. A well coordinated communication system for obtaining external emergency care support should be available as well.

Interpretation of Results—A properly administered exercise stress test should be accompanied by a sophisticated report to the referring physician. The interpretation should characterize: (1) The patient's overall clinical response to the procedure. Was it normal? Were symptoms or signs precipitated? (2) The quality of the ECG response. The ECG may have remained essentially unaltered, or specific abnormalities may have occurred. (3) The adequacy of the systolic blood pressure, diastolic blood pressure and pulse pressure responses. (4) The slope of the heart rate response per MET together with documentation of the peak heart rate level reached and its relationship to the age adjusted peak level. (5) The work capacity in MET's, and a comparison with anticipated norms.

The foregoing should be accompanied with a summary explaining the results together with a listing of any additional diagnoses that are appropriate as a result of the evaluation. If the patient was referred for evaluation in preparation for an exercise reconditioning program, the report should be accompanied by an exercise prescription (Figure 1).

Exercise Prescription

Physical activity has now been demonstrated to offer the clinician diagnostic and evaluative potential. As a result of the advances in cardiac rehabilitation, it has been demonstrated to have therapeutic value as well. Although an exercise pharmacopeia has not yet been developed, inroads have been made through the concept of developing an exercise prescription. The prescription should detail the heart rate levels to be monitored during exercise; the indications and contraindications for exercise in a given individual; any anticipated side effects; the frequency and duration of exercise sessions; and the indications which might affect a patient's response to exercise (see Chapter 18). A sample exercise prescription is shown in Figure 1.

EXERCISE PRESCRIPTION

Patient's Name: *John Doe*   Date: *June 10, 1977*

Peak Heart Rate on Exercise Stress Test	—*150 beats/min*
Exercise Heart Rate	—*Low 98 beats/min; High 128 beats/min*
Frequency	—*3 times per week*
Duration	—*15 minutes of intermittent activity for 3 weeks; increase to 30 minutes for next 3 weeks*
Indications	—*Myocardial infarction Work capacity below 6 MET's*
Contraindications	—*Symptoms at rest*
Potential side effects	—*Ventricular extrasystoles precipitated by exercise test*
Next exercise stress test	—*6 weeks (July 18, 1977)*

Signed: *John Doe, MD*

Figure 1. A sample exercise prescription.

The key to an exercise prescription is the peak heart rate reached during the exercise stress test. The prescription is constructed so that the heart rate during physical training is maintained above 70% yet below 85% of the peak value. The former insures that a training effect will be induced and the latter provides a margin for safety as well as insuring that the conditioning program is aerobic and not anaerobic in character.

The guidelines are easier to establish for the symptomatic patient, because he can use the symptom as a warning sign or indication for stopping an activity. The asymptomatic patient must develop insight as to the feelings he experiences at the appropriate heart rate levels.

Although considerable refinement remains to be done on formulating and structuring the exercise prescription, it is a concept of increasing importance, and this author encourages physicians to begin utilizing it in clinical practice.

Reconditioning Programs

It is generally recommended that cardiac patients be placed in a controlled environment for at least the first phase of physical reconditioning and rehabilitation. Many programs have been structured so that patients can be reconditioned in a health care facility located in a hospital or a clinic. After a desired level of conditioning has been achieved, patients can be referred to a community program conducted in a YMCA, Jewish Community Center or school gymnasium. Many patients will require a home program because of job requirements, transportation problems or individual preference.

Medically Supervised Programs—It is preferable to begin physical reconditioning programs for cardiac patients in a facility in which medical supervision can be assured. This is accomplished by equipping a facility with exercise equipment which can be used to adjust the workload to achieve the prescribed heart rate levels. A five-center research study identified as The National Exercise and Heart Disease Project (NEHDP) [4] and sponsored by the Rehabilitation Services Administration (RSA) of HEW has developed a model facility. In their program, each facility is equipped with a motor-driven treadmill, bicycle ergometer, a 9-inch high step, rowing machine, hand crank and arm wheel. The instruments are arranged so that leg work and arm work are alternated. A cardiotachometer is placed at each station, and the patients attach electrodes and cable to themselves on entering the facility. They plug the cable into the cardiotachometer at each exercise station, and the observer monitors the heart rate so as to maintain the prescribed level. This is accomplished by increasing or decreasing the workload appropriately.

These training sessions include a 5-minute period of warm-up prior to initiating the prescribed exercises; 2 minutes of recovery occur between each exercise station; and the session terminates with a 5-minute cool down. In NEHDP exercise at each station is maintained for 4 minutes.

It is recommended that a patient attend the physical activity program three times per week. Initially, sessions may last only 15 to 20 minutes, but eventually about 45 minutes is required. A major problem in clinical practice and for insurance carriers is to determine the proper duration for medically supervised and regimented exercise programs. Although a definitive answer is not available, this author currently recommends a minimum of 3 months following which the multiple stage exercise test is repeated. For those subjects who achieve a work capacity in excess of 8 MET's and in which the cardiovascular responses are judged appropriate, I recommend that the exercise prescription be updated, and the patient transferred to a community based program. For the remainder, approximately 20% of a starting group, another 3 months of medically supervised exercise might be warranted. If after six months a patient shows no evidence of achieving a conditioning effect, the medically supervised program should be terminated. These patients should not be referred to a community program, and many may, in fact, require a different mode of therapy or intervention.

The training facility should be well lighted, temperature and humidity controlled, and equipped with an emergency cart and a defibrillator. The model described above can handle six subjects at a time.

Community Facilities—Those subjects who have been reconditioned and whose clinical status and exercise stress test responses suggest that the risk of sustaining a new cardiac episode is low can be referred to a community facility. The staff of the community facility should be trained in the principles of exercise training, cardiac rehabilitation and emergency care, and they should have close communication with the rehabilitation program director.

Patients are advised to participate at the community facility three times a week. Patients should maintain a diary of their health and medical status, and should learn to document their heart rate and rhythm before and after each exercise session. In the community facility they graduate from the instrument approach used in the hospital or clinic to physical activities which can include games, walking, jogging, swimming and other sports.

These patients should be re-evaluated with an exercise stress test at 6-month intervals. Any new symptoms should be reported to their physician at once.

Home Programs—Many patients request a home program in preference to group programs. While probably not as desirable as group programs, there have been individual reports of success. A home program utilizes the same principles and requirements as the other types of approaches, but the amount of instrumentation is limited. Patients can use the guidelines put forth by the American Heart Association [5] or the Canadian Fitness Program.[6] Many will invest in a bicycle ergometer on which they can read or watch a television program while cycling in place. Good instruments are available at a reasonable price.

Comments on Exercise Regimens

It has been adequately demonstrated that selected cardiac patients respond to regular physical activity in a manner similar to presumably healthy subjects (see Chapter 24 and 25). Since the goals of physical reconditioning and rehabilitation are to enhance the cardiorespiratory system, the recommendations of most authors have stressed the principles of aerobic conditioning and endurance. This form of training is accomplished by repeating rhythmical exercise over an extended period of time at a threshold between 60 and 80% of a subject's aerobic working capacity. The most commonly performed aerobic exercises are walking and jogging, but other examples include cycling, skipping rope and rowing.

During the embryonic development of cardiac rehabilitation programs, the greatest emphasis was directed toward aerobic exercises which trained large muscle groups, because it was known that this would produce the optimal changes in work capacity. It is now recognized that physical conditioning is not transferrable from one group of muscles to another, and that if total conditioning is to be achieved, the exercise program must involve all muscle groups. The multiple machine method used in NEHDP is designed to condition upper and lower extremities.

Muscle groups which should receive particular emphasis in reconditioning programs include the strap muscles of the neck, the pectoralis major and minor muscles and the biceps. If these groups are properly reconditioned the incidence of noncardiac chest pain is decreased significantly, and it is much easier to clarify whether chest pain is cardiac in origin.

Effects of Physical Activity

It has been clearly demonstrated that regular physical activity reduces the level of systolic blood pressure, heart rate and double product at rest and at comparable levels of submaximal work [7] (see Chapter 4, 9, 15, 24 and 25). Peak values are not affected, but the workload at which they are reached is increased significantly. The end result is that the cardiovascular system is benefited by reducing the myocardial oxygen requirement for any given level of submaximal effort. These changes are translated into the life situation because all physical tasks are performed at less cost to the cardiovascular system. As discussed by Folkins in Chapter 20, there is evidence that the conditioned patient may also adapt to emotional stress more adequately.

A second category of benefit is that symptoms are diminished, and therefore, a sense of well-being develops. The decrease in symptomatology is not a reflection of altering the disease state *per se*, but is probably directly related to the increase in work capacity. Symptoms tend to correlate with the diminution of cardiovascular and/or overall physical reserve. Thus, the lower an individual's work tolerance, the greater his frequency of symptoms. This critical threshold has not been defined but seems to approximate 6 MET's and less. This is of interest because a patient whose cardiovascular status is rated Class I (NYHA) is usually capable of achieving a threshold of 7 MET's or greater. Therefore, a goal for cardiac rehabilitation is to achieve workloads of 7 MET's or greater following reconditioning. The foregoing suggests it is possible to be healthy and physically fit; unhealthy and physically fit; unhealthy and unfit; or healthy and unfit. Cardiac rehabilitation programs have developed a population of individuals who are unhealthy by virtue of having manifested coronary heart disease but are fit for most routine tasks and many avocational tasks by virtue of their being reconditioned.

A host of other effects has been ascribed to physical reconditioning programs. Many are not as well documented as are the cardiovascular and work capacity changes, but they should be mentioned. These include an improved work attendance, decreased rate of rehospitalization, enhanced income status, improved psychological status, and more enjoyment of sexual activity.

The effects on morbidity and mortality remain to be determined by longitudinal studies of randomized population groups.

Anecdotal Patient Experiences

Since cardiac rehabilitation is still in a state of evolution it is appropriate to reflect on some examples of individual variability which have been observed among participants in physical reconditioning programs.

Work Capacity Pre- and Post- Myocardial Infarction—Only a few patients have been stress tested before and after suffering a myocardial infarction. This author reported on the findings of a 54-year-old man who entered an adult fitness program in 1963. Prior to entering he performed a near-maximal stress test. He possessed several risk factors, *ie*, hypertension, obesity, and an elevated cholesterol level. Six weeks later he sustained a myocardial infarction from which he recovered uneventfully. Following recovery, he volunteered to help develop a physical reconditioning program for cardiac patients. When re-evaluated 6 months after myocardial infarction his work capacity of 13 MET's exceeded that of 9 MET's measured in his so-called healthy state. Thus this subject demonstrated that physical reconditioning resulted in a greater level of work performance following myocardial infarction than was possessed prior to illness. This subject maintained a capacity of 12 to 14 MET's for the next 14 years.

Denial—One of the problems that must be dealt with by physicians and patients is that of denial. It has been demonstrated that rehabilitation outcomes in terms of return to work are better for deniers than for nondeniers. However, deniers may use their defense mechanisms inappropriately, and thus jeopardize themselves and the rehabilitation program.

One patient took time out from his exercise in the gynmasium one day to report that he had telephoned the president of a savings and loan company to complain about a service charge. When it was suggested that he was upset, the patient stated, "I wasn't bothered at all." This statement of denial was accompanied by a burst of ventricular tachycardia which spontaneously remitted. Several weeks later this same individual was monitored while playing volleyball. During the last minute of play, he had another episode of ventricular tachycardia documented *via* telemetry. When he left the playing court, I asked how he felt. "Great," he replied. Then after a pause, he related that he had a little light headedness late in the game. When asked why he wasn't going to report it, he said, "It didn't last as long as other episodes I experienced previously." Although nothing catastrophic occurred, this was an example of how denial can be used inappropriately.

Another patient once told me about his visit to Dr. Gottheiner's program in Israel. When I asked how his wife felt about that type of program, the patient responded rather abruptly, "It doesn't matter what she thinks." His cardiac rate monitored *via* a continuous tachometer, increased dramatically from 70 to 140 beats/min. This observation was followed by some light and neutral conversation, and the same stimulus reapplied with exactly the identical heart rate response a few minutes later.

Workaholics—Many patients enter cardiac rehabilitation programs because they are motivated to regain and retain fitness. Some develop a concept that physical fitness will ensure improved health and longevity. They then develop the concept that level and intensity of work are synonymous with improved health. One such patient who was convinced of this philosophy was observed jogging at a rate of a mile every 6.5 minutes. This was slightly alarming to the observer because his work capacity indicated that his aerobic rate should be nearer to 8.0 minutes per mile and because he had a visible paradoxical pulsation on the anterior chest wall. When asked why he didn't slow down, the patient responded, "I don't understand you, Doc. The Bible says that people who work hard should be rewarded. Why do you want to punish me?" Obviously, this orientation can be dangerous to the program and the patient.

These are simple, thumbnail examples of types of problems that can go unnoticed in physical activity programs unless the staff is sensitive to certain symptoms and signs. They also suggest the concept that cardiac rehabilitation requires a total appreciation of each and every subject.

Emphasis on Physical Activity

To date the emphasis in cardiac rehabilitation has been directed toward physical measurements and physical activity. Speculation about this indicates that this emphasis is, indeed, appropriate because rehabilitation as a process implies physical restoration and because patients, in general, visualize their cardiac disorder as a physical rather than a nonphysical impairment. This is not to say that a multitude of other factors is not important as well. Rather, it is necessary to emphasize that for the cardiac rehabilitant the major need he perceives is the need to perform. For him, performance is equated with an ability to work comfortably. The patient knows that to work comfortably he requires a certain degree of myocardial integrity and a certain level of physical fitness. Observations available to date indicate that if physical restoration is achieved and physiological reactions to this life-threatening disorder are reduced (patients modify their dietary, smoking and drinking habits concomitantly), their overall social, vocational and recreational rehabilitation seems assured.

The Future of Cardiac Rehabilitation

It appears that myocardial infarction and its serious physical, physiological, social and vocational consequences are going to remain with Western society for an indefinite period of time. Organized approaches to longitudinal and comprehensive care utilizing exercise stress testing and medically supervised physical activity programs have enhanced the treatment and rehabilitation of selected patients. It must be surmised, therefore, that there is a patient and social need for the rehabilitation program, and that further refinement to incorporate it into routine patient care will continue.

Needs in Cardiac Rehabilitation—The foregoing does not suggest that all the answers are known. There is much to be learned and accomplished. For instance, little effort has been directed toward the rehabilitation of patients with angina pectoris and/or aortocoronary bypass surgery. These subjects should benefit from these principles as well.

Thus far, in the United States at least, patients of higher economic means and greater educational achievement have selected this method of therapy. Surely, there is a need to explore the requirements of skilled workers and blue collar workers. There is a definite need to integrate the medical rehabilitation system with the vocational rehabilitation system.

Lastly, there is a need to explore ways in which those patients with limited work capacities can be helped in order to make their lives more productive and comfortable.

References

1. Wenger NK, Hellerstein HK, Blackburn H, et al: Uncomplicated myocardial infarction. Current physician practice in patient management. *JAMA* 224:511-514, 1973.
2. Ellestad MH: *Stress Testing, Principles and Practice*, Philadelphia: F. A. Davis, 1975.
3. Gooch AS: Exercise testing for detecting changes in cardiac rhythm and conduction. *Amer J Cardiol* 30:741-746, 1972.
4. Common Protocol, National Exercise and Heart Disease Project: A Study of the Effects of Prescribed, Supervised Physical Activity on Myocardial Infarction Patients, Department of Health, Education and Welfare, Washington, DC, 1972.
5. Committee on Exercise, American Heart Association: *Exercise Testing and Training of Individuals with Heart Disease or at High Risk for its Development: A Handbook for Physicians*, 1975
6. *Royal Canadian Air Force Exercise Plan for Physical Fitness*, New York: Simon & Shuster, 1976.
7. Naughton J, Hellerstein H, Mohler I: *Exercise Testing and Exercise Training in Coronary Heart Disease*, New York: Academic Press, 1973.

INDEX

Index

Note to the reader: Please bear in mind that this index is based on major subject headings, and does not include scattered comments. Also, although there are several topics listed directly under "Exercise," please remember that the main topic for every listing is "Exercise."